HORMONE DECEPTION

HORMONE DECEPTION

How Everyday Foods and Products Are Disrupting Your
Hormones—and How to Protect Yourself and Your Family

D. LINDSEY BERKSON

FOREWORD BY JOHN R. LEE, M.D.
author of *What Your Doctor May* Not *Tell You About Menopause*

PREFACE BY JOHN MCLACHLAN
Director, Center for Bioenvironmental Research, Tulane
and Xavier Universities

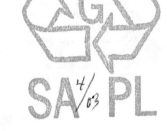
CB
CONTEMPORARY BOOKS

Library of Congress Cataloging-in-Publication Data

Berkson, Lindsey.
    Hormone deception: how everyday foods and products are disrupting your hormones—and how to protect yourself and your family / D. Lindsey Berkson ; foreword by John R. Lee, preface by John McLachlan.
      p.   cm.
    Includes biographical references and index.
    ISBN 0-8092-2538-7
     1. Reproductive toxicology.   2. Endocrine toxicology.   3.
Environmental toxicology.   4. Food contamination.   I. Title.
RA1224.2.B47   2000
618.1—dc21

Interior and cover designs by Monica Baziuk
Interior illustrations by Precision Graphics

Published by Contemporary Books
A division of NTC/Contemporary Publishing Group, Inc.
4255 West Touhy Avenue, Lincolnwood (Chicago), Illinois 60712-1975 U.S.A.
Printed in the United States of America
International Standard Book Number: 0-8092-2538-7

01 02 03 04 05 06 LB 20 19 18 17 16 15 14 13 12 11 10 9 8 7 6 5 4 3 2

Dedication

My father died two weeks before this manuscript was due. Before the funeral I was talking with the rabbi about my father and all the stories that intertwined our lives, and I remembered this. . .

My father had given up his law practice to join his family's scrap metal business. In the early 1960s, my father and his brother realized that the billowing smoke from their smelting furnaces was polluting the air. At the time, there were no government regulations requiring that furnaces be altered to prevent pollution. However, with much cost out of his own pocket, my dad insisted on reconstructing the furnaces to stop the contamination. I asked him why he spent all that money when he didn't need to. He answered, "I care. No matter the cost, do what is caring and right. It always makes a difference."

He was my prime inspiration in writing this book. I dedicate my efforts to his memory.

Contents

Part 3

What to Do About Hormone Disruptors

Foreword

JOHN R. LEE, M.D.
Author of *What Your Doctor May Not Tell You About Menopause*

Hormone disruption may not be new, but the high incidence of it we now see *is* new, and the extent is so great that we must consider it a twentieth-century epidemic. The age of puberty (menarche) is dropping. PMS afflicts at least 30 percent of premenopausal women; breast cancer incidence is not only rising, but its onset is earlier than ever before. Infertility and early miscarriage due to luteal phase failure are common, and sperm production in men is falling. Hysterectomy for relieving heavy, irregular periods is performed on more than 550,000 U.S. women annually. The signs that something has gone wrong with our hormones are all around us. Humans are not the only victims. We know that certain wildlife populations are dying out due to procreation problems secondary to petrochemical exposure. Evidence is mounting daily that hormone disruption due to the petrochemical menace (xenobiotics) is a major factor in a wide variety of illnesses affecting many animal species including humans.

Worse yet is the obvious fact that our old paradigm of casual estrogen replacement and the use of synthetic progestins and birth-control pills is not the answer. For too long we have ignored the concept of hormone *balance*. Fortunately, a more successful paradigm is emerging from research in cancer etiology, the new understanding of hormone-binding proteins, hormone-receptor sensitivity, gene modulation, specific nutrients, and the importance of heterogeneity. A specific hormone's effect is not simply the result of its presence but is the result of a dynamic relationship to stress, genetics, nutrition, and complex interaction with other hormones such as all the sex steroids, adrenal steroids, thyroid, and insulin, to name a few.

Any new paradigm emerges as a result of the leadership of those who dare to explore new concepts and who have the insight to synthesize the information. In this regard, a few lead the way. Not only do they "see" problems and solutions better than most of us, but also they have the ability to communicate their vision of biochemical concepts and treatment options with extraordinary clarity. This new book by Lindsey Berkson complements the evidence compiled by Theo Colborn and the authors of *Our Stolen Future* and extends it into the realm of human medicine. Petrochemical hormone disruptors pervade our human environment. To ignore them is to invite disaster. *Hormone Deception* is an important step in helping us understand them and, hopefully, to eventually solve the problem they present.

Foreword

J. V. WRIGHT, M.D.
Author of *Natural Hormone Replacement for Women Over 45*
and *Maximize Your Vitality and Potency for Men Over 40*

"It's enough dealing with my own hormone cycles. Now I've learned that an enormous variety of environmental chemicals—from plastics, detergents, solvents, pesticides, dioxins, and industrial by-products like heavy metals—can literally infiltrate my hormone system and change the way it works. I could get anything from PMS to cancer! It feels creepy—like my health could be slowly hijacked by common but hidden environmental chemicals without me even knowing it!"

This reaction came from a woman with whom I shared Dr. Berkson's book. It'll likely be your reaction, too, when you've read the overwhelming mass of evidence presented. Fortunately, having laid out the problem, Dr. Berkson gives us solutions and practical measures we can all take to protect ourselves and our families from "hormone disruptors." This combination makes *Hormone Deception* one of the most valuable health books of our generation.

Preface

JOHN A. MCLACHLAN, PH.D.
Weatherhead Distinguished Professor and Director, Center for Bioenvironmental Research, Tulane and Xavier Universities

One of the most compelling issues at this time is the interaction between us and our environment. While we have a significant impact on the globe, we exist within a complex set of signals that connect species on a monumental scale. Our place in this signaling system is only now starting to be understood.

One of the most potent of signals, which literally changes the way humans and animals develop, is the female sex hormone estrogen. Estrogens are associated with normal development of the reproductive system in embryos, not only in humans but also in all other animals such as lab mice, cats, dogs, and even birds and alligators. In addition to this powerful effect on the attainment of our reproductive capacity, estrogen is involved in the onset of puberty in girls, preparation of the uterus for development of an embryo, bone and heart health in women, and even perception of pain. In a way not yet understood, estrogens also are associated with breast cancer.

In 1979, while working as a scientist at the National Institutes of Health, I organized a meeting of researchers and health policymakers to explore whether or not chemicals introduced into the environment were acting like estrogens. Little did we know at the time what an important question we were asking. Over the last two decades, the concept that environmental chemicals can mimic our own sex hormones has been firmly established. Literally hundreds of meetings and thousands of scientific reports have been devoted to understanding this important environmental fact that is central to our reproduction and development and, indeed, to those of most other species on earth. Since hormones like estrogen are part of one of the body's major signaling networks, the endocrine system, chemicals that mimic or alter our hormones are known as endocrine-disrupting chemicals.

It is of central importance to all of us that we know what these chemicals are, how they work, how we may be exposed to them, and what the effects might be on our health. While complex scientific issues are often difficult to understand, such understanding is necessary for us to make the right choices.

In *Hormone Deception*, Lindsey Berkson does a marvelous job of making complex environmental and health issues understandable. She writes with passion, wit, and understanding. Her book is one of those rare volumes that balances a need "to do something" with the available scientific information. Dr. Berkson brings the skills of an experienced writer to a topic of significant personal concern; her own experience with hormone deception is both well documented and profound. I am proud, on the twentieth anniversary of the first meeting on estrogens in the environment, to be asked to write the preface to this timely and accessible treatment of the topic.

Acknowledgments

Hormone Deception is the result of six years of research and writing, and a lifetime journey to get me to the place where I could tell this story. It has not been a project for one lone woman. Endocrine disruption bridges so many fields—neurotoxicology, reproductive toxicology, comparative evolutionary biology, and molecular biology, to name a few—that to delve into these subjects I needed the assistance of numerous dedicated specialists. Many scientists, doctors, and others generously gave their time for interviews, comments, and review of various drafts of the manuscript. These amazing human beings are out in the world trying to make it a safer and better place. They do not want another DES-type tragedy to happen, like the one I have been living. Despite the help of the experts, I take full responsibility for any refutable interpretations and unseen mistakes.

Dr. John McLachlan's groundbreaking work on the long-term effects of exposure to estrogens in the womb is the backbone for much of our present knowledge on endocrine disruption. I consistently heard from others that he was busy and impossible to reach. Yet he gave me hours on the phone, nights in a row, late after his working day. He and Dr. William Toscano kindly invited me to speak at the Center for Bioenvironmental Research at Tulane and Xavier Universities, in front of a number of folks whose papers I had been reading for years. It was exciting and scary. They believed in my efforts enough to offer me a consulting-scholar position with them on endocrine disruption, which I accepted.

Dr. John R. Lee is a pioneer in the field of hormones and graciously reviewed the whole manuscript and provided vital input on progesterone, unopposed estrogen, and hormone disruptors.

I met Dr. Bob Moore, a researcher from the University of Wisconsin, because he was wearing an anti–death penalty T-shirt at a conference I was attending. One of my former roommates is a public defender in New Mexico, and getting rid of the death penalty is her goal. Dr. Moore offered citations, articles, time, and support, as well as friendship.

Dr. Allen Silverstone's conversations stretched my viewpoint; he spent many hours getting me papers, reviewing work, and hashing over different perspectives. His contributions were instrumental in adding to this work.

Dr. Dan Sheehan and Dr. Frederick vom Saal were inspirations who gave much time, thought, article references, and counsel. They made themselves and their work available. I can't thank them enough.

Dr. Wade Welshons, Dr. Dan Vallero, and Dr. Dennis Lubahn are great thinkers and talkers and didn't yell at me when I E-mailed, faxed, and called on them again and again. Their patience and input were vital to my understanding and writing. Dr. Wayne R. Ott sent so much material over my fax, he almost broke it. He gave tirelessly of support, comments, and incredible firsthand information on how the EPA has evolved. Dr. Lance Wallace gave hours of interview and comments for the chapter on exposure in the home. He, John Roberts, and Wayne Ott all have dedicated their lives to the landmark work that will help us make our homes safer.

Dr. Linda Birnbaum is one of the most articulate people with whom I have ever spoken. She helped convey information about the mechanism of endocrine disruption and freely gave of her time in interviews and manuscript comments. I bugged her with numerous E-mails, and she agreed to read whatever I sent, so I sent the whole manuscript. She kept her word and earned my eternal gratitude.

Dr. John A. Katzenellenbogen, Ph.D., Swanlund Professor of Chemistry at the University of Illinois, read through the manuscript and gave critical as well as humorous comments, which improved both the text and my spirit.

Dr. Bruce Blumberg was supportive intellectually and emotionally, as both of us lost our fathers during the writing of this book. Dr. Oliver Putz shared deep conversations on hormones, science, and confusion, all of which brought more clarity.

Dr. Retha Newbold, from the National Institute of Environmental Health Sciences and a sincerely kind-hearted woman, helped me understand what is happening with *in utero* estrogen exposure and guided me on some important personal treatment decisions.

I want especially to thank Dr. Jonathan Wright. He has been a colleague and friend for decades. His pioneering work in the clinical application of nutrition in medicine, along with his researching skills, was a major influence in my life. That he agreed to be the medical consultant for this book was tremendous joy and support to me. His comments and encouragement helped bring this project to fruition.

Dr. Craig Dees is an innovative and entertaining scientist, dedicated to eradicating breast cancer, who willingly spent hours conversing with me. Drs. Ana Soto and Carlos Sonnenschein gave hours of interview on their groundbreaking work on plastics and endocrine disruption and provided a number of important research leads.

Dr. Tudor Oprea, both an M.D. and a Ph.D. in molecular physiology, has been a long-distance help. Working in Sweden, he acted as a reviewer and consultant. Because of his interaction with this project, he has gone on to write and present papers on endocrine disruption to the medical community.

Dr. Christine Greene has been a tremendous support. Originally a colleague, she ended up being a dear friend—from giving me a hand to hold and a house to stay in during surgery at Stanford to accompanying me to Fairfax, Virginia, for the Endocrine Modulation conference.

Polly Short at the World Wildlife Fund came through with sending us Dr. Brouwer's not-yet-published article that was instrumental in understanding current positions on hormone disruptors and thyroid hormones. I appreciate that Dr. Brouwer gave permission for me to have the article before publication. Dr. Michael Smolen, a senior scientist who has been working with Theo Colborn for many years, read the first chapter and offered numerous suggestions.

Dr. Pat Costner gave freely of her time and provided citations to help with many facets of this book. Dr. Alan Gaby carefully reviewed the manuscript and helped with some aspects of the research. Dr. Leo Galland started out being someone whose lectures I admired and, along with his wife, has become a dear friend. He reviewed this manuscript and offered invaluable critique and encouragement.

Speaking with Janet Raloff and reading her elegant science journalism contributed to this project. Talking to Gary Cohen was like meeting a sage in a mountain cave and reading poetry while the sun sets. He is an activist's activist who makes my heart warm with hope.

Dr. Michael Gallo was helpful in personal conversations at the Endocrine Modulation conference and was able to get me the hard-to-find early French research that linked DES with breast cancer in rodents. Dr. Thomas Gasiewicz gave freely of his time and work. His paper on dioxins was a scholarly piece that contributed valuable information.

Dr. Generosa Grana is an oncologist I met at a conference who let me publish her comments. Dr. Earl Gray was helpful in discerning the available research. Dr. Gordon Gribble granted an interview, reviewed the chemical chapter, and sent much research. Dr. Stephen Safe gave freely of time and debate and sent many helpful articles.

Dr. Walter Crinnion shared invaluable research, time, and expertise on the topic of detoxification. Dr. Susan Schantz gave hours over numerous phone calls and sent very helpful articles.

Dr. Bernard Weiss gave hours in interview time and sent well-written papers that helped clarify endocrine disruption in cognitive behavior. Dr. Joseph Jacobson kindly gave me time for an interview as well as reviewing the section on behavior and intelligence.

The people in Dr. Herbst's group at the University of Chicago gave time and counsel and sent information on diethylstilbestrol, more commonly known as DES. The DES Action group—the mother and daughter team of Pat and Nora Cody—were helpful in their meticulous reading of the DES chapter. I had long heard of Judith Helfand's work before I met her. She has taken the DES lemon and made lemonade.

I want to thank Dr. Kurt Davies, Dr. Richard Willes, and all their dedicated coworkers at the Environmental Working Group for their important research. Dr. Devra Davis's staff at the World Resources Institute sent information for the breast cancer chapter.

Dr. John Gierthy gave enlightening discourse on associated subjects; we both are dance fanatics and have become E-mail pals.

I thank Doug Meffert for plowing through the manuscript under a deadline and offering much help.

I also want to thank Dr. Herman Adlercreutz, Mirabai Bush, Dr. Mark Cline, Dr. Tom Crisp, Greg Friedman, Lois Gibbs, Elaine Hiller, Dr. Claude Hughes, Dr. Craig Jordan, Dr. Pavel Langer from Slovaki, Dr. John McCarthy, Dr. Donald C. Malins, Colin Meiklejohn, Dr. Mark Messina, Dr. David Pimental, Dr. Susan Porterfield, Amanda Sherman, Dr. Daryl Sumner, Dr. Shanna Swan, Dr. Wulf Utian, Dr. Lon White, and Dr. Mary Wolff, who all gave me time for discussion and comments. Both Drs. Irva Herty Picciotto and Bill Toscano kindly edited their vital contributions to this book.

Special thanks to the American Lung Association of Seattle for their "Master Home Environmentalist Program," the editors from the *Environmental Health Letter* for "Refining Our Understanding of Risk: Chapter 1: Endocrine Disrupters," and the librarians at the University of New Mexico Medical School for assisting me in my research.

I also want to thank Janet Steinberg, Rusty Crutcher, Marcia and Roger Hirsch, Joan Ellis, Sheila Lewis, and Stephen Weiss for their emotional support throughout this process. Dr. Keith Block and Mark Mead are constant supports and voices of wisdom and expertise on women's health.

Special thanks to a number of caring readers: David Ingersol, Rama Paine, Radha Baum, Vicki Stamm, Joan Ellis, Susan Friedman, and Linda Freedman. Greatly appreciated are Wendy Warner and Laura Ware for transcribing many hours of taped interviews and conference notes. If I have inadvertently left out anyone who has contributed to this book, I apologize.

I especially want to thank my agent, Meredith Bernstein, and my dear editor, Judith McCarthy, both of whom believed in this project through thick and thin.

And last, but most important, is Parvati Markus. She is an editor and friend whose contribution has been invaluable in writing this book.

It is important to point out that government scientists stated their personal perspectives and opinions; their views do not necessarily represent those of their agencies or institutes.

Introduction

Hormones. We all know what hormones do—they make men masculine and females feminine. They make us fertile, support pregnancy, make us crave chocolate, put pimples on our teenager's chin, and bring about The Change.

How about those first copies of *Playboy* you find underneath your son's bed? What's at work here? Hormones. Or one reason it's harder for women to lose weight than it is for their husbands? Hormones. Hormones play our lives like instruments, constantly influencing and fascinating us. Hormones tell our bodies when to start developing breasts or producing sperm. Hormones direct the cells in the fetus, guiding them to become cells of the reproductive organs, cells of the brain or the various glands, cells of all the particular tissues of our bodies.

Betsy says she's living in hormonal hell. "My daughter is picking fights, then locking herself in her room like she does every month right before her period. My sister is staying with us, and she's an emotional wreck because she just had a miscarriage. I'm starting to have hot flashes, and my doctor wants me to take hormones because my mother had osteoporosis. I sit down to relax with a magazine, and I'm reading that maybe I should take testosterone to restore my fading sexual desire. I'm beginning to think hormones rule my life!"

In a way, Betsy is right. Hormones (which are named from a Greek word meaning "to urge on") do exert a powerful influence over many facets of our growth and development, our sexual and reproductive capability, our behavior and intelligence, our energy, and our memory and aging. Hormones regulate puberty, fertility, pregnancy, and menopause. There's a reason the ancient Greeks called the main female hormone "estrogen." The word *estrus*—when a female animal goes into heat—comes from *oistros*, meaning "frenzy."

When our hormones send us into a frenzy, they can do more than urge us to sidle up to that cute cowboy at the bar or to eat another handful of chocolate-covered almonds. Hormonal imbalance can contribute to diseases like endometriosis and breast or prostate cancer. However, it's not only our natural hormones that can wreak havoc with our lives. Sometimes the pharmaceutical hormones we take for birth control, fertility, and to stop those @#! hot flashes can also disturb our hormonal balance, leading to health problems. As if this weren't already confusing enough, now there's another aspect to hormones that we must learn to take into consideration if we're going to stay healthy ourselves as well as raise healthy families.

WHY YOU SHOULD CARE

Certain chemical compounds can act like hormones once they get inside our bodies. This means that our health is now influenced by hormonal factors that come from outside our bodies. Therefore, in order to have a thorough understanding of your own hormonal situation or any hormonal treatments, you now need to take into account your exposure to hormone disruptors. This information is particularly important if you are planning to become pregnant, are caring for young children, or are thinking about taking birth-control pills, fertility treatments, or hormone replacement therapy.

It appears as though exposure to hormones, particularly estrogen or estrogenic compounds (or others not yet studied), can affect many of the factors that are involved in your child's growth and development. Even very low dosages of estrogenic chemicals can irreversibly alter the programming that takes place in the womb that will ultimately play a major role in how your child's body, mind, and emotions will turn out in later life.

Certain manmade chemicals, many of which are found in the household products we use regularly and in the foods we consume every day, are under suspicion. We are exposed to these compounds through the air we breathe and the food and water we ingest or absorb through our skin. Called *hormone disruptors*, these particular compounds can mimic our natural hormones, creating imbalance, or they can alter the way our natural hormones are supposed to work in the body.

The question of hormone disruptors has become so important that Congress mandated the Environmental Protection Agency (EPA) to examine the issue of hormone-disrupting chemicals. More than 500 studies are in progress on different aspects of hormone disruption. In some of these studies, chemical compounds that have the ability to disrupt the hormone system are being examined in relation to:

- reproductive system abnormalities—such as smaller penises or misshapen wombs

- infertility—one American couple out of five or six currently has trouble conceiving. Infertility grows more common with increasing age; about one-third of couples in their late thirties are infertile.

- female health problems like endometriosis, fibroids, and menstrual and breast disorders

- learning and behavioral problems—such as lower IQ scores and hyperactivity in children

- immune system deficiencies and thyroid disorder

- increases in the rates of certain cancers—breast, prostate, testicular, and other reproductive system cancers

In other words, hormone disruption can possibly affect everything from lowered sperm counts to our ability to fight off disease. It can alter or determine our and our children's destiny.

The last thing we need is something else to be paranoid about. Don't worry. *Hormone Deception* gives usable guidelines for reducing your exposure and thus protecting your health and that of your family.

One undeniable human proof of hormone disruption is the physical damage sustained by the children of women who were given diethylstilbestrol

(DES), a potent synthetic estrogen, while pregnant. I am a DES daughter. The DES taken by my mother upon her doctor's advice while she was pregnant with me (both of them acting with my best interests at heart) led to my lifelong health problems and prompted the direction my life would take as a researcher and educator on women's health issues. Despite having lived an exemplary healthy lifestyle—often growing my own food; eating whole grains and organic vegetables and fruits; exercising diligently; meditating; and working with my emotional "stuff"—I have had eight female surgeries, had a damaged uterus that could not support birth, and had to fight breast cancer. Now we know that the problem of hormone disruption goes far beyond DES.

I have worked in the field of health for many years, as well as constantly working on healing myself. The hormone disruption that has so severely impacted my life has given me a passion for this subject matter and led to my present position as a consulting scholar with the Center for Bioenvironmental Research at Tulane and Xavier Universities. *Hormone Deception* is a result of my commitment to make women aware of what I believe are the potential problems posed by hormone-disrupting chemicals and what we can safely do. Scientists tell us that the ones most at risk of being affected by hormone-disrupting chemicals are the fetus in the womb and the developing child. We need to know what is happening so we can find ways to keep ourselves, our children, and our grandchildren healthy. We have a right to be educated about the topic so we can make responsible decisions. And we need to know that there are simple and often inexpensive ways in which we can protect ourselves and our families from exposure to hormone disruptors (see Part III).

There are those who believe that ignorance is bliss. I disagree. We live in a day and age when we cannot afford to live unconsciously. As a matter of fact, we can greatly enhance our ability to lead healthy and fulfilling lives, and to have healthy children who grow up to be "all that they can be," if we are willing to be aware of the challenges that confront us. Awareness is always the first step to healing both our personal health and the health of the world around us.

In the course of working on this book, I interviewed more than sixty inspiring people who are studying endocrine (hormone) disruption from many different angles. Highly regarded and extremely busy scientists gave me a lot of their precious time as I badgered them in person, on the phone, or through frantic E-mails because they, too, want you to understand what's happening with endocrine disruptors.

The Importance of Hormone Disruption

Hormone disruption has become such an important issue in the United States and throughout the world that various groups and agencies have made the study of endocrine-disrupting chemicals a top priority. Congress has begun by mandating the EPA to come up with ways to identify and test hormone-related toxicants that are already on the market and in the environment for their potential to disrupt the endocrine system. The EPA responded by creating EDSTAC (Endocrine Disruptor Screening and Testing Advisory Committee; see Chapter 12) in October 1996. An estimated $5 billion will be needed to carry out EDSTAC's recommendations. Endocrine disruption is one of five priority research areas of the Committee on the Environment and Natural Resources within the Executive Office of the President. In other words, our government is taking the threat of hormone disruption very seriously.

Worldwide interest in the topic has given rise to a number of gatherings of eminent scientists and researchers. In 1991 a group of international experts gathered to look at the problems hormone disruptors pose for all life on earth. They concluded, in the Wingspread Statement: "We estimate with confidence that: Some of the developmental impairments reported in humans today are seen in adult offspring of parents exposed to synthetic hormone disruptors released into the environment."

Another gathering in 1995 in Erice, Sicily, for a work session on endocrine-disrupting chemicals, issued a statement that said (in small part): "A variety of chemical challenges in humans and animals early in life can lead to profound and *irreversible* abnormalities in brain development at exposure levels that do not produce permanent effects in an adult." The Erice consensus statement continues: "Endocrine-disrupting chemicals can undermine neurological and behavioral development . . . and may be expressed as reduced intellectual capacity and social adaptability as well as impaired responsiveness to environmental demands," all of which can "change the character of human societies and destabilize wildlife populations."

What does this mean in simple English? Exposure to hormone disruptors in the womb and during infancy may keep some children from developing to their utmost potential. No wonder it's of such importance to understand what is happening.

HOW TO USE THIS BOOK

Hormone Deception is the result of many years of diligent research. It is divided into three parts for easy reference. Feel free to skip around, reading what is most interesting and important to you.

This book offers new insights into the hormonal "soup" and an exploration of the compounds that can disrupt our hormones. Once you understand the problem, there are steps you can take—ways to protect yourself and your loved ones at home, school, or work from the possible effects of hormone disruption. Out of this understanding comes a practical list of what-to-dos in relation to diet, your home, and the way you may choose to utilize pharmaceutical hormones.

Here are some examples of what will be covered:

- Assessing your risk
- Why men are from Mars and women are from Venus in relation to hormone disruptors
- How a child's IQ may be affected while still in the womb
- The fruits and vegetables most contaminated with hormone disruptors
- The latest information about the soy controversy
- Consumer product information (and how product names can mislead you)
- Steps for ridding yourself of toxins
- Shocking news about baths and showers
- Herbal and nutritional remedies for specific menopausal complaints

Part I offers an introductory explanation of hormone disruptors, as well as describing the role of estrogen and other natural hormones in regard to our health. Chapter 4 shows how the daughters and sons of mothers who took DES, the first synthetic estrogen, are the canaries in the mine of hormone disruption.

Part II shows how the fetus in the womb and infants are the most vulnerable to hormone disruption, and how these compounds can affect the health of some of our children in relation to childhood diseases, puberty, sexual identity, behavior, and intelligence. Women's health issues—including fertility, pregnancy, menopause, endometriosis, and cancer—are examined. Reproductive abnormalities in men, such as lowered sperm count and abnormal penile development, are also discussed, as well as diseases that affect both men and women.

Part III is an encyclopedia of practical suggestions, covering the food we eat, the water we drink, and a room-by-room tour that provides guidelines for minimizing our exposure to hormone disruptors in our home. Methods of detoxification—ways to get this stuff out of us—are discussed. Part III also looks at the ways in which we can help and shows that consumership is a powerful tool for change.

Appendix A goes into detail about the various chemicals that are known and suspected hormone disruptors. Appendix B explains natural hormone replacement and hormone potentiators, alternate ways of treating menopausal symptoms. Appendix C includes lists and charts that are referenced in earlier chapters. Appendix D is a list of resources for further information.

Sometimes life seems very complicated and the issues that confront us can appear overwhelming. Don't give up hope. We can make a difference, individually and collectively.

I attended a lecture by one of our present-day spiritual leaders in which he said that he is often asked if we are facing Armageddon or the dawning of a new Golden Age. His answer was that it really doesn't matter one way or the other. What we need to do is exactly the same in either case: quiet our minds, open our hearts, and work to relieve the suffering around us. This book is an attempt to help prevent and relieve the problems that have been inadvertently created by our quest for progress.

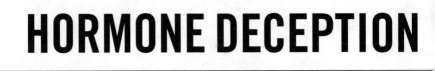

HORMONE DECEPTION

what are hormone disruptors?

What does my story as a DES daughter have to do with your health and that of your children? You're not exposed to the types of potentially dangerous substances I'm talking about, are you?

Perhaps you think that you already know enough about protecting your health. You eat a moderately good diet and go to the gym a few times a week. You've started to cut down on caffeine and alcohol, and cigarettes went out the window a long time ago. You probably don't feed your baby soda pop in her bottle. Read through the following list of questions and see how many pertain to you.

ASSESSING YOUR EXPOSURE RISK

- Did your mother take prescription DES or another synthetic hormone when she was pregnant with you?
- Do you consume a diet high in animal fats (over 30 percent)?
- Do you dust and vacuum your home less than twice a week?
- Do people walk on your carpets with street shoes?
- Do you shower without turning on the bathroom exhaust fan?
- Do you hang recently dry-cleaned clothes in your bedroom closet?
- Do you eat nonorganic, commercially grown food? Canned foods and drinks?
- Do you microwave food in plastic containers or cover foods with plastic cling wrap?
- Do you use pesticides on your lawn and garden or foggers or bombs in your home?
- Do your pets wear flea collars?
- Do you use clothes-washing detergent?
- Does your new car have a strong new-car smell?
- Do you use commercial air fresheners in your home or car, deodorizers in your bathroom?
- Do you use any solvents or chemicals in your work, home, or hobbies, or have you been exposed to these in the past?
- Do you park your car in a garage attached to your home?

Chances are you answered yes to at least a few of these questions. Each of these situations can introduce hormone disruptors into your body. Don't panic. The purpose of this book is not to create fear. The purpose here, first of all, is to make you conscious of your exposure to hormone-disrupting chemicals and to show how your health or your children's health may be affected and, second, to demonstrate that you can take steps to reduce your exposure.

This first section of the book provides basic information about hormones and hormone disruptors so you can better understand this important topic.

Hormones—Messengers of Life

*When you think about it, **life is about messages**. What I am referring to here are the natural chemical messages that come from our genes and become the instructions for the next generation: how to grow, how to develop, how to mature from fetus to adulthood. **These messages are life itself.***

— J. P. Myers, U.N. Conference on Environment and Development, March 14, 1997

A pregnant woman holds her hands gently over her swollen belly, already loving the unborn child who lives within her. It is our ultimate image of safety and nourishment—the time of protection within the womb, before we are buffeted by the world outside. And yet we now know that all mothers are passing more than nutrients and love along the fetal lifeline. Not stopped by the placental barrier, certain chemical compounds—called hormone disruptors—are being transferred from mother to infant.

Everyone in the world is exposed to these compounds and can be affected by them. We all are exposed to background levels of man-made chemicals—what we get through our normal day-to-day living—even in the relative safety of our own homes. There is not a single person on earth who does not have residues of at least a dozen chemical compounds in his or her body, and the numbers can go much, much higher. The hormone disruptors that a woman has stored in her body, plus any new exposures that take place while she is pregnant or nursing, get passed on to the fetus in the womb and the infant suckling at the breast. This is what happened to me; the DES (synthetic estrogen) my mother took to ensure a safe pregnancy was passed on to me in her womb.

MY STORY

In my early twenties I once took a job as a fashion model on the *Queen Elizabeth II* cruise ship. I woke up one night to find the sheets soaked through with bright red blood. I thought I was dying. The ship's doctor gave me an injection to help control the bleeding. This was one of the worst episodes of a repetitive situation that had been happening since I hit puberty at age nine and began menstruating.

For as long as I had my uterus, except for short periods of time when I would try a new nutritional program, I suffered with severe pain at the time of ovulation and serious hemorrhage-like bleeding and pain during menstruation. Whenever I told a doctor or nurse about my symptoms, I was reassured that excessive bleeding and pain were simply part of life for some women. These symptoms would not kill me. I should be more stoic. They would go away when I got pregnant and, if not by then, certainly when I became menopausal.

I began to experience breast pain, breast and ovarian cysts, and benign growths in my cervical canal that required multiple surgeries. Because nutrition proved to be more helpful than anything else, I earned a master's degree in nutrition (following joint degrees in psychology with an emphasis on neurobiology and theater/communications), then went through four and a half more years of schooling in nutrition and natural healing techniques so I could help other women with their health problems.

Every time I had another question that no one could help me with, I became a nutritional sleuth and searched the peer-reviewed medical literature for answers. This was in the 1970s, when very few people talked about nutrition and women's problems. I found that consuming more soy and whole-grain products, eating more vegetables and less red meat, taking certain vitamins, and avoiding coffee, tea, and alcohol reduced my pain. I would heal myself for periods of time.

For eleven years I was in a team practice with a cardiologist and internist specializing in nutrition. Many women would come to me with problems similar to those I had experienced. After using the protocols I prescribed, based on scientific research and programs I had tried on myself, many of these women became healthier. The irony was that these women improved and stayed healthy. As a DES daughter, I did not.

Today, many people are experiencing an increasing number of problems with their reproductive organs, fertility, and immune disorders. More women than ever are at risk for breast cancer and endometriosis. More men in Western countries have lower sperm counts, and the incidence of testicular and prostate cancer has increased. More children than ever are being diagnosed with behavioral problems, as noted by the fact that prescriptions of Prozac for children between the ages of eight and eighteen have gone up by more than 200 percent in the last several years.

Something is going on here.

More than 87,000 chemicals have entered the marketplace since World War II, very few of which have been sufficiently tested to determine whether or not they present risks to our health. My chemist friends get upset when I use the word *chemical* to refer only to man-made chemicals. All the processes in our bodies are started and regulated by natural chemical reactions. However, in this text I use the word *chemical* to refer to synthetic chemicals—the ones the chemists create in their laboratories. When I am referring to a natural chemical or chemical process, I will say so.

When we look at the weight of evidence—read all the scientific laboratory studies that have been conducted, see what has happened to DES children and to wildlife, and check the statistics for cancer and other diseases—it makes plain common sense to be as careful as possible about chemical compounds that act or are suspected of acting as hormone disruptors.

To understand hormone disruption, we first need a basic understanding of hormones and how they work.

SIGNALS OF LIFE

Birds do it. Bees do it. Alligators and petunias, fruit flies and polar bears do it. The baby in the womb does it. A teenager with pink hair, a 100-year-old woman blowing out her birthday candles, and an Olympian carrying the torch all do it. So do you and I. Every living thing that's bigger than one cell does it. Every organism operates through the same mecha-

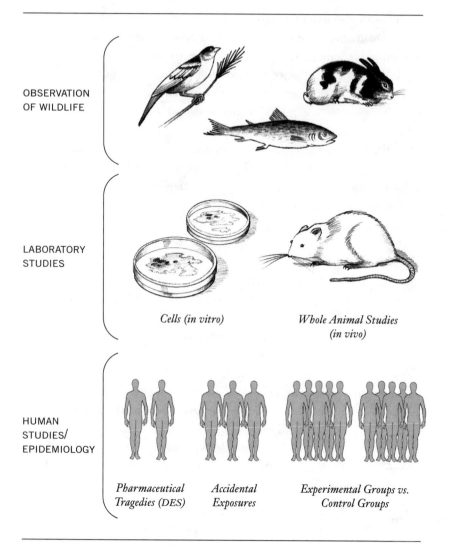

OBSERVATION OF WILDLIFE

LABORATORY STUDIES

Cells (in vitro)

Whole Animal Studies (in vivo)

HUMAN STUDIES/ EPIDEMIOLOGY

Pharmaceutical Tragedies (DES)

Accidental Exposures

Experimental Groups vs. Control Groups

FIGURE 1.1 *Where We Get Our Data*

nism of signal and response that has changed very little over the last 400 to 500 million years or so.

One cell sends out a signal and another cell receives the message. It's so simple, yet this is how *magic* happens throughout biology—how life develops and gets directed.

There are signals that decide which end of the earthworm will become its head and which end will be the tail. There are signals that direct plant roots to communicate with bacteria to take nitrogen out of the soil so the plants can thrive. Cells in the human brain send out signals called neurotransmitters. These messages leap across gaps and are received by other cells. "I got it!" you yell with delight as you suddenly figure out the solution to a problem that's been bothering you.

The cell-to-cell signaling system was firmly established long before plants and animals split off from each other on the evolutionary path and it has remained basically the same ever since. This is called evolutionary conservation—meaning the signaling system has been basically the same throughout evolution. All life is based on sending and receiving these signals. The messages we are concerned with in this book are the ones in humans and animals that come from the endocrine system. They are called hormones.

THE BODY'S MESSENGER SERVICE

The signal-response mechanism is used in many different ways in the body. Our immune, nervous, and endocrine systems all work through this cell-to-cell process. These systems control development and aging—the way we grow from an embryo to a fetus to an infant to a child to a teenager to an adult, all the way to old age.

The endocrine system, which is responsible for sending out hormonal signals, runs a very efficient messenger service. An endocrine gland sends out a small amount of a hormone carrying an important message. The hormone jumps on its trusty bicycle and rides through the bloodstream until it finds the correct address—the cells of a specific organ or tissue (called *target tissues*) that are meant to receive the message. The hormone finds a place to park, called a *receptor*, located either at the cell surface or inside the cell, and delivers its message. The signal has been delivered from one cell to another.

Now there is a response. Central headquarters in the cell takes the message and runs with it. The message is copied and translated into orders, which are sent to various parts of the body. For example, the pituitary is an endocrine gland that sends signals to the ovary, which then sends E-mail messages to the uterus and, in response, the uterus sheds its lining.

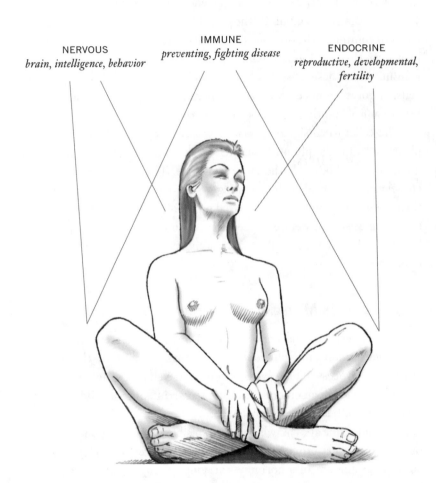

NERVOUS
brain, intelligence, behavior

IMMUNE
preventing, fighting disease

ENDOCRINE
reproductive, developmental, fertility

THE BODY HAS THREE MAJOR SYSTEMS: NERVOUS, IMMUNE, AND ENDOCRINE. ALL THESE
SYSTEMS INTERACT AND INFLUENCE EACH OTHER. IN OTHER WORDS, THEY "TALK" TO
EACH OTHER CONSTANTLY.

FIGURE 1.2 *How Body Systems Work Together*

You suddenly realize why your daughter has been eating candy bars and slamming doors for the past few days.

The signal-response mechanism—where one cell secretes a message and another cell receives it and produces a response—is a widespread phenomenon. A few days before a woman ovulates, the hormone estrogen sends a signal to the endometrial cells inside the uterus that urges the cells to grow thicker so the uterus is ready for pregnancy to occur. This same mechanism of signal and response occurs in the mating of sea urchins. An urchin releases molecules called pheromones that reach another sea urchin and bind to receptors, telling its chosen partner that it's time to clink their underwater wineglasses and mate.

Natural Hormones

Hormones are organic compounds that are secreted by the various cells, tissues, and organs of the endocrine system. Natural hormones, the hormones our bodies make, are usually short-lived, staying in the bloodstream for only a few minutes or at most a few hours. Just long enough for them to deliver their message. After the hormone delivers its message, enzymes from the liver break up the hormones into pieces that are either flushed out as waste or reused to build other molecules.

Natural hormones are so potent that they can produce very dramatic changes in cell activity with very small amounts, known as parts per billion or even parts per trillion, so minute that only extremely sensitive tests can measure them. One part per billion (ppb) is like putting a pinch of salt into 10 tons of potato chips. Most hormones, including estradiol (the body's most potent estrogen), insulin, and adrenaline work in amounts that are measured in parts per trillion (ppt). This is like placing one drop of water into a six-mile-long train with 660 tank cars!

Despite their tiny amounts and the fact that they work in the body for only short periods of time, hormones are absolutely essential for regulating the different biological processes in the body and can have long-lasting effects. Some endocrine actions are immediate, like the "butterflies" we feel in our stomach when we're nervous. Other hormonal actions are long-term. Growth and reproductive cycles happen over months (such as the menstrual cycle in women) or years (such as the process by which a child grows into an adult).

There are hundreds of hormones acting throughout the human body that we know about so far. For example, adrenaline is a well-known hormone, responsible for the fight-or-flight response. The hormone insulin helps regulate blood sugar. Thyroid hormones (thyroxine and triiodothy-

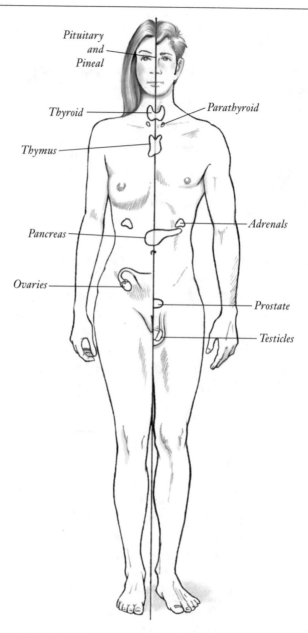

HORMONES ARE PRODUCED IN GLANDS (INCLUDING OVARIES, TESTICLES, PANCREAS, PITUITARY, ADRENAL, THYROID, PARATHYROID, AND THYMUS) AND RELEASED INTO THE BLOODSTREAM TO URGE RESPONSES IN VARIOUS TISSUES.

FIGURE 1.3 *The Endocrine System: Where Hormones Come From*

ronine) are needed for overall metabolism and brain development. Testosterone is responsible for libido and certain behaviors (like leaving the toilet seat up).

ANCIENT CELL PHONES

If the endocrine system is the body's messenger service, the hormone itself delivers the actual message. When the endocrine system works properly, the right message is sent by the endocrine glands, which secrete a hormone that travels through the bloodstream, and the message is received by special proteins called receptors. A receptor looks a little like an open pouch or the shape of a tiny womb. Receptor sites have frequently been compared to locks, waiting to be opened by a hormonal key. When a hormone enters the binding site and snuggles into the pouch, the hormone is said to be *bound* to the receptor.

The receptor is *usually* located in the cell's nucleus, the central command zone. The hormone's message gets delivered to the DNA. The DNA is like an archival library, containing all the genetic information within a cell. Then the genes carry out the instructions contained in the message. Gene function is turned on and off to produce a variety of rapid responses and long-term effects in the body.

Hormones integrate all systems in the body and urge the body to regulate, through the action of the genes, among other things:

- metabolism (the extraction of energy from nutrients)
- sexual development and reproduction
- mental processes
- growth and maintenance
- many aspects of our development before birth

Development is a word you will read frequently in this book. In humans and mammals, it refers to the growth and basic processes that take place, from the fertilization of the egg by the sperm through the entire step-by-step course of evolving into a mature living being. In a developing fetus, the endocrine system regulates cell division (growth) and organ differentiation (cell specialization)—the basic processes that set the stage for who we will become—and affects all parts of the body, including the brain.

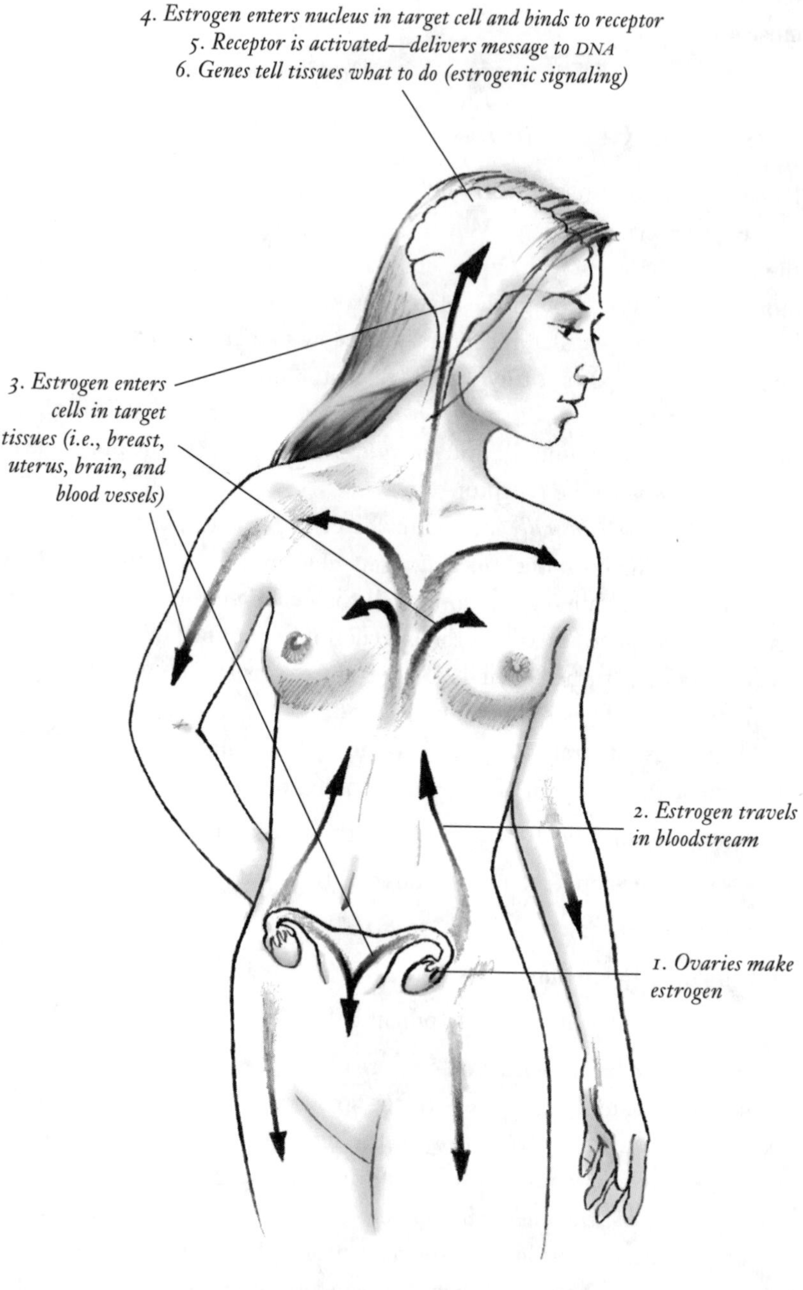

4. Estrogen enters nucleus in target cell and binds to receptor
5. Receptor is activated—delivers message to DNA
6. Genes tell tissues what to do (estrogenic signaling)

3. Estrogen enters cells in target tissues (i.e., breast, uterus, brain, and blood vessels)

2. Estrogen travels in bloodstream

1. Ovaries make estrogen

FIGURE 1.4 *How a Hormone Works: Example—Estrogen*

It's a very competent and effective setup. Messages are sent and received and the body complies with the orders contained in the messages. It's a system that's worked exceedingly well for a very long time.

Up until recently.

Getting the Wrong Message

For the last fifty years, man-made chemicals used in the external world have been entering our bodies, where they are participating in an age-old signal/response system that has not had time to adapt to them. Hormonal signals always used to come from *inside* our bodies or from natural substances, such as the estrogens in plants, that have evolved along with us.

The signal/response system in vertebrates is hundreds of millions of years old, while endocrine-disrupting chemicals have only come into widespread use since the end of World War II. Our bodies haven't had enough time to take into account these alien messengers, coming from *outside* our bodies, which are now pervasive in air, land, and water, and to make the necessary evolutionary changes that would protect us from these substances.

All this points to what can go awry. If something is wrong with the signal, the body will respond to the wrong message. In other words, an unnatural signal may create an inappropriate response. What science is discovering is that hormone disruptors can bind with receptors and send messages the same way our natural hormones can. But these particular messages can significantly *alter* normal cell function and growth.

Body systems like the immune, nervous, and endocrine systems are not separate and distinct entities. Their functions overlap, and there are receptors for signals from each of the systems in many different parts of the body. For example, the intestinal tract has receptors for the immune and nervous systems as well as receptors for estrogen and possibly other hormones in close proximity to one another. This cross-talk among our various body systems may be why we lose our appetite or get diarrhea before we have to speak before a crowd or take an important test.

In fact, hormone disruption may very well turn out to be just the tip of the iceberg when we finally learn how chemicals from the environment are acting inside the integrated whole of our bodies. In a machine, if one part is damaged or altered, the functioning of the entire engine can be disrupted. If someone threw a wrench into the engine of your beautiful new Jaguar, chances are your automobile would have trouble. Likewise, an incorrect message sent by a chemical that mimics a hormone can tell the genes to turn on when they should be turned off, or vice versa. Creating a disturbance at any one point can throw things off balance anywhere else in the body.

A DEFINITION OF HORMONE DISRUPTORS

Hormone disruptors are chemicals (or mixtures of chemicals) from outside the body that can interfere with the development or function of body systems in humans and wildlife, especially in their offspring, and may lead to irreversible adverse health effects.

THE QUESTION IS . . .

In wildlife, when hormone disruptors enter an animal's body, these "wrong messages" have been shown to mimic, amplify, or block the working of the animal's own hormones. What happens? Male fish start making female egg proteins. Female gulls, called "gay gulls," start nesting with other females. Panthers are born with undescended testicles. Male alligators have such small penises they cannot reproduce. Research experiments with laboratory animals also show the effects of endocrine disruption on mammals.

But has endocrine disruption been proven in humans?

Many scientists believe that the weight of evidence points to endocrine disruption as a human reality. Until recently, there has been little solid cause-and-effect proof of health effects in humans except for the "experiment" with DES. However, hormone disruptors *have* been linked with specific health conditions in humans. For example, pesticide exposure to the pregnant mother has been shown to have a definite effect on children's neurological behavior. Other chemical compounds can even cause lowered intelligence. Endometriosis (a painful reproductive tract problem that contributes to female infertility) has been associated with exposure to dioxins (airborne hormone disruptors). But scientifically confirming the link between hormone disruptors and human health would mean doing experiments that deliberately expose humans to chemicals, which, of course, wouldn't be ethical or desirable.

Why then, you wonder, should possible health effects based on a scientific theory concern you?

AND THE ANSWER IS . . .

Scientists use the word *theory* differently than the lay public, which uses the word to mean little more than a guess or an untested idea. In the scientific definition, a theory is a more or less verified or established explanation that accounts for known facts or phenomena, such as Einstein's theory of relativity or Newton's theory of gravitation. (And, looking at our bodies as they age, we all accept that gravity is real.) There are scientific theories that chemicals can cause cancer or that electrons are part of an atom. Natural selection is a theory. We tend to think of these things as facts, but scientists call them theories.

In wildlife and laboratory animals, endocrine disruption is a solid theory, offering a well-tested explanation for what is being seen. The Food and Drug Administration (FDA) and other government agencies review the testing done by the manufacturers, who test chemical products through animal trials. If animal testing is good enough for determining the safety of products that will ultimately be used by humans, we should be listening to what wildlife problems and the results of animal testing in the laboratory are telling us about hormone disruption.

In fact, research based on animal testing may even be underestimating the effect of estrogenic compounds. Most commercially available laboratory animals have been bred for large litter size and vigor, which has now been shown to make them more resistant to estrogen. Thus, experimentation on most laboratory animals may be greatly underestimating the effects of estrogenic compounds.

In many ways, the hormonal system in animals and humans is very much the same and has been so for a long evolutionary time. Still, some people believe that the results from laboratory or animal studies don't necessarily apply to humans. In other words, if exposing pregnant mice to a certain chemical results in their babies being born with damaged reproductive systems, what difference does that make to us? After all, they're only mice.

Actually, many scientists believe that the endocrine disruption that is observed in wildlife and in laboratory studies has direct implications for humans. Commonalities across species in the hormonal mechanisms that

GOD AND SCIENCE

As Dr. Frederick vom Saal, a professor of biology at the University of Missouri, puts it: "Way before DES was used on five million women in the U.S., it was clear from animal studies that DES would be damaging to fetuses. But we have this absolutely bizarre notion that humans are separate from the rest of life on Earth. You will hear physician after physician say, 'But that's an animal. What relevance does that have to humans?' You *can* believe in religion and believe in God and believe in creation *and* believe that God created a template for life. Just saying that we have similar systems to animals doesn't negate that there could be a God.

"At the molecular mechanistic level, we are dealing with a system that is identical across all vertebrates, not just mice and humans—a system that essentially hasn't changed in the last 300 million years of vertebrate evolution. This is a remarkably conserved system evolutionarily because it's so critical to life. So if a chemical can disrupt the endocrine system by acting as an estrogen in a fish, for instance, the likelihood is that it will do that in humans. Endocrine disruption in fish has to be a concern with regard to human health. Not just mice, not just birds or reptiles, it's all of them. They're all sentinels for our health because these chemicals are in all likelihood operating on systems that we all share."

---

control development and function mean that any adverse effects we observe in wildlife and in laboratory animals may also happen in humans. On the other hand, one study has shown that animals can differ in their response to the same chemicals and warns that sweeping generalizations may not accurately portray a chemical's effect on all animals. However, if a chemical can disrupt the endocrine system by acting like a hormone in an alligator, a fish, or a panther, the likelihood is that it will act like a hormone within the human body, although the effect we see in the human may be different from the effect in the animal. The same chemical that may cause smaller penises in alligators may cause lower sperm counts in men. When we see mice with early puberty, for example, it is a serious concern that cannot be dismissed before long-term, accurate studies are performed.

WHY WAIT?

There is a problem with long-term accurate scientific studies that would provide scientific "proof"—they take a very long time.

Think about cigarettes. Smiling doctors used to appear in magazines and on television in the 1950s and 1960s, reassuring the public that the medical profession endorsed smoking as a wise way to relax, to digest, and to face life's trials. Then scientists began to suspect that smoking caused health problems. Over the years, numerous studies were run. Many showed a correlation between smoking and lung cancer, as well as other health problems such as emphysema. Yet other studies showed no cause for alarm.

This is the way science works, carefully and cautiously, compiling evidence over an extended period of time. It took forty years and more than sixty studies to get warnings out to the public that, in fact, cigarettes constitute a health hazard. At present, the accepted theory is that cigarettes do contribute to lung cancer as well as many other diseases. However, for decades, millions of people still smoked and got ill, all because the connection between cigarettes and disease, though suspected, had not yet been proven.

What is going on with endocrine disruption is big—so big that if we are afraid to ask questions, we very well may miss the answers. Why wait another twenty to forty years until the final word is in before we take preventative action on hormone disruptors?

We have a right to know what is happening, in language we can understand. Very few people can read a scientific study and comprehend what is being said, let alone what is being implied. We need to take this growing body of information out of the hands of professionals alone and place it in the hands of everyday folks—the people who buy the groceries and feed their families, microwave quick meals, take their kids to dentists, use hormone replacement therapy—the people who need to know how to minimize the risks for breast cancer, the people who understand the danger in waiting years and years for more studies to be funded and carried out in order to prove conclusively the correlation between hormone disruptors and damaged health in humans.

That's you and me.

Alien Hormone Messengers

The hypothesis is that multiple chemicals in the environment trick the body, trick this developing embryo into thinking that it's getting a signal, a normal signal . . .

— Dr. Lou Guillette, Department of Zoology
at the University of Florida

The scientific evidence presented in this book shows that hormone disruption is being observed in wildlife, in laboratory studies, and in humans. But I *know* about hormone disruption because it happened to me. When my mother was pregnant, she was given a dose of diethylstilbestrol (DES), the first synthetic estrogen ever marketed. My mother's doctor believed that DES would prevent miscarriage and enhance pregnancy. A very potent estrogenic chemical (meaning it acts like an estrogen), DES got into my cells when I was in my mother's womb and sent very destructive messages. It disrupted my developing reproductive system, giving me "female" problems, which ultimately resulted in my inability to have a child. And I suspect that DES exposure in the womb was a causative factor in my getting breast cancer in my forties. If DES was the only culprit, it would be enough to simply stop using it. But the problem is far broader than this one chemical.

I have been a health-care practitioner and a diligent academician and researcher on women's health issues for several decades. And I'm concerned about the fact that most people know very little about hormone

---

WHAT ARE THEY CALLED?

Here are some of the different terms used to describe hormone disruptors:

- *Hormone disruptor* or *endocrine disruptor* is used broadly to label man-made chemicals or naturally occurring substances like phytoestrogens that produce possible alterations of the endocrine system functions. When we use either of these terms, we are referring to a foreign substance (as opposed to the natural hormones made by our bodies) that in some way affects our hormone system and therefore our health (although we always must remember that not everyone is adversely affected). The term *hormone disruptors* is somewhat of a nickname for this class of compounds that disrupt the endocrine system—more formally known as *endocrine-disrupting compounds* or EDCs. In some countries, such as Japan, the preferred term is *environmental hormones*.

- *Xenohormones* is a term that indicates these hormonal substances are foreign to our bodies, coming from chemicals in the environment—also called *environmental hormones, hormone-related toxicants* (poisons), *environmental contaminants,* and *xenobiotics*. The terms *hormone mimics* or *hormone impostors* refer to xenohormones that alter the endocrine system by acting like hormones.

- *Environmental estrogens, ecoestrogens,* and *xenoestrogens* are endocrine disruptors that specifically mimic or affect the hormone estrogen. *Phytoestrogens* are a class of naturally occurring substances in plants that act like weak estrogens.

- *Anti-estrogens* or *anti-androgens* are endocrine disruptors that block or cancel out the normal effects of the female (estrogens) or male (androgens) hormones.

- *Endocrine modulators* is a term recently used by some authors to describe endocrine disruption without implying that it necessarily leads to irreversible adverse effects.

- *Environmental signaling* is a general term for messages coming from outside the body. Many environmental chemicals might disrupt signaling processes, but not all do it by interfering with hormones.

---

disruptors and the ways in which these chemicals can send the wrong messages to our bodies.

Alien hormone messengers—in the form of man-made chemicals—have entered our environment in overwhelming amounts over the last fifty years. These synthetic chemicals enter our bodies through the food we eat, the water we drink and bathe in, and the air we breathe. Some of these chemicals have the ability to masquerade as hormones. They ride freely through the bloodstream, not subject to the rules and regulations that guide natural hormones, and bind with hormone receptors. They deliver a message to central headquarters. Responses take place, even if the orders are inappropriate. Hormone disruptors may:

- mimic the natural hormones in our bodies, such as estrogens
- antagonize (block) our natural hormones, such as androgens (male hormones), thyroid hormone, and progesterone
- alter the way in which natural hormones are produced, eliminated, or metabolized
- modify the number of hormone receptors we have and thus the amount of hormonal signaling in our bodies
- stimulate the release of hormones or other natural substances that affect the balance of our hormones in our bodies

WHERE ARE THESE HORMONE DISRUPTORS COMING FROM?

The man-made chemicals that can disturb the endocrine system within our bodies are the by-products or building blocks of fuels, pesticides, detergents, and plastics—the regular stuff of life as we enter the new millennium. Normally we don't think at all about the synthetic chemicals that have given us our modern lifestyle. Today's technology makes our lives easier, fuller, and more fascinating. How different would our lives be without a computer, TV, telephone, microwave, automobile, or disposable diapers and fast food?

Since World War II, approximately 87,000 new chemicals have been synthesized in the United States alone. New ones are always being invented, at the rate of at least 2,000 a year. These chemicals are used in thousands of different ways, from making plastic more pliable, to lengthening the shelf life of groceries and shrink-wrapping foods, to inventing new fabrics and new medicines. Chemicals have been responsible for some great strides forward, giving us the ability to prevent or fight the diseases that used to wipe out large segments of the population, allowing us to live longer and better. There is no way we will turn back the clock, nor would we want to turn away from the progress that has given us so much. How-ever, we cannot be blind to the consequences of this progress.

The chemicals that we discuss in this book that are either known or suspected hormone disruptors are part of an ever-changing list. The Office of Toxic Substances is called upon each year to review about 2,000 new chemical products, many of which are suspected of being harmful. How many of these chemicals actually disrupt our endocrine systems? No one knows. Are they harmful to everyone or just to supersensitive indi-viduals or babies in the womb? No one knows. How many of these chem-icals act to turn on or off thyroid or adrenal function? Our sex hormones? No one knows. At present, tens of thousands of man-made chemicals are used, yet their effects on the endocrine system have been studied for only a few of these. Up until now, the estrogenic activity of most chemicals has been detected by accident, not by intent.

What scientists and researchers have become increasingly concerned about in the last decade is that these endocrine-disrupting compounds are more a part of our food and daily lives than anyone ever imagined. Hor-mone disruptors are so intricately woven into the web of modern life that all women, men, and children carry within their bodies a chemical legacy

HOW MUCH OF THIS STUFF IS OUT THERE?

According to statistics from the 1997 Toxic Releases Inventory Public Data Release from the EPA Office of Toxic Substances:

There were 2.58 billion pounds of listed toxic chemicals (not just hormone disruptors) released on site.

62.9%	into the air
10.3%	into the water
10.4%	underground
16.4%	into landfills and dumps

All within one year. All within the United States alone.

Off-site releases add another 461.1 million pounds of toxic chemicals to the environ-ment.

that may be altering the wonderful hormone signaling system we share with other species.

A century ago, this chemical legacy didn't exist. Now, anywhere from a dozen to 500 chemicals can be found in measurable quantities in the body fat of every living human. (Different studies cite different numbers, although I've found no studies that say there are people with *no* chemical residues in their bodies.) These chemicals are found even in people who live in remote and presumably pristine wilderness more than a thousand miles away from major sources of pollution. From the North Pole to the South Pole, on every continent and in every ocean, hormone-disrupting chemicals are found in air, soil, water, plants, and animals, including humans. And many of these chemicals break down into compounds

---

NIMBY (NOT IN MY BACK YARD)

Most people date the chemical revolution to the 1920s or earlier, when industry geared up. However, the revolution accelerated with the war against bugs. Diseases carried by insects were killing American soldiers faster than the enemy in 1943 when a Swiss firm applied for a patent on a new insecticide, dichlorodiphenyl-trichloroethane (DDT). The U.S. government dusted millions of soldiers and refugees with "the miracle white powder" to prevent malaria and typhus. Its inventor, Paul Mueller, was awarded a Nobel Prize—in medicine. Nearly five billion pounds of DDT were applied indoors and out after it was introduced. By 1944, scientists found residues of DDT in human fat, and a few years later in human breast milk. Much later, of course, DDT became known for its adverse health effects. Its use was eventually banned in the United States. But just because the pesticide is banned in the United States doesn't mean it isn't still manufactured here and then exported to other parts of the world. There are as yet no effective alternatives in certain circumstances, and it is still critical to malaria control. Mexico and Brazil use about 1,000 tons a year. In 1992 U.S. manufacturers shipped more than 300 tons of the mosquito killer to Peru.

At least 1,950 tons of other pesticides whose domestic use had been banned or discontinued were exported in 1992. In 1993 and 1994, domestically outlawed pesticides were exported at the rate of more than 9 tons per day. And this was just a quarter of the roughly 250,000 tons of recorded pesticides to leave the United States in any given year.

KNOWN AND SUSPECTED HORMONE DISRUPTORS

TYPE	SOURCE
PLASTICS	
Phthalates—class of chemicals used as plasticizers (to make plastics more flexible). Some of the hormone disrupting phthalates are diethylhexyl phthalate (DEPH), butyl benzyl phthalate (BBP), di-n-butyl phthalate (DBP), and diethyl phthalate (DEP).	Plasticizers are used in food-packaging materials, car parts, toys, blood bags, inks, nail polish, and on and on.
Bisphenol A—BPA is a component of plastic. It is one of the top fifty chemicals in production. Coats metal products (like tin cans and bottle tops) and water supply pipes.	Used in polycarbonate plastics, dental sealants, and composites.
DETERGENTS	
Alkylphenolic compounds (APES) and nonylphenols (NPES)—class of chemical surfactants that dissolve and remove oils and grease and make products more water soluble.	Some commercial detergents, personal products (hair dyes, shampoos, shaving creams, cosmetics, spermicides), latex paints. Also used as stabilizers and antioxidants in plastics.
POPS (PERSISTENT ORGANIC POLLUTANTS)	
Dioxins (family of seventy-five compounds) and furans (135 dibenzofurans). Most potent is tetrachlorodibenzo-p-dioxin (TCDD).	Created when plastic, especially PVC, and other chlorinated compounds are manufactured or are burned in older incinerators.
Polychlorinated biphenyls (PCBS)—class of 209 compounds	Previously used as electrical insulator, adhesive, and lubricant. Production is banned but it's still used in sealed equipment in other countries.

TYPE	SOURCE
POPS (PERSISTENT ORGANIC POLLUTANTS) *CONTINUED*	
Polyvinyl chloride (PVC)—vinyl, most widely used plastics. Often mixed with phthalates.	Children's toys, teething rings, flooring, etc.
Pesticides	Both active and inert ingredients can be endocrine-disrupting compounds.
OTHER ENDOCRINE-DISRUPTING COMPOUNDS	
Polycyclic aromatic hydrocarbons (PAHS)	Come from incomplete combustion of petrochemical products, wood, and tobacco.
Heavy metals—lead, cadmium, and mercury	Lead—lead crystal, plumbing, PVC, batteries, old paint, tin cans Cadmium—NiCad batteries, stabilizers in plastics, fossil fuels Mercury—fluorescent lights, pesticides, dental fillings, seed coatings

(metabolites) that are sometimes more potent than the original chemicals themselves.

Hormone-disrupting compounds come from:

• **Pesticides** (an umbrella term for herbicides, fungicides, and insecticides—a $30 billion a year industry)—used on food crops and home gardens and found in flea collars for your pets, lice shampoo for your kids, or even under the foundation of your home.

• **Plastics**—both in their manufacture and disposal. Every four years there are 1 trillion pounds of plastic made in the world. When certain plastics are burned in incinerators (for example, medical waste like IV bags burned in hospital incinerators), they can release **dioxins**, which are potent hormone disruptors.

• **Plasticizers** (*phthalates*, pronounced *thalates*)—compounds added to some plastics to make them more flexible. Sitting in your new car inhaling that new-car smell, you're actually breathing in the phthalates that are used in polyvinyl chloride (PVC) in different car parts. Eventually, your car dashboard will crack when there are no more phthalates in there. Another example is the PVC (polyvinyl chloride) cling wrap that is used in supermarkets to wrap wedges of cheese and meat. Plasticizers are used in synthetic leathers, adhesives, caulking, and cosmetics, and as a carrier and dispersant for insecticides, repellents, and perfumes. They are also used as a component of paper and paperboard that comes in contact with liquid, fatty, and dry foods. Phthalates slowly leach from plastics and are now found throughout the environment, including the ecosystems of rivers and oceans. *Bisphenol A* is a building block of polycarbonate plastics. It may leach into our bodies from food and beverage packaging, including baby formula bottles, and from the lining of tin cans and from dental sealants and composite fillings.

• **Pharmaceuticals**—including birth control pills, hormone replacement therapy, fertility drugs, and synthetic estrogens (similar to DES), which are used in almost every feedlot in America.

• **Persistent Organic Pollutants** (POPS)—which are among the longest lasting chemicals ever produced. They are all chlorinated or brominated. Chlorine or bromine molecules, when added to substances, make them more stable and more persistent.

Polychlorinated biphenyls (PCBs) were used in transformers and other electrical equipment until they were banned. There are 209 different types of PCBs and the ones that are the most toxic and most persistent in our bodies and the environment are the ones that are fairly heavily chlorinated. Their concentrations increase in the body as we get older.

Dioxins and *furans* are a large family of chemicals—seventy-five halogenated (chlorinated or brominated) dibenzo-p-dioxins (PCDDs) and 135 dibenzofurans (PCDFs)—that are not intentionally produced, but are released into the environment as a by-product of chemical processes involving chlorine. Of the seventy-five dioxins, tetrachlorodibenzo-p-dioxin (TCDD) is the most potent and best studied.

PVC (polyvinyl chloride), or vinyl, is one of the most common of all plastics, used in everything from flooring to children's toys. The manufacture of PVC generates large quantities of dioxin, and burning PVC plastic can create dioxins, especially in older incinerators. New, high-tech incineration does not produce dioxins. PVC plastic has been called one of the single most environmentally damaging and least recyclable of all plastics.

• **Detergents** (*Alkylphenol ethoxylates*, APES)—along with their derivatives, the commonly used *nonyl phenol ethoxylates* (NPES), which are surfactants that are manufactured from petroleum. A *surfactant*—short for surface active agent—is a chemical that functions in cleaning products to dissolve and remove oils and grease and to make water penetrate more readily. Ordinary household products, like laundry detergents and cleansers, spermicides, nail lacquers, cosmetics, and hair products, can contain APES or their cousins, NPES, which are also used as industrial detergents in the textile and paper industries, as degreasers for engine parts, and as detergents for cleaning wool.

INDUSTRY STANDARDS

Dr. John McCarthy, the vice president for scientific and regulatory affairs for the Trade Association of Pesticides said, "I believe firmly and strongly that the system we have is a system of high integrity, particularly with the good laboratory practices and government inspections. Believe me, major companies don't want to get the wrong answers. They don't pay their scientists to get the answers they'd like to get."

Dr. Daryl Sumner, a Ph.D. in toxicology who is on a medical school faculty, said that "federal requirements are very strict. Data must be submitted to the EPA and then the EPA reevaluates the data. There is never any pressure from management to make a study come out a certain way. Industrial scientists are always aware of these accusations and, if anything, don't take kindly to being told how results should come out."

Then again, what about biting the hand that feeds you? Some scientists may be swayed because they receive money from the chemical or pharmaceutical industries for giving lectures or consulting, or their research may be funded through industry. For example, since 1997 nearly half the articles evaluating drugs in the *New England Journal of Medicine* were written by scientists who worked as paid advisers to drugmakers or received major research funding from them. Most medical journals these days don't require the authors of studies to stay independent of industry.

THE SCIENCE OF POISONS

To learn how chemicals affect us, scientists called toxicologists study different compounds to determine the amount at which they would act as poison in our bodies. *Classical toxicology* is defined as the "science of poisons." It dates back to the Greeks and Egyptians and is based on how much was needed to kill. Dr. Bernard Weiss (a neurotoxicologist and professor of environmental medicine and pediatrics at the University of Rochester Medical Center) says, "Think of the images that such a definition evokes: Lucretia Borgia in her kitchen, hunters dipping arrowheads in curare, preparations to defend against chemical warfare. It conjures up visions of lethal incantations like the opening scene of *Macbeth*." There's the story of Emperor Claudius's wife, who had to sample the emperor's food before he would eat it. She desensitized herself with low doses of a poison, then spiked the emperor's food with it. As usual, he let her taste the food first. She was fine; he died.

Rather than trying to figure out how much of a substance will kill, *contemporary toxicology* is concerned with discovering the impact on health of low environmental exposures whose outcomes may not be known until decades after exposure takes place.

Some alkylphenols such as BHT and BHA are used to prolong the shelf life of food and to retard oxidation. Four hundred and fifty million pounds of alkylphenols were sold in the United States in 1990. They are degraded during sewage treatment; the resulting compounds are weakly estrogenic and have been found in drinking water.

In other words, endocrine-disrupting chemicals are everywhere. (See Appendix A for a full examination of these chemicals.) One source is from foods typically found in U.S. supermarkets. When a pregnant woman consumes these foods, along with other hormone disruptors she has stored in her body from the environment, some of the fat-soluble chemicals get transferred to the fetus. In a lactating mother, the chemicals may be concentrated in the breast milk and transferred to the baby.

Did loud alarm bells go off in your head when you heard the words *breast milk*? Hormone-disrupting chemicals are known to contaminate our most perfect food—mother's milk. Tests of mother's milk have shown it can contain higher levels of contaminants than are permitted in cow's milk sold in grocery stores (although breast milk is still considered the best food for babies).

The federal government does not screen chemicals for safety before they are sold, although they do test pharmaceuticals for human use. Only between 1.5 and 3 percent of chemicals have been tested to see if they cause cancer; almost *none* have been tested to see what they do to the endocrine system. In other words, a man-made chemical is considered innocent until proven guilty. And it is up to the manufacturers themselves—those who design and produce these chemicals (and reap the profit)—to determine whether or not their products pose a risk to our health or to the environment.

How Hormone Disruptors Differ from Natural Hormones

If hormone disruptors mimic our own hormones, aren't these chemicals basically the same as our natural hormones?

No, they're not.

Natural hormones are short-lived, staying in our bodies only for the amount of time necessary to do their jobs. They don't accumulate in the tissues and are easily broken down and eliminated by our bodies.

The same seems to be true for phytoestrogens. These plant compounds are either flushed out or changed and absorbed into the body in a (usually) beneficial way. Synthetic estrogens, like those in birth-control pills, fertility drugs, or hormone replacement therapy, remain in the body longer than natural estrogens. However, they are not nearly as long-lived as pesticides and other environmental compounds that can act like hormones.

On the other hand, many hormone-disrupting chemicals are not easily broken down by the body. They remain intact inside living organisms and can accumulate within our tissues. Most are lipophilic, meaning they are attracted to fat and don't dissolve easily in water. This means that hormone disruptors aren't easy to flush out of the body; instead, they take up residence in our fat cells and may stay there for many years, even decades. In a woman's body, fatty tissue is concentrated in the breast, ovaries, and placenta during fetal development, but it is also found in other organs, including the brain, and it is used throughout the body for padding and insulation and as caloric reserves. During stress or yo-yo cycles of weight loss, some of these substances can be released from the fat cells and redistributed; during pregnancy and breastfeeding, they can be passed on to offspring.

Another difference is that EDCs (endocrine-disrupting compounds) are far more flexible than natural hormones. They are like molecular acrobats that can make themselves fit into various receptors.

Chemicals, by themselves, are not good or bad. Generally, they are cheap to produce and highly effective. It wasn't until they had been used for decades that some of their health and environmental effects surfaced. Endocrine disruptors are part of a complex set of interlocking problems in our modern life. In this book, I'm not trying to brand any particular group as the villain in the story of endocrine disruption. Chemical manufacturers and industry are providing ways to improve our lives as well as finding ways to maximize their profits. Nowadays some chemical manufacturers are trying to find more natural chemical products that benefit us (and them) without producing major risks.

HOW HORMONE DISRUPTORS DIFFER FROM CLASSIC POISONS

Endocrine disruptors are very different from the poisons toxicologists have worked with in the past. Why? Because we are talking about hormonal activity, which is totally different from discussing toxicity.

Traditionally, toxicologists have believed that "the dose makes the poison," which means that the higher the dose, the more likely it is that a substance will do damage. At high enough dosages, all chemicals are toxic. For example, too much vitamin A can be poisonous. As a corollary, conventional wisdom says that if a lot is bad, then less will be safer. Many of those who work in the field of risk assessment and toxicology are still guided by these old rules. However, the endocrine system responds to tiny quantities of hormone messengers: minute amounts of endocrine disruptors can elicit a response and cause changes. Frederick vom Saal, a noted scientist in the field, has a different perspective. He starts from the level at which estrogens and environmental estrogens act in the body—called the physiologic range—so he works from the bottom up while toxicologists work from the top down. He calls it bottom-up toxicology.

Scientists are looking at hormone disruptors as having a whole range of possible effects, from behavior and IQ problems to infertility and

---

THE GRASSHOPPER EFFECT

We know that chemicals volatilize (go into the air) more easily in the warmer latitudes. Through what's been called the grasshopper effect, these chemicals slowly but surely move to the colder latitudes. For example, persistent organochlorines increase in sea water as they move north. (As a side note, it is interesting that there is more incidence of breast cancer in the northern part of the United States than in the south.)

There are global air patterns that pull up material from the south in a swirl pattern that lasts 30 years. This means a slow mini-whirlwind can maintain pollutant exposure for three decades. There is a similar 30-year cycle in water. There are no manufacturing companies in the pristine northern regions of Canadian land masses, so how to account for elevations of certain chemicals in many native peoples of the northern regions of Canada? Dr. Bernard Weiss said, "Where does it all come from? Well, folks, it's coming from us. It's coming from the south and migrating north."

---

endometriosis. Up until now, health risks usually have been defined as cancer, birth defects, or death—the endpoints that are still used by government health agencies as a guide to decide safe doses and exposure to various chemicals. With endocrine disruptors, a number of different questions have to be considered:

- What is the hormonal activity of the molecule by itself and in combination with other chemicals?

- How is the chemical metabolized by the body? Does it produce metabolites (chemical offspring) that act differently from the parent compound? A good example of this is the pesticide methoxychlor, which itself has very little estrogenic activity and is relatively short-lived in the body, but which is metabolized in the liver into a compound that is a strong estrogen with high estrogenic activity. In another example, DDT has two major metabolites that act differently from each other. One is estrogenic and the other is anti-androgenic (blocks male hormones); both have similar endocrine-disrupting results.

- What was the dosage at which the chemical was tested? Testing only high dosages of chemicals for their safety in humans could seriously underestimate the risk of chemical exposure at a low dose. What will the chemical do as a hormone at a million times lower dose? Dan Sheehan, a research biologist with the National Center for Toxicological Research, says his lab finds effects at any dose of hormone disruptors, no matter how low. While low doses may evoke strong responses, higher doses of hormones or hormone disruptors may overwhelm and deactivate a system. Hormones are active when they occupy only a very small proportion of the available receptor sites, but when too much hormone enters the system, the system begins to shut off—it down-regulates. This means the high dose may have different effects than low dosages or do nothing at all.

WHAT'S OUTSIDE IS INSIDE

Since the chemicals outside of us are now omnipresent inside us, we cannot talk about endocrine-disrupting chemicals without setting them in the

CLASSICAL TOXICOLOGY
LINEAR RESPONSE

*Classical poisons where
"the dose is the poison"*

CONTEMPORARY TOXICOLOGY

*Hormone disruptors have
varying responses at
different dosages*

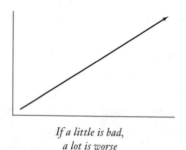

*If a little is bad,
a lot is worse*

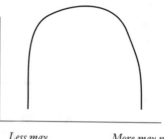

*Less may
be worse*   *More may not
be as bad*

FIGURE 2.1 *Dose-Response Differences*

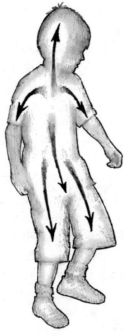

Most of the natural signals that direct hormonal activity come from inside our bodies.

Unnatural environmental signaling (signals from man-made chemicals in food, air, water, and everyday products) is coming from synthetic sources outside our bodies.

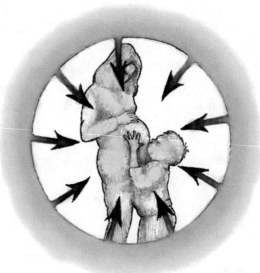

FIGURE 2.2 *Signals (Outside vs. Inside)*

context of the *environment*. We need to rethink what we mean when we talk about the environment. Many things, from hair dye to the pesticide-laden manicured greens of our golf courses to processed foods such as commercially colored and fat-laden ice cream, contain chemicals that are known or suspected hormone disruptors. However, the environment that affects our health is not only what surrounds us in our first home—the womb—and also in our houses, our towns, or our nations, although those are significant. Endocrine disruptors travel on global air and water currents and end up thousands of miles away from their place of origin. Chemicals used anywhere in the world—even those banned in America—can reach us.

Each year we breathe 10 million pints of the atmosphere into our lungs, air that might have circulated from India or China, Zaire or Australia. Snow that looks white and pure could be transporting pollutants that have blown in from distant lands. When the snow melts, the pollutants seep into water and soil. High mountaintops are full of chemicals that arrive via the air, snowfall, and cold condensation.

Even when levels in the water, air, or soil are low, the concentration of a chemical in animals at the top of the food chain may be high enough to cause adverse effects on behavior, reproduction, or disease resistance and thus endanger that species. A hormone disruptor can enter the food chain at any point in the environment, get stored in the body faster than it is broken down or excreted (bioaccumulation), and become more concentrated as it moves up the food chain (biomagnification). This means that animals at the very top of the food chain, through their regular diet, may store much more of the chemical than was present in organisms lower in the food chain. So the herring gull eating a diet of trout from the Great Lakes can have a chemical in its tissues that is 25 million times more magnified than it was in the plankton at the bottom of the sea. The pollution can be concentrated in the sediment and in the body of the organisms, yet the water from the lake can test clean for the chemical!

It's a spaceship Earth problem. We all share a common ecosystem and must all accept the responsibility for our effect upon it. Our planet is a relatively closed system—energy is coming in from the sun and we're losing heat, but everything we make and do stays with us. We can never go back to living in isolation from those who live in other areas of the world. In an intimate dance, we affect the environment with our technological cul-

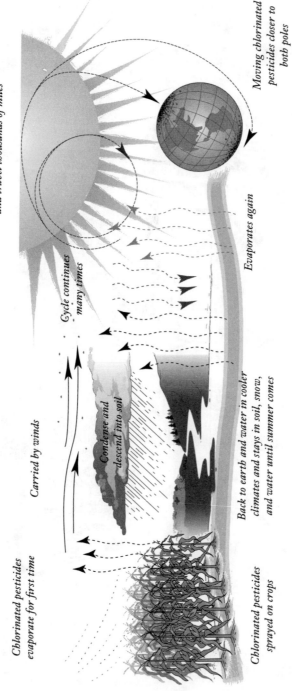

Some wind and water mass mini-whirls of contaminants can last up to thirty years and travel thousands of miles

Moving chlorinated pesticides closer to both poles

Cycle continues many times

Carried by winds

Evaporates again

Condense and descend into soil

Back to earth and water in cooler climates and stays in soil, snow, and water until summer comes

Chlorinated pesticides evaporate for first time

Chlorinated pesticides sprayed on crops

FIGURE 2.3 *How Chemicals Travel Around the World*

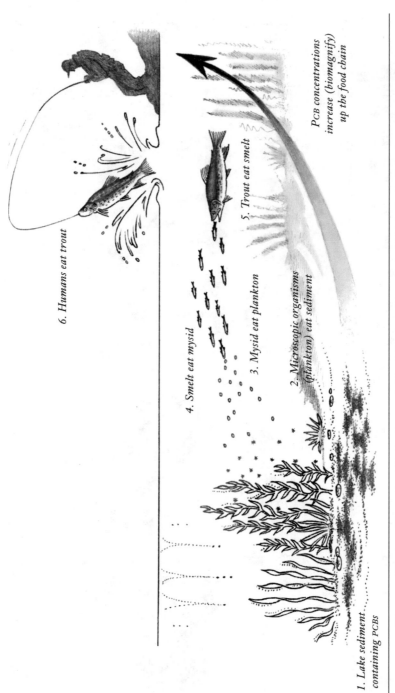

6. Humans eat trout

5. Trout eat smelt

4. Smelt eat mysid

3. Mysid eat plankton

2. Microscopic organisms (plankton) eat sediment

1. Lake sediment containing PCBs

PCB concentrations increase (biomagnify) up the food chain

FIGURE 2.4 *Biomagnification: Example of Lake Ontario's Food Chain (Adapted from Our Stolen Future, Dutton, 1996.)*

ture, and, in turn, endocrine-disrupting chemicals have the potential to affect us all. We could call it the shadow side of technology.

Dr. Theo Colborn is the director and senior scientist of the wildlife and contaminants program at the World Wildlife Fund and a coauthor of *Our Stolen Future*. She was the first person, with visionary prowess, to synthesize the vast literature on the problems wildlife were experiencing and to recognize that many of the effects that were being observed were related to disruption of the endocrine system. Colborn has said the topic of global exposure to hormone mimics is so huge that it is a *moral* issue even more than a scientific one.

All About Estrogen

If Shakespeare had been a chemist, he would have loved estrogen, a hormone fit for comedy, tragedy and a sonnet or two. . . . And just when scientists think they've got estrogen figured out, the hormone turns Puckish, mocking their assumptions and rewriting the script.

—Natalie Angier, "New Respect for Estrogen's Influence,"
The New York Times, June 24, 1997

Before we can fully comprehend how chemicals may act like hormones and why hormone disruption is an issue that deserves attention, we first have to know about hormones and the biochemical role they play in our bodies. In this chapter we look at the hormone estrogen in particular, not because it is bigger and better than any of the other hormones in our body and not because it is the only hormone that chemicals may mimic, but because environmental estrogens have been the focus of most of the research on hormone disruption to date.

Estrogen is one of the hormones most responsible for programming the way all our bodies grow and develop; it actually organizes our development in utero. It's like a VCR that programs how the movie of our life will play itself out. Estrogens in the womb also program how we will respond to other hormones when we are adults, both those in our bodies and those from our external environment. Environmental estrogens stimulate more female hormonal activity in our bodies than we would have from just our natural hormones. Some scientists have called this abnormal elevation of estrogenic activity in the body through hormone disruptors the feminizing effect of technology.

THE SEX HORMONES

Estrogens and progesterone are the feminine sex hormones (steroids) essential for life. The active ingredient from ovarian secretions was isolated in the 1920s and called estrogen because it is produced when female animals are in heat (estrus). Estrogen is not a single substance; it is an umbrella term for a class of 60 hormones and hormone metabolites with similar estrogen-like actions, of which estrone, estradiol, and estriol are the most famous.

Estrogens are the hormones responsible for many of the physical attributes we associate with the female body—the appealing curves and softness of women and their ability to give birth. Natural estrogens cause specific cells to enlarge, divide, or make proteins. Think of the many changes that take place at puberty in girls:

- the accelerated growth and development of the vagina, uterus, and Fallopian tubes
- enlargement of the breasts
- growth of the bones and underarm and pubic hair
- darkening of the nipples and aureole

Estrogens control reproductive cycles and pregnancy, prepare the breasts for lactation, and influence skin, bone, the cardiovascular system, the immune system, and even the brain, including memory.

Steroid hormones are basically made from cholesterol, which comes in part from our diet and mostly from the cholesterol that's made in our bodies by the liver. Far from being the bad guy, cholesterol is actually a vital component of our bodies. It is cholesterol in excess, especially a fraction called LDL, that has been associated with problems.

Cholesterol is transformed through a series of steps into the precursor of estrogen, which is produced in the ovaries, adrenal glands, and fat cells. The production of natural estrogen varies with gender, age, and reproductive cycles. Women produce more than men, especially when pregnant. Postmenopausal women typically have much less estrogen, though not as little as we once thought. And estrogens are smart hor-

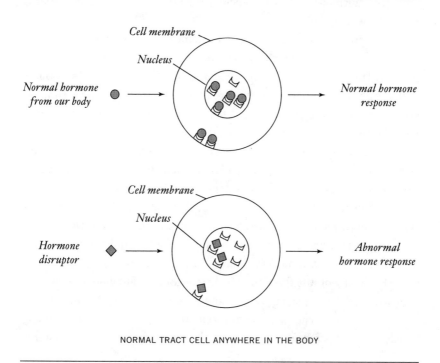

FIGURE 3.1 *Hormone (or Hormone Disruptor) Binding with Receptor*

mones. During times of famine, when it would be undesirable for a woman to be pregnant, estrogen production slows down to prevent fertility.

Androgens are the classic masculine hormones, but they operate in women too. Androgens contribute to bone growth and the production of protein, especially in muscles, as well as promoting the development of male sex characteristics. Both estrogens and androgens are fat soluble, making them nimble swimmers, able to easily swim through cell membranes. They bind with receptor sites in the nucleus of a cell, where they can turn on or turn off the functions of certain genes.

Vive la Difference

Unless we're from Pluto, instead of Venus or Mars, we recognize that men and women are physically different. Basically, it's a result of specific genes along with hormonal balance, especially the ratio of hormones in the fetus when it's developing.

Most people think of estrogen as the female hormone and testosterone as the male hormone, but this is not the whole picture. Men and women both have male and female sex hormones. It is the variation in the amounts of the sex hormones that is at the core of why a man burns three times as many calories pushing a supermarket cart down the aisle as a woman does, and why her voice is higher than his.

Even though men and women have their own ratio of hormones, research is showing that men depend on the female sex hormone estrogen (as well as androgens) for the development of their maleness as much as women depend on estrogen for their femaleness. There is so much overlap, with both men and women leaning on estrogen to help them be all they can be, that one doctor stood up at a conference and said to the hundreds of scientists and media present, "Life itself is estrogen dependent."

Estrogens, not just the Y (male) chromosome, contribute to making a man a man. All of us start out the same—as a developing bundle of cells in the womb with rudimentary reproductive organs for both male and female. Then, at six weeks of gestation, the sex-determining process starts.

MEN AND ESTROGEN

Estrogen is most definitely not just a female hormone. Estrogen is:

- found in high concentrations in semen
- essential for sperm to be concentrated enough for fertility
- present in males in low concentrations in blood
- found in the testicles in higher amounts than female blood estradiol levels

Male reproductive tissues have estrogen receptor sites, and animal studies suggest that estrogen is needed for normal sexuality in both males and females. In the developing fetus, a specific ratio of estrogens to androgens must be maintained for proper sexual differentiation to occur, and the hormones must be activated at particular times. In other words, for a male to become a male and a female to become a female, male and female hormones must be present in the mother in the right amount at the right time between fertilization and birth.

TURNING MALES INTO FEMALES

Dr. David Crews heads a lab in Texas where he studies turtles. The sex of some turtles, like crocodiles, alligators, some lizards, and some fish, is determined by the temperature inside the incubating egg. At low temperatures, the animals hatch out of the eggs as males. A few degrees higher and they hatch out as females. In the lab, they've learned that what is happening is that, as the temperature is raised, the amount of estrogens that the fetuses are producing is increased. The researchers have shown that if estrogens are painted onto the eggshells, when the eggs are incubated at a temperature that usually produces males, instead of males the eggs will hatch out females. Similar findings have been reported by Dr. Michael Fry in birds. Fry and his coworkers also painted two kinds of PCBs on turtle eggs and got "gender bending" at amounts comparable to average levels of PCBs found in human breast milk in industrialized nations.

If the fetus is to be a girl, no male chromosome is present. If it's to be a boy, the genes carried on the fetal cell's Y chromosome instruct cells to make male gonads. This elbows the budding female organs out of the picture. The male organs produce testosterone. Some scientists think that testosterone travels through the fetal bloodstream into the developing brain, where it is transformed by an enzyme (aromatase) into estrogen (estradiol). The dose is everything. Just the right amount of testosterone makes just the right amount of estrogen, producing the cellular events that lead to masculine development.

One cheeky irony of life is that how masculine a man is as an adult is partly the result of his having had optimal amounts of estrogen in his brain at a certain time during his stay in the womb. Amazingly minute differences—parts per trillion or parts per billion of a few sex hormones—literally affect the making of men or women. Most certainly this new understanding of how estrogens and androgens work together emphasizes just how fundamental estrogen signals are in directing the development of life. Even though all the sex hormones dance to a syncopated beat that creates the rhythms of life, estrogens may very well turn out to be the conductor waving a baton to maintain the essential harmony of the tune.

As a side note: part of fully becoming male is producing a hormone that makes the sprouting female organs regress. The gene Wnt-7 alpha (and perhaps other Wnt genes) that allows the male fetus to respond to this hormone may be one primary target of DES. Other hormonal disruptors may be found to affect this gene or related genes.

ENVIRONMENTAL ESTROGENS

Most estrogens are made inside our bodies. Estrogens that come from outside the body include both natural compounds and synthetic chemicals:

- *Phytoestrogens* are natural compounds (isoflavones, lignans, coumestrans, and others) in plants that produce a weak estrogen-like action in the body, which has been associated with *mostly* beneficial effects. Plants have been making phytoestrogens for more than 400 million years. Unlike synthetic estrogens, naturally occurring phytoestrogens spend very little time in our bodies and are not stored in fat or tissue. Soybeans, mung beans, clover, whole grains, and many fruits, nuts, and vegetables contain some of these phytoestrogens, which can occupy receptor sites that otherwise would have been available to bind with more potent estrogens, thus acting as a protection for the body. This may be one reason that lifelong vegetarians have a lower risk for estrogen-dependent health disorders such as breast cancer.

  Some foods are turned into phytoestrogens during the process of metabolism in the intestines. A round of therapeutic antibiotics can knock out this intestinal ability for several months. Some people (called responders) convert plants into phytoestrogens in the gut better than do others, and various factors play a role, such as the amount of meat and carbohydrates in the diet. Sometimes soy may not be beneficial (see "The Soy Controversy" on page 229).

- *Synthetic estrogens* are drugs made by pharmaceutical companies. These estrogens have had their molecular structure altered so they can be patented and sold. Estrogenic drugs, such as birth control pills and the estrogen component of hormone replacement therapy, are more stable and remain in the body longer than natural estrogens. However, they are not nearly as persistent as pesticides and other eco-estrogens.

- *Xenoestrogens* are environmental compounds that usually come from petrochemicals and other chemical sources. They have varying estrogen-like activity. Many of these chemicals are very persistent, meaning they can stay in the environment for many years, often decades, allowing a much longer period of possible exposure to humans. Some xenoestrogens are not as long-lived, but we are exposed to them on almost a daily basis. Xenoestrogens are hormone disruptors and are discussed throughout this book.

ESTROGEN RECEPTORS: WE'RE ALL CONNECTED

We hear from spiritual sources and environmental advocates that we are all connected. Now we're also hearing it from science. In the last decade, the study of comparative developmental biology has uncovered unexpected sameness throughout multicellular life forms. The endocrine system is one striking example. The hormone signaling system has come down to us from the ancestor of all vertebrates. Humans today have estrogen receptors that are nearly the same as estrogen receptors from 400–500 million years ago. In fact, the estrogen receptors in alligators and fruit flies are more similar to the ones in our bodies than different hormone receptors in humans are to each other. To me, this screams about the interrelatedness of all life forms.

It was once thought that estrogen would bind mainly with estrogen receptors in the female organs—the breasts, uterus, and ovaries—and perhaps some was sent to other places like bone cells or hair follicles. Now we know that estrogen receptors have real estate all over the human body, with receptors lining the blood vessels and present in the brain, bones, liver, kidneys, adrenals, and eyes. In the male, the prostate gland has estrogen receptors. Sperm may even be assisted in their urgent desire to enter eggs by the action of estrogen.

There are between 20,000 and 50,000 estrogen receptors per cell. In normal healthy tissue, the highest number of estrogen receptors is around 20,000—the number found in some uterine cells. The number of estrogen receptors varies according to cell type.

For decades, researchers had assumed there was only one type of estrogen receptor, called estrogen receptor alpha (ER∂). Now it turns out that there is another smaller receptor through which estrogen can convey its message—*estrogen receptor beta* (ERß). This receptor happened to be identified by two different research teams at approximately the same time. Dr. Siesta Mosselman and coworkers from The Netherlands found this new estrogen receptor in humans, while Dr. Jan-Ake Gustafsson and his colleagues at the Karolinska Institute in Huddinge, Sweden, identified this receptor in rodents.

ERß closely resembles the alpha receptor: both bind strongly with estradiol and both act as genetic switches, turning some genes on and some genes off. It now looks like there may even be multiple forms of ERß. However, there are some important differences between these receptors, and more data is being collected all the time.

Alpha seems to be more the reproductive receptor, meaning it is found predominantly in the breast, the uterus, and abdominal fat. Beta seems to be the nonreproductive receptor, found mostly in the brain, in early embryonic life, and in blood vessels (there are, of course, many exceptions). Both alpha and beta are required for normal functioning in the ovaries. Phytoestrogens, for example, bind much more to ER beta receptors than to ER alpha receptors, and more research will unveil further differences. Both receptors occur together in the brain, liver, bones, and testes. Most tissues have both types of estrogen receptors, but usually one or the other type predominates. They can exist in the same tissues but in different cells and in different ratios at different times. It may be that ER alpha is the "bad guy" (but one we need to live with nonetheless) and ER beta is the good guy, and the balance between the two types of estrogen receptors dictates normal or abnormal growth. We just don't know yet.

The discovery of the beta receptor has resolved some of the questions that puzzled scientists about estrogen and could lead to exciting breakthroughs in the treatment of estrogen-dependent diseases. It may help to explain how estrogens, and man-made chemicals that mimic estrogens, are able to act on so many different tissues. For example, bisphenol A (a chemical used in the plastic liners of most food and drink cans) is eight times more likely to bind with the beta receptor than to the alpha receptor. This means that bisphenol A is much more potent than testing originally showed because testing of the chemical's estrogenicity was at first only performed on alpha receptors.

Dennis Lubahn's group at the University of Missouri thinks they have evidence of a gamma estrogen receptor. Another scientist, Ellis Levin, M.D. (Chief, Endocrinology and Metabolism, Department of Veterans Affairs, Medical Center, Long Beach) feels there is rigorous evidence of yet another receptor called membrane ER that lives on the surface of a cell rather than inside the nucleus. He believes this receptor stimulates nitric oxide, which ultimately protects the blood vessels against heart disease.

CHEMICAL SABOTEURS

Dr. Thomas A. Gasiewicz is a professor of environmental medicine at the Medical Center at the University of Rochester School of Medicine. He says: "Let's say that to run hormones, it's like using electricity. You need to turn lights on and off to get things done at the appropriate time. But when dioxin [a hormone-disrupting compound] combines with a receptor site, it keeps the light switch turned on all the time. It's supposed to be turned off once in a while, but now this no longer happens. When it stays turned on during critical times of development when it should actually be turned off, reproductive and other factors of development are affected. When alterations occur during critical times, these effects may often be *irreversible*."

Dr. Wade Welshons, a professor of veterinary biomedical sciences at the University of Missouri–Columbia, says: "One of the issues which has already come up in the last ten years and in the last several for environmental endocrine disruptors is the idea and the proof that estrogens at physiological levels during fetal development have *permanent effects* on that development. If a compound is estrogenic, if you've identified it as being potentially estrogenic, the only thing that matters any more is will its concentration in the cell be high enough to occupy receptors or not? Because if there is enough of it to bind to receptors, no matter what effect it has, it will be abnormal."

Future research might reveal a link between EDCs acting through these receptors and heart disease.

Dr. Toran-Allerand and coworkers at Columbia University's College of Physicians and Surgeons have found substantial evidence for yet another estrogen receptor, which she calls ER X. It lives on the surface of a cell in the plasma membrane, but is different from the receptor found by Levin. Toran-Allerand's research focuses on how this ER affects nerve cell signaling in the brain.

Not only are there new receptors to deal with, but it's also been discovered that estrogen works in more than one way to send its signal. All this research shows that we are just beginning to scratch the surface of the mechanisms in the body through which chemicals can enter and affect different estrogenic signaling systems. Other receptors are also starting to receive attention, such as androgen, thyroid, vitamin, and even insulin receptors.

THE LOOSE POUCH

For a substance to act like an estrogen, simply speaking, it has to be carried in the blood, get out of the clear liquid of blood and into the cell, and be present near estrogen receptors in sufficient concentration to occupy and affect some of them. It turns out that our estrogen-receptor sites are flexible locks that are easily activated by a wide variety of keys. The molecules don't even have to have a structure similar to our natural estrogen, although many chemicals do.

It is the womblike shape of the receptor itself that allows so many different molecules to enter, nestle in for the winter, and bind with it. In the words of some scientists, this womb has "wobble," meaning it is flexible and accommodating. The receptor pouch is so accommodating that it has been called promiscuous, perhaps an appropriate term for a protein molecule that's been around for the last 400 million years or so. (Dr. Earl Gray, a reproductive toxicologist with the EPA, suggests that androgen receptors may be even more promiscuous than estrogen receptors. Dr. Jeff Cobb, a principal research scientist at Glaxo Wellcome, said the insulin receptor involved in diabetes has huge wobble and is even more promiscuous.) It looks like receptors in the nucleus have lots of room to mate with a wide variety of compounds.

Many different estrogenic compounds can unlock the receptor gateways in our bodies just as if they were molecules of our own estrogens—and the receptors don't seem to care. The bigger they are and the more wobble they have, the more the receptors invite a wide variety of hormonelike chemicals to come on in. The only thing that matters to the receptor is the hormone signal, and it's not concerned about where that signal comes from—in-the-body (endogenous) hormones or environmental (exogenous) sources such as xenoestrogens. The receptors are happy singing that old Stephen Stills song, "Love the One You're With."

Once the key is in the lock, the key-and-lock together—the hormone or hormone mimic together with the obliging receptor—can call on the DNA and send messages that turn our gene functions on and off. Hormone disruptors that gain entry into the human body can act like saboteurs who enter a top-secret government installation and download a virus into the communications software. This is the way a hormone disruptor like the synthetic estrogen DES and its breakdown products, which have a high

ADDITIVITY AND SYNERGY

We are not exposed to only one chemical at a time. Instead, we have multiple exposures each day and over time, so low levels of various chemicals may be present and active in our bodies at the same time. Each item may contribute just a little, but the overall effect is *additive.* Some xenoestrogens add their effects to any natural estrogen present.

Synergy means that the mixture of chemicals works together to produce a greater effect than the sum of the individual chemicals. A chemical tested by itself may not show an estrogenic response until it is mixed with another chemical. Suddenly the first chemical may become more potent in its estrogenic effect. Dr. Ana M. Soto at Tufts University combined 10 different estrogen mimics, each at one-tenth the dose required to produce a minimal response. She found that the combination was 10 times more potent than expected. However, synergism is considered very tricky to test and some scientists are not certain that it has been adequately proven.

---

affinity with the estrogen receptor, wreaked havoc with the reproductive system of many DES daughters like myself.

Throughout this tangled tango, in which hormones or hormone impostors partner with receptors, there are complexities on top of complexities. As many scientists at conferences about hormone disruptors love to quote: "The devil is in the details."

There are a number of complicating factors in the hormone/receptor dance.

- The same uterine, breast, and bone cells that have receptors that accept estrogens also contain receptors for other hormones, such as progesterone and androgens, and receptors for some vitamins.

- The same hormone, at a different dose, can bind to different receptors. For example, if estradiol is around in high enough dosages, it can bind to progesterone receptors and androgen (male hormone) receptors as well as to estrogen receptors. A number of estrogenic chemicals have been shown to interact with androgen receptors.

- Estrogen can work differently in different parts of the body. This is the key to all hormonal regulation. For example, estrogen can bind to a receptor in the breast tissue and signal an action to turn *off*, while it can bind to a receptor in uterine tissue and signal an action to turn *on*.

- The receptor doesn't only interact with a hormone or a hormone impostor. It can also interact with other players that may help turn on, amplify, or turn off signaling. These other players are called by a variety of names: coactivators, corepressors, second messengers (like cyclic AMP), or other transcription factors (such as FOS and JUN). They may even be able to cause signaling without a hormone or hormonelike substance around. It's as if the people in the stands at a football game were able to score a goal without any help from the team on the field.

- Sometimes a chemical that is tested outside the body won't appear to be a hormone disruptor, yet inside the body it can be metabolized and change its form so it does become an EDC. For instance, DES has a metabolite nicknamed DQ, which appears to bind irreversibly to the estrogen receptor and stimulate it continuously, which means it would continue to turn on the genes. In another example, vinclozolin (a fungicide used on many common fruits and vegetables) breaks down into two metabolites, M1 and M2, which have been studied for endocrine disruption and have been found to bind to the androgen receptor and block its signaling.

- Even a weak estrogen given at a critical time can produce irreversible effects. Weak environmental estrogens may also *synergize* with stronger natural estrogens. This is accomplished through several mechanisms. For example, even though some environmental estrogens are weak by themselves, when they get into our body they fraternize with our own hormones and become stronger.

According to Dr. Wade Welshons: "The estrogen receptor is probably the single strongest indication of whether or not a hormone-disrupting chemical will have an effect. You don't know if it will be estrogenic or anti-estrogenic and certainly there are some compounds that can bring about different qualities of estrogenic response. But either way, if compounds interact with a receptor, they have to bring about a response of some sort. Natural estrogens are present in the body all the time. If substances from outside enter the body and add to, subtract from, or alter natural hormone signaling, some functions in the body are bound to change."

This is just some of the beauty and complexity of the hormone system and part of the frustration in understanding how hormone disruptors work. "No matter how complicated something is, if you look at it in just the right way, you can make it even more complicated," says George Stancel of Texas Medical Center in Houston. Or as another scientist said during a heated exchange over endocrine disruptors at a meeting, "For every complex problem there is a simple answer . . . that is wrong!"

ESTROGEN'S DANCE PARTNERS

In the normal working of the human body, estrogen dances with other hormones, meaning there are always lead and follow partners. To ensure that estrogen doesn't always take the lead, the body produces natural controls. When these controls are not functioning properly, we may wind up with higher levels of estrogen in our bodies—our natural estrogen plus whatever estrogenic signaling we're getting from xenoestrogens and phytoestrogens. Our contemporary lifestyle contributes to how many times estrogen's name gets written on our dance card.

Anti-androgens: In order for estrogen to stay in balance in the body, it must be in a correct ratio with the male sex hormones. If something is blocking the production of androgens, which is what certain endocrine disruptors can do, there will be a higher ratio of estrogens to androgens in the body. For example, in Lake Apopka, Florida—which was the site of an accidental dump of pesticides—Dr. Lou Guillette has shown that male alligators were being born with penises that were too small for successful mating, there was reduced fertility, and more females than males were being born. Scientists originally thought the pesticides that caused these problems were estrogenic hormone disruptors, but it turned out that the chemicals were actually having an anti-androgenic effect. It was the blocking of male hormones that allowed too much estrogen to adversely affect the alligators' reproductive health.

Progesterone: This is a powerful hormone that balances the effects of estrogen. It helps regulate changes that occur during menstruation and it influences the mammary glands during pregnancy. It is necessary for the survival and development of the embryo and fetus. Progesterone appears to have anti-estrogenic actions: it can plug up estrogen receptors and it can block the metabolism of some chemicals in the body so that it prevents the parent compound from turning into more active (and possibly more destructive) metabolites.

A number of hormone disruptors inhibit progesterone. Animal studies in primates show that some environmental estrogens suppress progesterone synthesis. Also, a high level of estrogen in the body can make xenoestrogens bind to progesterone receptors and can plug up the receptors, not allowing our natural progesterone to send its message. Thus, if some hormone disruptors inhibit progesterone and others inhibit androgens, the overall trend appears to be heavily weighted toward more estrogenic signaling and feminizing effects in the body.

Progesterone is made by the ovaries and adrenal glands as a result of ovulation. It used to be that the production of progesterone started to roller-coaster several years before menopause, which used to occur in the majority of women in their mid-forties to early fifties. But now, according to John R. Lee, M.D., through juggling home and career, eating poor diets, and exposure to xenoestrogens, many women cease ovulating regularly or sometimes completely in their early thirties. (Working women, don't worry; the cause of non-ovulatory cycles is not really known yet.) During non-ovulatory cycles, the ovaries still make enough estrogen to rebuild and shed the uterine lining so that periods appear normal. This means many women have no idea that their bodies are not producing enough progesterone and their progesterone levels may be inadequate to act as a metabolic balance against estrogen.

Other hormones: The secretion of estrogen is regulated by three other hormones which are produced by the pituitary gland: follicle-stimulating hormone (FSH), luteinizing hormone (LH), and prolactin. Prolactin (as well as thyroid hormone and progesterone) may affect estrogenic signals. On the other hand, excess estrogen may inhibit the levels of these hormones or how these hormones function. To complicate matters even more—the body seems to love diversity and complexity—some human and animal studies suggest that endocrine-disrupting chemicals may act like or indirectly affect both thyroid hormones and prolactin. What was once an harmonious fox-trot between these hormones may turn into an out-of-control roller derby.

Other molecules can also signal the hormone system. Dr. John McLachlan says, "Data and opinions from five or six different labs around the world have shown that different kinds of signaling molecules, like growth factors, are actually able to influence or able to stimulate an estrogen-like response."

Liver function: This is very important for helping the body get rid of estrogen. The liver combines estrogen with certain molecules (sugar or protein) to prepare it to be excreted out of the body. If the liver is too busy struggling with overconsumption of alcohol, a deficiency of B vitamins, or trying to detoxify drugs and pollutants, it may not be able to eliminate enough estrogen.

Friendly bacteria: After the liver binds estrogen to a sugar molecule, the compound enters the intestines before being excreted in the feces. "Bad guy" bacteria can destroy the binding and free the estrogen so it gets reabsorbed back into the body through the gut wall. In essence, the person becomes exposed to the same estrogen twice. A good balance of probiotics (intestinal-friendly bacteria such as L. acidophilus and others) normally helps to minimize this double whammy. The balance of good-guy to bad-guy bacteria can be jeopardized by eating a junk-food diet, especially one high in fat, or by multiple rounds of antibiotics. New research is suggesting that a certain family of antibiotics, the cephalosporins, perhaps acted upon by intestinal microbes, may themselves act as endocrine disruptors.

Melatonin: During the dark nighttime hours, this hormone is produced by the pineal gland. One hypothesis suggests that melatonin is one of the naturally occurring regulators of estrogen in the body and that excess electromagnetic fields (EMFs), which are invisible lines of force surrounding all electrical wiring and devices, can suppress or shut down the production of melatonin.

With the advent of electricity, we now stay up during nighttime hours under artificial light, thereby decreasing our natural production of melatonin. Even low-level EMFs, which are impossible to avoid, may suppress melatonin. Other implicated factors in the reduction of melatonin are alcohol consumption—even moderate amounts of alcohol raise estrogen levels in premenopausal women—and junk-food diets, which may calcify the pineal gland and decrease its secretion of this hormone. Get the picture? A party animal who regularly stays up late, drinks heavily, and munches on doughnuts while fretting about her bills may wind up with estrogen out of balance with the estrogenic dance partners.

THE PROBLEM WITH UNOPPOSED ESTROGEN

Unopposed estrogen is estrogen that does not have stable dance partners. Dr. Peter Ellison of Harvard University has studied ovarian hormone levels in various populations. He found that in the Western world premenopausal estrogen levels are generally at an extreme high end of the spectrum and should be considered abnormal, especially when compared to other cultures.

An abnormally increased exposure to estrogen throughout an individual's life results in an elevated estrogen body burden, which is a major factor in increasing the risk of estrogen-dependent illnesses (illness that is caused and/or exacerbated by the presence of estrogen). Remember that very tiny amounts of a hormone can create big changes. Estrogen exposure is known to be a requirement for many breast and uterine cancers and other types of reproductive tract cancers and certain immune diseases. And we now know that many natural and man-made chemicals can act to increase estrogen-like activity or can block the other hormones that help maintain normal estrogen levels.

There is plenty of opportunity for a modern woman to be exposed to too much estrogen throughout her life. Here are some of the ways:

THE PULSE GENERATOR

GnRH is a hormone that is considered a pulse generator. GnRH pulses once an hour throughout most of a woman's life. It affects everything from the release of eggs to fertility to the production of sex hormones to the beginning of puberty and menopause. In tests on monkeys, the two major factors that turned off the GnRH generator were chronic stress and excess estrogen. The GnRH generator is exquisitely sensitive to estrogen. Small amounts of extra estrogen seem to adversely affect the timing of puberty, fertility, and even hot flashes in postmenopausal women. Another factor appeared to be low caloric intake. Young girls who diet severely in order to look like models may be adversely affecting their GnRH system.

- **Early onset of menstruation** (before age eleven)—The earlier a woman starts menstruating, the more menstrual cycles she will have and therefore more exposure to estrogen.

- **Perimenopause** (starting in thirties or forties)—a woman may get her period but not ovulate. Ovulation is what produces progesterone. Insufficient progesterone causes surges of estrogen and unopposed estrogen.

- **Late onset of menopause** (after age fifty-five)—Again, more opportunity for cycling estrogen in the body.

- **Hormone replacement therapy**—Either long-term (ten to fifteen years or more) or current use of HRT brings more estrogen into the body. If a woman starts menopause in her mid-fifties and/or drinks and takes HRT, this may increase her lifetime exposure to estrogen.

- **Birth-control pills**—These can expose a woman to too much estrogen, especially with long-term use.

- **Postmenopausal obesity** (body mass index more than 30.7 kg/m)—Fat cells make their own estrogen from circulating adrenal hormones. Thus, women with more fat have more estrogen. Obesity is associated with elevated levels of testosterone and lower levels of protective hormone binding proteins, both of which can lead to more available free estrogen.

- **Alcohol abuse**—Regular consumption of several alcoholic drinks per night or more than fourteen drinks per week is associated with statistically significant increases in the levels of several hormones in premenopausal women, including estradiol.

Dr. John R. Lee, in his book *What Your Doctor May Not Tell You About Menopause*, has proposed that a new syndrome be recognized—estrogen dominance. He writes, "A key to hormone balance is the knowledge that when estrogen becomes the dominant hormone and progesterone is deficient, the estrogen becomes toxic to the body."

It seems that many women suffer from, especially in the ten- to fifteen-year period *before* menopause, an excess of estrogen that causes estrogen dominance symptoms and illnesses. Problems in women that have been associated with excessive estrogenic signaling include:

- breast and uterine cancer
- fibrous breasts
- menstrual disorders, such as painful cramps or excessive blood flow
- premenstrual syndrome (PMS)—which affects 40–60 percent of all women in the West
- endometrial polyps—little warts that grow on thin stalks on the lining of the uterus
- endometriosis
- ovarian problems such as cysts
- immune disorders
- difficult menopause
- problems of infertility

Estrogen-related problems in men include:

- lowered sperm counts

NOISY CROSS-TALK: THE MECHANISM OF ENDOCRINE DISRUPTION

Endocrine disruption is "a cause, not an effect," according to Linda Birnbaum (head of experimental toxicology at the EPA). She graciously explained as simply as she could: "The job of the endocrine system is to keep *homeostasis*—physiological and chemical balance within the body. The job of each hormone is to act as a communicator in this process. Signals are submitted by one cell in a tissue to control and make effects in other cells in other tissues. And there are many different hormone systems, of which estrogen is just one. Hormonal perturbations can occur in the adrenal glands, the thyroid, reproductive system, pineal gland, and on and on. And all of these can affect estrogen. They don't act in isolation.

"The focus of the endocrine system is to integrate, so if you perturb one hormone system, you are likely to perturb multiple hormone systems because they all talk to each other and they talk to each other at multiple levels of organization and multiple levels of biology. Endocrine disruption is therefore a mechanism whereby there could be a toxic or aberrant effect."

- undescended testicles
- testicular and prostate cancer
- congenital abnormalities of the penis (called hypospadias)
- immune disorders
- breast cancer

Although estrogen has been the hormone most studied in relation to hormone-disrupting chemicals (which is why we are emphasizing it in this book), we have to remember that estrogens are not the only hormones in our bodies. There are hundreds of hormones. If a number of these different hormones are as delicately choreographed as estrogen, imagine what may be happening in our bodies as hormone disruptors signal incorrect messages to the endocrine system.

PROGESTERONE RESISTANCE

We've all seen a cartoon of a light bulb suddenly lighting up over someone's head. As I read and reread the hundreds of scientific articles piled all over my home, I began to see that some studies associated hormone disruptors with poor progesterone functioning. Then one day my researcher sent me a study of about twenty-five women with breast cancer—most with a history of unopposed estrogen problems such as fibroids and endometriosis—who were found to have normal levels of progesterone in their blood, but the progesterone was not functioning normally in their bodies. The researchers called this progesterone resistance and suggested it could be an important factor in cancer. The light bulb lit up. I saw a pattern emerging: ecohormones may be upsetting the balance between our natural progesterone and estradiol, and it is this balance that affects our health.

It is well documented that environmental estrogens can bind to estrogen receptor sites and cause estrogenic signaling. But hormone disruptors, especially as they increase in amount in the body, can also bind to progesterone sites, which may block natural progesterone from fulfilling its job description. The amount of progesterone a woman has in her body may appear to be normal when measured in the blood, but the hormone doesn't have the chance to send its message. This results in an imbalance between progesterone and estrogen, which may be one way in which hormone disruptors contribute to the "estrogen dominance" syndrome.

Studies have long shown the protective importance of progesterone and the way ecohormones can affect progesterone. As far back as 1975, rats were given progesterone one-half hour prior to an injection of an estrogenic metabolite of DDT, which stopped the estrogenic effects of the metabolite. Monkey studies showed that an environmental pollutant—HBC (short for hexochlorabenzene)—suppressed progesterone during the phase when it is supposed to do its job (luteal phase). Then, in the mid 1990s, some scientists showed that dioxin could block the protective effects of progesterone in endometriosis (in mice). Also during the '90s, a relationship was found to exist between the timing of surgery for breast cancer patients (during their hormonal cycle) and their recurrence rates and survival outcomes. Some articles showed that if a woman was operated on during the luteal phase of her cycle (when progesterone was present), she had a better chance of beating the disease. This was such a strong association that one researcher wrote a paper in 1997 suggesting that it might be wise for women going in for breast cancer surgery to receive a presurgery shot of progesterone to offset the circulating unopposed estrogen. Research published in 1999 gave additional compelling evidence that premenopausal women have a better chance of beating breast cancer based on the menstrual timing of their surgery.

I faxed my ideas to Dr. John Lee. He said that the balance between estradiol and progesterone is more important than the levels of either hormone alone. A healthy ratio between estradiol and progesterone is 1:100–200. That is, progesterone concentrations (as tested in saliva) should be 100–200 times greater than estradiol for progesterone to act as a protection against unopposed estrogen.

Hormone disruptors can cause problems with progesterone. According to Dr. Lee, "Prenatal tissue development is exquisitely sensitive to xenobiotics. Exposure to xenobiotics during embryo life is known to damage follicle cells [cells that make eggs] in ovaries. . . . The result is that, even if a given follicle successfully ovulates, it may produce the necessary progesterone for only two to three days, rather than twelve to fourteen days of the supposed luteal phase of the menstrual cycle, or the six to eight weeks of early pregnancy. This is probably the leading cause of early miscarriages." Today, many young women seem to be producing less than optimal amounts of progesterone in their bodies. One study looked at twenty normal regularly cycling females (average age twenty-nine) and found that progesterone production was low in about a third of these women. Dr. Lee believes this is an indication of the prevalence of in utero follicle damage showing up later in life.

Dr. Lee also said that stress plays a role. Cortisol is a hormone that is released when stress levels go up. This hormone binds with progesterone receptors, thus blocking progesterone from getting its signal delivered. I found a study where patients had been treated with an estrogenic metabolite of DDT, which doubled the time that cortisol stayed elevated in the bloodstream. In other words, some hormone disruptors may be prolonging the time cortisol levels remain elevated in our blood, blocking progesterone receptor sites and, thus, indirectly decreasing the ability of progesterone to bind with its receptors and carry out its work. This may be contributing to a number of unopposed estrogen health problems.

The Canaries in the Mine

Until DES, *most scientists thought a drug was safe unless it caused immediate and obvious malformations. They found it hard to believe that something could have a serious long-term impact without causing any outwardly visible birth defects.*

—T. Colburn, D. Dumanoski, and J. P. Meyers,
Our Stolen Future (Dutton, 1996)

All my life I have had "female problems"—the kind related to unopposed estrogen—most likely due to the fact that my mother, like 5 million other women in the United States, was given DES (diethylstilbestrol, a synthetic estrogen) during her pregnancy with me. DES has been an instigator and motivator in my life. During the time I was researching this book about hormone disruptors and their possible association with numerous diseases, I was diagnosed with breast cancer and had three surgeries related to that and had another surgery to remove an ovary covered with endometriosis, both possibly results of my DES exposure. Thus, this book is both my work and my personal journey, mercilessly and miraculously intertwined.

Yet DES is more than just a personal issue, and far more than just an old story. DES was used as a drug to prevent miscarriage from 1938 to 1971, until a rare form of vaginal cancer was linked to DES exposure in the womb. The cases of vaginal cancers in DES daughters were thought to have hit their peak when these women were in their twenties. After that, specialists thought it was all over—DES had done its damage and retired. They were wrong. New cases of this deadly cancer, as well as other health issues, are still being found in DES daughters in their forties. The health effects found in DES daughters, DES sons, and DES moms are discussed throughout this book.

So the tale of DES exposure continues to be of contemporary significance—a warning beacon to all of us about synthetic hormones and hormone-disrupting chemicals. It warrants our respect and attention because DES is the only wide-scale human experiment we have had with hormone disruptors. Even though DES was a potent drug, more powerful than many EDCs, its effects on humans and its use in the laboratory convey vital information. It clearly demonstrates that human disease—including reproductive and developmental abnormalities, immune system malfunction, and cancer—may result from fetal exposure to estrogenic substances. And the problems manifested by children exposed to DES in utero echo what is being observed in wildlife and in the laboratory from other hormone disruptors.

Because the use of DES was so widespread and DES has been shown to be one of the most powerful synthetic estrogens known to date, it has become the model that has sensitized the scientific and medical commu-

---

THE MAN WHO SAW CLEARLY

Charles Dodds, who first synthesized DES in the 1930s, also studied groups of other substances that could mimic hormones. In essence, he was the first to study hormone disruptors. Decades before Theo Colborn recognized the phenomenon in wildlife and collated the results into a theory of hormone disruption, Dodds found that chemicals that looked like estrogens, and ones that didn't, could act like estrogens. By the mid-1930s he had implicated diphenyls (today called biphenyls)—which include DES, Bisphenol A (in some plastics), and some PCBS—as being estrogenic substances. Later he found that alkyphenols (certain detergents) also acted like estrogens. These same chemicals are now the focus of hot and heavy research as endocrine disruptors. The father of DES was, thus, the grandpa in recognizing estrogen-like activity in chemical compounds.

nities to the long-term effects possible from in utero exposure to an endocrine disruptor. We can best prepare for the future when we understand what has happened in the past.

THE HISTORY OF DES

DES was created in 1938—the very first synthetic estrogen—with a chemical structure that differs considerably from naturally occurring estrogen. (It looks a lot like the molecule for tamoxifen.) DES was more potent than natural estrogen and could be taken orally. The scientist who synthesized it, Charles Dodds, was an Englishman who didn't patent his discovery. It was therefore cheap to produce.

Originally utilized for conditions such as gastrointestinal disturbances, vertigo, and skin rashes (even acne), DES eventually came to be used for the prevention of miscarriages. Doctors at Harvard University did some studies on DES in 1945 and, believing it could reduce the risk of miscarriage, published a paper in 1947 extolling its virtues. Pharmaceutical companies were thrilled—here was an inexpensive drug endorsed by prestigious Harvard! Drug companies pushed the FDA to have DES approved for use during pregnancy, which happened in 1947. Why didn't it surprise me to learn that an FDA official involved in the approval of DES later became president of one of the first chemical companies to manufacture DES?

What was basically ignored, however, was the fact that *from the start* studies showed DES promoted cancer in lab animals. French studies in the late 1930s showed that mice exposed in utero to DES developed mammary cancer (cancer of the breast). In 1939 and 1940, other studies showed that mice exposed in utero to DES were born with malformed reproductive organs, and some got liver cancer. Even though different species of mammals are prone to different cancers, if animals exposed to a drug get *any* kind of cancer, this is a significant warning for humans.

Despite the fact that no controlled studies had been conducted to determine the effectiveness or safety of DES for use during pregnancy, drug companies blanketed the country with the news, inundating pediatricians and family doctors with word of the potential benefits brought about by modern science. DES was soon widely prescribed even for women with no apparent problems "to make a normal pregnancy more normal."

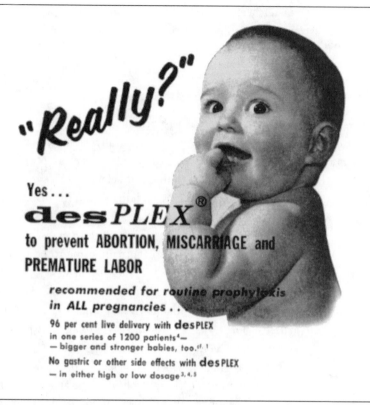

FIGURE 4.1 *A 1957 Advertisement.*

For more than thirty years, DES was given to an unknown number of pregnant women as pills, injections, and °vaginal suppositories, and it was the active ingredient in some vitamin tablets given to healthy pregnant women. It is estimated that nearly 10 million Americans were exposed to DES either during their pregnancy (DES mothers) or in the uterus (DES daughters and sons). The data available probably underestimates the number of in utero exposures of DES since many private physicians administered the drug and hospitals often did not keep records of "enhancement" treatments. Even if they did not receive direct injections of DES, many of our mothers ate DES-contaminated food before and during their pregnancies. We know that endocrine-disrupting chemicals are stored in fat cells, especially in breast tissue, and are released through breast feeding.

You May Be a DES Daughter or Son and Not Know It

Many children who were exposed to DES in utero still don't know that this could be one of the causes of the problems they face today. One study showed that 64 percent of DES-exposed daughters didn't know their mothers had taken the drug. Some DES daughters learn of their exposure after a pregnancy mishap. Mothers, after hearing of the problems with DES, often kept their knowledge as a guilty secret. Others never knew what it was they had been given by their doctors or hospital clinics, as was the case with my mother, since DES was manufactured by 267 companies under various trade names. (See list in Appendix C.)

When I sat in medical libraries and read the abundant literature about DES, I was amazed that it had been given to anyone at all. The use of DES for pregnancy-related problems was based primarily on two theoretical studies. The field of medical endocrinology was young. Though the studies were based on presumed effects rather than on clear-cut evidence, they were given a hearing by their colleagues.

None of the six other comparative studies following the publication of the initial studies on the use of DES demonstrated any beneficial effects for pregnant women. Though a few studies did report helpful effects, the great majority did not. Two huge reviews of the scientific literature, neither of which found that DES was effective in preventing miscarriages, were published in 1953 and 1958 respectively. As a matter of fact, it turned out that DES actually seemed to increase the rate of miscarriage.

The first person to take a look at DES and how exposure in utero might affect adulthood was Dr. John McLachlan, who is now the director of the Center for Bioenvironmental Research at Tulane and Xavier Universities. In the late 1960s and early 1970s, he had been working with DES, trying to assess the problems that in utero exposure could cause animals once they had matured. His boss at NIEHS thought McLachlan was way off the mark (and humorously showed him ads for other jobs). In that era, looking for problems from uterine exposure other than birth defects was thought by most scientists to be a waste of time.

In 1961 the first case of a rare vaginal cancer was diagnosed in a young woman. At Massachusetts General Hospital in Boston, a cluster of eight such cases was diagnosed. One of the mothers raised the question: was her daughter's cancer possibly connected to the DES she had taken while pregnant? Dr. Arthur L. Herbst detailed the association in a paper that was published in 1971 in the *New England Journal of Medicine*. When Dr. Herbst came out with his paper connecting these cases of vaginal cancer with DES, McLachlan was ready with his research to back up Dr. Herbst's hypothesis.

For the first time, people were connecting in utero exposure to a powerful estrogenic drug with problems in adult humans. By November 1971, 21 cases of clear cell vaginal cancer had been reported to the registry set up to monitor this disease. Only then did the FDA issue an alert advising against the use of DES during pregnancy, although the drug itself was never outlawed for use by humans. By 1981, there were more than 400 cases of vaginal or cervical cancer reported to the registry, two-thirds of which involved in utero exposure to DES or similar estrogens.

It is now well understood and scientifically proven that—for all its widespread usage—DES never worked. It never prevented miscarriages. By the late 1970s, reliable testing methods backed up active concerns about the long-reaching effects of drugs given to pregnant women. Many of the concerns were raised by DES Action, a national nonprofit organization founded in 1975 to represent mothers and children exposed to DES. In 1982 the DES Cancer Network was formed. Still, it was not until 1992 that the National Institutes of Health (NIH) convened the first meeting on the long-term effects of DES.

DES is still sold in many developing countries for a variety of reasons—suppression of lactation, menopausal symptoms—and there have been reports of continued use of DES as an anti-miscarriage drug in China, Mexico, and parts of Africa. My reproductive endocrinologist told me that a pregnant patient of hers went on vacation to Mexico, in December of 1998, and started to spot. She immediately went to see a local doctor who gave her a shot of DES. Of course, my doctor was horrified and had to consider how to tell this woman the implications, without scaring her or causing guilt—not an easy task.

FOOD FOR THOUGHT

Beginning in the 1940s, DES was also widely used as a growth promoter in poultry, hogs, and cattle, and thus was consumed by millions of people through the chicken, pork, and beef they ate. Americans were enjoying the abundance of peacetime after the scarcities of World War II. This meant eating lots of meat; many Americans ate it at every meal. Thirteen tons of DES were added every year to the environment through feedlots (a large plot of land where livestock, especially beef cattle, are fed and fattened prior to slaughter) and feedlot waste.

One of the consequences of adding DES to feed was that some exposed male agricultural workers suffered sterility, impotence, and breast growth. When high DES levels in poultry (some were found to contain 1,000 times the amount of DES necessary to cause breast cancer in mice) produced similar symptoms in consumers, the FDA banned the use of DES in chicken and lambs in 1959. It was, however, still touted as a wonder drug for pregnant women.

By the early 1970s, twenty foreign countries had banned DES, and many Europeans wouldn't eat American beef specifically because of its DES content. Today, Europeans still ban American beef because of the estrogenic growth-promoters that Americans feed their cattle. Estrogen-like compounds with similar activity (such as Steer-oid, Ralgro, Compudose, and Synovex) are still widely added to food lots. Switzerland, the only country that still tests for DES in meat, rejected thousands of pounds of U.S. beef in 1999 because it contained DES. Finding DES in meat shipped outside the United States raised fears that it may also be in our steak and hamburgers. The USDA has not tested for DES in meat since 1991.

By dumping DES by the tons into feed, it got into our food. It got into the waste. By various routes, DES got into the environment. Today, DES substitutes also get into the environment through these same routes. It is apparent that DES and its contemporary substitutes are an environmental exposure problem—a question of public health—not just a drug problem for individual women.

What Does Hormone Disruption Mean in a Human Life?

My mother's delight when she learned she was with child was overshadowed in early pregnancy by the spotting she was experiencing. Her family doctor was also concerned about the possibility of miscarriage, but, fortunately for her, this was an era of scientific breakthroughs. My mother's doctor prided himself on being up-to-date with the latest developments, and the Chicago hospital with which he was affiliated was known for its DES use. "My doctor told me I needed the injection of DES to prevent miscarriage. Of course I believed him," she told me. A seemingly healthy baby girl was delivered at term.

But something started going wrong at puberty, when I was only nine years old. I bled heavily and would writhe in severe pain for the first three or four days of my ten-day period. I bled more and more profusely as the years progressed. Weeks of relentless PMS would be followed by a week of near-hemorrhaging. My world seemed to center on my period. How bad would the bleeding be? Could I leave the house, let alone travel? Doctors reassured me and my mom that this "just happens" to some girls.

As a seventeen-year-old, I took an unforgettable trip to Europe. As I walked down the aisle of a bus, the Yugoslavians (holding baskets of live chickens on their heads) were pointing and whispering about me. It turned out that the whole back of my skirt was drenched in blood that had soaked through two extra-absorbency tampons and two extra-thick menstrual pads. One of my most vivid memories was sailing from England to Ireland. While the boat swayed, I noticed a pool of blood on the floor and looked at my leg, where a red tributary was flowing down toward the deck. Two slightly drunk men stared in unison at the puddle and then at me as I dashed for the "loo," shielding my back with a purse. After washing out the white and black polka-dotted skirt in the small dingy bathroom, I waited hours for it to dry, desperately trying to figure out what was happening and how to heal it.

Thus started my pilgrimage to doctors. They all said it was within normal range to hemorrhage like this, that it wouldn't last forever.

As an aspiring actress at age nineteen, living in a fifth-floor walk-up on the Lower East Side of Manhattan, I bled so badly during one period that I fainted from loss of blood while walking up the stairs. Someone called for help. Someone carried me down. In the hospital after surgery, I was diagnosed as having severe cervical dysplasia, considered a precancerous condition. This is when the cells lining the cervix (the opening to the uterus) are growing faster than normal, out of control. I had a cone biopsy to get rid of the bad tissue and was sent home, packed with gauze. I continued to bleed. I went back to the surgeon, who made a pass at me. I ran home, bleeding down my leg, jumped into bed and cried for days.

I made an appointment with another doctor, who told me that some girls bleed from excessive masturbation.

It all felt hopeless. Finally another doctor who examined me asked, "Did your mother take DES when she was pregnant with you?" I didn't know what DES was. The doctor explained that daughters born of mothers who were given DES often had a variety of anatomical changes, such as a piece of skin that looks like a hood over the clitoris, T-shaped uteruses, problems with menstruation such as decreased or increased bleeding, cervical dysplasia, and a rare form of vaginal cancer. I had all the symptoms of DES exposure except the cancer.

I asked my mother if she had been given diethylstilbestrol while pregnant. "How can you think I would have taken anything to hurt you?" my mother, hurt and angry, answered a question with a question. I dropped the subject.

The dysplasia wasn't cancerous, but the next three or four months were filled with such severe hemorrhaging I had to quit my life as an actress. A friend had offered to care for me in California, where I was introduced to yoga and nutrition. A nutritionist was the first person to suggest that regardless of what was causing my problem, I was most likely anemic from frequent loss of blood. How obvious! Why hadn't any of my doctors realized that? After only a week on a new diet—no animal products except raw goat's milk, iron-rich foods like raisins and dark leafy green vegetables, and calcium and iron supplements—I had more energy. Within one month I could walk without getting dizzy, digest food without stomachaches, and face menstruation without trepidation. There was less bleeding and pain.

I was so impressed that diet could have such a rapid influence where surgery and drugs had failed, I was prompted to go back to school for my master's degree in nutrition. After several years as a nutritionist and exercise instructor, I went back to school again for my fourth degree. I practiced for a decade, along with a cardiologist and internist, specializing in women's health.

In 1976 I had a lumpectomy for a fibroid adenoma in my right breast. For me, the 1980s were filled with constant severe pain—mid-cycle pain, pain right before my period, menstrual pain, and breast pain. I had so much breast pain, I needed to wear two bras and couldn't hug people without severe discomfort. In 1984 and 1986 I needed D&Cs (a surgical procedure on the uterus) to get the severe bleeding to stop. There was also the severe mittle schmertz (pain upon ovulation) that often lasted for a week and on numerous occasions was so intense that it literally knocked me flat on the floor. One time I lay on the floor of a movie theater unable to get up, even when they wanted to close the theater for the night.

"I bet I have endometrial polyps," I told the gynecologist.

"You're not fat, you haven't had a bunch of kids, I'll bet you a dinner that you don't," he replied.

He lost the bet.

I designed one of the first natural alternatives to hormone replacement therapy made from herbs and nutrients for women who are not candidates for synthetic hormones, such as some DES daughters. I wrote freelance columns on food for the *San Francisco Chronicle*, had a radio show on nutrition, taught relicensing courses for nurses and Ph.D.s in public health, lectured around the country on health for different professional groups, and held free weekly classes on health and nutrition for the public. I spent literally thousands of hours in medical school libraries searching medical journals for nutritional information that I shared with my patients. I saw wonderful improvements in the women I treated. Despite all the work I did helping other women, my own problems started to get worse again.

After several years of disabling pain, periods coming every three weeks, uterine cramps and hemorrhaging, and years of trying to cure myself with noninvasive therapies, in 1991 I had a hysterectomy, during which the doctors found severe adenomyosis (internal endometriosis that causes overwhelming pain, which is usually found to this degree only in women who have had numerous children), large fibroids, and numerous Fallopian cysts. Later I learned from DES researchers that adenomyosis,

---

DES POSTER CHILD

At one point during a telephone interview with Dr. McLachlan, he listed the conditions he had found in his laboratory experiments on animals exposed to DES prior to birth. With almost every one he mentioned, I said, "I had that."

Finally McLachlan said, "I wrote a paper on tubular cysts and published it in a scientific journal. Did you ever have tubular cysts?"

"Yes."

"That's it!" he said. "You should be the poster child for DES."

---

especially to the degree I had it, is very common in DES-exposed laboratory animals.

The anesthesiologist for the hysterectomy told me that my uterus was so big—the size of a cantaloupe—and malformed that it "didn't look human." It had indented on all my organs. I went to the pathology lab and took photos of it. The pathologist said it was the most disfigured and painful-looking uterus he had ever seen. I was glad to have it removed. At last, I felt, my health problems were over. Although I would never have a child, at least there would be no further bleeding and pain.

I thought I was home free. I could take all my past experiences and help other women. Some years later, I read an article in *Science News* about endocrine disruptors and their similarity to DES. I began to read everything I could find about hormone disruptors and knew I was meant to write this book.

In the early stages of research, I was struck by the fact that all of the conditions found in my uterus and tubes were frequently observed in test animals exposed to DES in utero. For many years, I had assumed I was a DES daughter; now I had to know for sure. I pressured my mother until she agreed to request microfiche records from the hospital where she had received medical treatment during pregnancy. She read the pages to me over the phone. "See honey," she said, "there is no DES mentioned here." I had her send the records to me. She hadn't realized that DES stands for diethylstilbestrol. She hadn't recognized the whole word. Yet there it was in black and white—the day she had received a single injection of diethylstilbestrol during the first trimester of pregnancy. It was official: I was a DES daughter.

A few months later, I felt a lump in my breast.

I had just had a completely healthy breast exam several months earlier. I returned to the doctors. They said the lump felt benign, let's wait. I didn't want to wait. We retook mammograms and ultrasounds. They didn't show anything abnormal. The doctors suggested I wait a month or two, which didn't feel right to me. I opted for a biopsy, which came back inconclusive. This meant I now needed to have the lump removed.

Although I had refused a general anesthesia, I had been given an injection of something that made me groggy. I was shaking my head, trying to hear what the surgeon was whispering in my ear.

"Have you started yet?" I asked

"We have it out already."

DES STORIES

While I was going through treatment, I met a nurse at a clinic in Bellevue, Washington. When I told her my story, she said, "I can top that." She explained she had five sisters. All six of them were DES daughters. Everyone, including herself, either had cancer or had experienced a catastrophic pregnancy.

While I was writing this book, the following events happened:

1. I met a woman who had been diagnosed two years previously with a small precancerous lump in her breast. The top doctors in Los Angeles said to just cut it out and she would have a 98 percent chance of having no further problems. When I met her, she was fighting for her life. I asked if by chance she was a DES daughter. "Yes," she said, "why do you ask me that? No one else has." She died while I was writing this book.

2. One of my roommate's friends called me, wanting to read a draft of this chapter. I asked why. She said, "I had cervical cancer six years ago and thought I was fine. I was just diagnosed with ovarian cancer last week. I'm a DES daughter, too."

3. One of my close friends is a medical doctor in California specializing in women's health. She told me two women in their 30s had come to see her, both with diagnoses of breast cancer. Knowing about my situation, she asked if they were DES daughters. They both were. They wondered why she was asking them that question.

4. When I interviewed Dr. Craig Dees, a noted scientist who is working on new causes and treatments for breast cancer (including screening methods that don't use radiation), he told me: "I had two lab technicians in their 30s who were DES daughters. One died from breast cancer. The other had a catastrophic pregnancy and had to stay in bed for months, which caused severe money problems. The baby was born premature, which caused stress and more money problems. The mother was depressed and anxious and, when the child was one, she killed herself."

   Dees then emphatically stated, "I directly attribute the deaths of both these young women to DES, and you can quote me on that."

These stories are called anecdotal accounts in medicine. What they tell me is that we need to keep better track of children of DES-exposed mothers and see what is really happening to us.

He was saying some more words. What were they? I kept shaking my head, trying to understand him.

"It's a carcinoma. You have cancer, do you understand? It's cancer."

I lay my head back down on the gurney. I have cancer. I have breast cancer. Why me?

But my very next thought—knowing I was a DES daughter, knowing I'd had all these other problems—my very next thought before I closed my eyes was "Why not me?"

A HEALTHY BABY GIRL

Judith Helfand is a DES daughter who happened to get a job working on a film crew that was shooting a movie about DES. The director insisted that anyone who was a DES child get a check-up. Judith balked. She had just had her yearly exam and was fine. The director held his ground, so she reluctantly went and got another gynecologic workup. This was how she learned that she had clear cell adenocarcinoma (CCA), the rare form of cancer that DES daughters were prone to get. At twenty-five years of age, Judith had to have a radical hysterectomy.

While recuperating from her extensive surgery and grieving for the children she could never have, Helfand decided her story was public and political. "It's not a private thing we're going to keep in our own house," Helfand says on the videotape that became part of her autobiographical documentary film, *A Healthy Baby Girl*, chronicling her experience with cancer caused by DES.

Judith uses her film to forge links between her concrete story of DES and the long-term implications of other synthetic chemicals. She finds the common threads among toxic exposure, family health, and corporate responsibility and seeks to raise awareness. After all, she says, "we already have an experiment [DES] that not only is chemically proven, but we have something else to show—long-term impact to our lives, families, emotions, and what we hold to be most personal, our relationships." (See Appendix D for further information on Helfand's campaign and video.)

AND THE "GOOD" NEWS IS

Some aspects of the DES experiment on humans and the animal and laboratory research with DES are actually good news. Most DES sons, even those with testicular abnormalities, have no problem with fertility. Half of DES daughters have no problems with pregnancy. It all seems to be a matter of timing—at what point the fetus was exposed in utero—and underlying minor genetic glitches. It is obvious that the timing of exposure to a hormone disruptor is critical.

John McLachlan's research on how DES and chemical estrogens are related to cancer has shown that if mice are given DES before puberty they have a higher risk of getting different cancers of the reproductive system. If DES is given to mice after puberty, these mice don't have any increased risk of getting cancer, which means that many of the exposures we receive throughout our lives will, in all likelihood, not cause us serious problems. This is why many scientists don't buy into the doomsday approach to hormone disruptors, why they don't believe we will all become sterile and the human race become extinct. *Not everyone is affected.* Of course, if you or your children are, that fact isn't all that comforting.

Are Things That Different Today?

I sometimes stop to wonder about the decades of the 1940s, 1950s, and early 1960s. Women listened to what their doctors recommended. They stopped breastfeeding their babies and instead fed them formula in bottles. They took pills or injections during pregnancy, not really knowing what they were being given. They were told that smoking was a great relaxant. People did not think to question either the medical model or the doctors themselves. And what about the drug companies? By 1947 the people making the decisions at the drug companies were aware of many animal studies that indicated DES posed the threat of cancer, that it could cross the placental barrier, and that DES caused malformations in the offspring of exposed pregnant mice. However, DES was sold until 1997.

What is considered "true, customary, and procedural" in medicine for drugs, treatments, and surgeries changes about every seventeen years. The DES used to treat miscarriage two decades ago is not prescribed now, at least not in the United States. The Dalkon shield is no longer used. Aspirin is no longer recommended for children. Smoking is not considered a healthy relaxant. The idea of what is best changes.

Presently, Prozac is one of the most widely prescribed drugs on the market for depression and weight loss and is even used as a veterinary medicine for pets with neuroses. Made by Eli Lilly, Prozac is one of the world's bestselling drugs. It is being prescribed in record amounts to children. Approximately 2.5 percent of young children and 8 percent of teens are affected by depression. Yet a Canadian research team proposed in 1992 that Prozac, when given to rats in dosages equivalent to the dosages given to humans, enhanced the growth of preexisting cancer. Both Canadian and U.S. officials wanted to replicate the research before they took any action.

If you were a cancer patient suffering from depression, wouldn't you want to know that some studies suggest Prozac increases the rate and aggression of any cancer that is present in the body—even if the information comes "only" from animal studies?

Dioxin, a known hormone disruptor, can cause extra tissue over the vaginal opening in a somewhat similar way that DES daughters can have extra tissue hooding the clitoris. Thomas A. Gasiewicz, from the Department of Environmental Medicine at the University of Rochester Medical Center, says dioxins affect developing tissues in the embryo, fetus, and child, and these developmental effects may persist into adulthood.

Dr. Bob Moore, a toxicologist at the University of Wisconsin who has studied the effects of in utero exposure to dioxin, has said: "I think there is genuine and honest skepticism about whether endocrine disruption is a serious problem for humans, although I suspect that some of these skeptics are the same sort of people who would conclude they should stay in the coal mine even after the canary dies because no humans have keeled over yet, and besides, the mine hasn't exploded."

How Hormone Disruptors May Affect You

It seems that certain people are more sensitive to toxins in the environment than are others. Do you know someone who has to leave a room if anybody nearby is wearing perfume? (Perfume, once made from the essence of flowers, is now mostly a chemical concoction.) Of course, one of the most sensitive groups of people is children, who have less well-developed immune systems than do adults. And the most vulnerable of all is the fetus in the womb, especially during the first trimester of pregnancy.

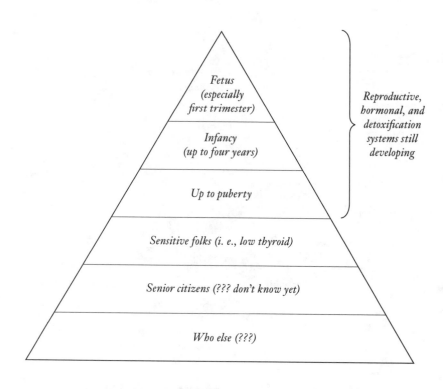

FIGURE II.1　*Populations Most Vulnerable to Hormone Disruption*

Laboratory studies, extensive observations of wildlife, and human pharmaceutical tragedies like DES are all warning signs that some vulnerable populations will be affected by hormone disruption, resulting in irreversible harmful effects. Since endocrine disrupters are a recently recognized phenomenon, we do not yet know all the illnesses or problems that may eventually be associated with these chemicals and their metabolites. However, even though the phenomenon is relatively recent and controversial, we should still be aware of the possibilities.

We've seen how complex the problem of endocrine disruption is and that proving cause-and-effect is going to be a long arduous process if it's even possible at all. More and more scientists, activists, and government officials are now leaning toward what is called the weight-of-evidence approach for evaluating the potential danger of hormone disruptors. The weight of evidence about hormone disruption is based on:

- an integrated body of data from laboratory experiments, wildlife studies, and epidemiological studies (studies on large groups of people to understand causes of disease)

- the recognition that adverse health effects in animal species do imply a real potential danger for humans

- the recognition that chemicals act in mixtures, making it impossible to evaluate safety by simply testing individual chemicals

- accepting that all epidemiological studies are limited because they cannot be completely controlled, but this does not invalidate their findings

- the recognition that hormone disruption of biological processes may manifest in many different ways in an individual, not just as a single disease

- the recognition that hormone disruption in the developing fetus or child may lead to subtle end points such as altered behavior and intelligence, immune and nervous system dysfunction, as well as reproductive problems and illnesses such as cancer. Subtle end points refer to effects that are usually seen later in life and are harder to identify. Also, while these end points may be subtle for an individual, they may not be so subtle on a population basis. For example, a five-point drop in IQ may not make a major difference in an individual, but a five-point downward shift in the IQ of a population means far fewer geniuses and many more intellectually challenged people.

As Dr. Wade Welshons says:

*The kind of experimental **proof** that people want can never be obtained in humans. It would require a controlled experiment and, of course, that's unethical everywhere on the planet. You can't intentionally treat pregnant women with these compounds to determine the effects on the fetus, so the standards used to judge the effects of endocrine disruptors have to be a little different from the ones you would use in evaluating experimental science* *based on work in animals or tissue cultures. This is why regulatory agencies are shifting to the idea of* weight of evidence—*what do the data or experiments tend to indicate? And in the last several years the weight of evidence has certainly shown that estrogens at physiological levels during fetal development have permanent effects on that development.*

This section of *Hormone Deception* examines the various effects of endocrine-disrupting compounds on different segments of the human population.

In the Womb and at the Breast

If we design a compound to be toxic to an insect cell, why does it surprise us when we find out that the same compound is toxic to a human cell? We've always thought the issue was mass—that these things could be toxic to an insect without having significant effects in a much larger human. But how big is an embryo?

—Dr. Lou Guillette

Women carry and nurture within their bodies our future generations—the innocent fetuses who are the most vulnerable of all when exposed to hormone disruptors. The substances that a mother has been exposed to throughout her life, and some of what she takes in during her pregnancy, become the legacy of the next generation. So the womb is really the first environment with which we should be concerned. In many ways, the fetus and the developing child are the focus of this book.

Up until the time of puberty, children are still developing and therefore appear to be more susceptible than adults to exposure from environmental toxins. The fetus is the most susceptible and can be affected by hormone disruptors while in the womb. For example, according to Dr. Earl Gray, the fetus is especially vulnerable to dioxin because it has a different distribution of Ah receptors (the receptor that receives dioxin's signals) than does the adult.

A group of international experts who gathered in Erice, Sicily, for a work session on endocrine-disrupting chemicals issued a statement that said (in small part): "A variety of chemical challenges in humans and animals early in life can lead to profound and irreversible abnormalities in brain development at exposure levels that do not produce permanent effects in an adult."

Passing Along Hormone Disruptors

While a mother-to-be is watching her belly grow rounder and joyfully picking out baby names, she and the fetus and the placenta are interacting with each other on a daily basis. The mother feels safe knowing that her baby is protected by the placenta (the organ that surrounds the fetus and attaches to the mother, controlling metabolic exchanges), but it is not actually a perfect barrier protecting the unborn from many pollutants. The placenta can reduce the amount of some of the chemicals that travel from the mother to the fetus, but not all. Dr. Walter Rogan demonstrated that DDE levels in the umbilical cord blood of newborns are about one-third the DDE level in the mother's blood at the time of birth. A Japanese study released in April 1999 showed higher levels. These researchers found that umbilical cord blood (as well as the placenta and breast milk) had dioxin at 90 percent of the level that was in the mother's bloodstream. There is no question but that some pollutants are indeed getting through to the unborn child.

Once pollutants do cross the placenta, the fetus has far fewer resources for getting rid of toxins than does the mother. The unborn baby doesn't have a fully functioning liver or kidneys that can clear out pollutants, so when chemicals get in, most of them cannot get out.

From the embryonic stage to the time of puberty, the body is still developing, meaning that hormone disruptors have the opportunity to create problems that may not be visible at birth or during youth but may manifest when the child is older, even many decades later. Because the effects of the hormone disruptors that are passed from mother to child may not surface until the child reaches sexual maturity or beyond, it becomes extremely complicated to connect cause and effect.

Endocrine disruptors are potentially so powerful that a woman can receive one harmful exposure during her pregnancy that may affect the health of her child years down the road, as in the case of DES, while not harming the mother at all. This is known as transgenerational exposure.

THALIDOMIDE BABIES SHATTER PLACENTA THEORY

Does the word *thalidomide* ring a bell? It was a prescription drug given to pregnant mothers with morning sickness in the early 1960s that produced offspring with flippers instead of arms and legs. Before thalidomide, medical experts believed that the placenta acted as a complete protection for the developing baby from harmful outside influences. The thalidomide tragedy shattered that theory.

Many other children who were exposed to thalidomide in the womb had perfectly fine limbs, but instead had problems with heart and organ malformations, brain damage, deafness, blindness, autism, and epilepsy. Some were spared any ill effects. It appeared to be the timing of thalidomide ingestion rather than the dose that influenced the babies' deformities. While some of the mothers with limbless children had taken only two or three thalidomide pills during their entire pregnancy, ingestion occurred between the fifth and eighth weeks when the babies' arms and legs were developing.

An interesting note is that eleven out of 380 children born to thalidomide victims in the United Kingdom have limb defects, a figure which is five times higher than the usual rate for the general population. If proven, this would mean the drug caused genetic damage in at least two generations.

At this point in history, every pregnant woman in the world has endocrine disruptors in her body, some of which are transferred to her baby before birth and through breastfeeding. This includes not just a pill or a shot she may have received during pregnancy, but the body burden resulting from the mother's total lifetime exposure before she became pregnant. Even though the mother may be completely unaffected by her adult exposure to endocrine disruptors, her children may develop problems.

A pilot study performed at the Center for Women's Health at Cedars-Sinai Medical Center in Los Angeles, California, measured amniotic fluid from routine amniocentesis procedures. Thirty percent of the women had detectable levels of PCBs, DDT, and lindane as well as estrogenic compounds, such as phytoestrogens from foods. Dr. Larry Needham said the degree of concentration of in utero exposure is sufficient to be a cause for concern. Future studies will look at thirty-five other compounds in amniotic fluid.

A FREE RIDE

During critical times such as pregnancy, a mother's body has extremely high levels of estrogen. Fortunately, 99 percent of the estrogen a pregnant woman makes is attached to sex hormone-binding globulin (SHBG). When estrogen rides piggyback on these blood proteins, it is said to be bound. Estrogen that is bound does not cross the placental barrier, so the estrogen cannot enter the body and brain of the developing child. The estrogen that is not bound is referred to as free estrogen as it is able to pass freely into cells and bind with receptors. Free estrogen is thus the biologically active estrogen that can get into a cell and send a signal to start estrogenic activity. Only 0.2–0.3 percent of a mother's estrogen is free and can get into the fetus.

At this time, it is thought that most xenoestrogens do not bind with these blood proteins. DES, for example, is not bound at all to the sex hormone-binding proteins in blood. Xenoestrogens, therefore, circulate freely and have access to places where natural estrogens cannot tread. Even if these chemicals are much weaker than natural estrogen outside the body, their potency increases inside the body because of their unrestricted travel capabilities.

Environmental estrogens can travel across the placenta and enter the growing fetus. These ecoestrogens can store in the placenta, which has a large fat content, and slowly release toxins to the developing fetus. So although these substances might not be nearly as potent as natural hormones when they are tested outside the body, xenoestrogens are relatively more potent within the body than testing would suggest—parts per trillion can have an influence. When a compound like DES is introduced into the body and doesn't bind with the blood proteins, it can be as much as 100 times more potent than natural estradiol in the fetus. In another example, bisphenol A, by not binding to SHBG, has higher activity levels in the fetus than when tested in the lab.

As a side note, it appears that women (so far the studies have only been on women) who carry more fat around their middle (apple-shaped people as opposed to the pear-shaped ones) have lower amounts of these protective proteins (SHBG), which keep our natural hormones at safe levels. (Diets high in saturated fat may also decrease SHBG levels in the body.) Abdominal fat is associated with higher risk for diseases such as diabetes and heart disease. These women may also be more at risk for exposure to EDCs.

A Brief Lesson in Biology

We start from a dot and eventually we become a complete adult—a complex and challenging developmental process. Our genes take us from that union of the single sperm and egg (when two sets of chromosomes meet, mingle, and mate) and program us into becoming a brown-eyed, curly-haired, 5′7″ person with freckles.

The cell is the basic unit of life. Each cell is surrounded by a membrane, which protects the inside of the cell from the outside environment. Inside the cell is the nucleus, the information and control center (like the control deck where Captain Kirk and Spock sat on the starship *Enterprise*) which is protected by its own membrane. The nucleus of the cell is the home of DNA (deoxyribonucleic acid), which encodes the essential blueprint for who we are—the archival information that is used for building and maintaining life. Between the nucleus and the outer cell membrane is

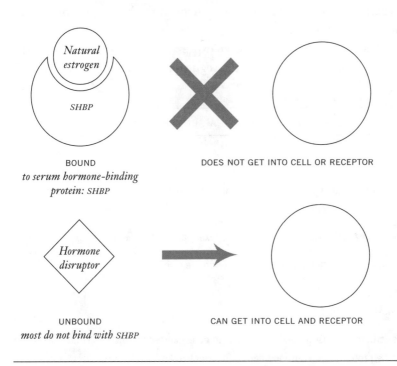

BOUND
*to serum hormone-binding
protein:* SHBP

DOES NOT GET INTO CELL OR RECEPTOR

UNBOUND
most do not bind with SHBP

CAN GET INTO CELL AND RECEPTOR

FIGURE 5.1 *Bound vs. Free Estrogen*

the cytoplasm (a watery substance in which most of the chemical activity of the cell takes place), which is where proteins are formed. Proteins are the building blocks for body tissues and also act as enzymes, substances that promote natural biochemical reactions.

Together with protein molecules, DNA is organized into structures called chromosomes. In humans, there are forty-six chromosomes, with each cell containing two complete sets of chromosomes, one from each biological parent. Lined up along part of the chromosomes are the basic units of heredity, called genes. Each gene determines one function. There may be thousands of genes on one chromosome. The genome—the master set of instructions or genetic blueprint for making a human—is composed of at least 100,000 genes, of which only about 200 are now known.

DNA cannot leave the nucleus. It is like the queen bee who holds the master plan, but she speaks Italian while the workers bees, the proteins, only understand Portuguese. Therefore, the genetic blueprint needs to be transcribed and translated into marching orders for the proteins before anything can get done. Once the translation is complete, the gene faxes its instructions to all the appropriate proteins in the body. This process is called gene expression.

Whether or not a gene is ever expressed depends on a regulatory sequence. It is here, as a link in the regulatory system of genes, that hor-

---

LET'S GET THIS STRAIGHT: A GENETIC GLOSSARY

DNA—knows everything, can't *do* anything

Genes—the sequence of DNA (on the chromosomes) that receives the hormonal message and turns on or off accordingly

Gene expression—the orders get copied, faxed, and translated for the proteins

Proteins—receive the orders and actually do the work

Genetic damage—direct damage to DNA; results in mutations that are passed along to the next generation

Classic hormone disruption—alterations in gene expression; the orders are sabotaged and the proteins carry out modified or incorrect tasks

---

mones ultimately deliver their message. This is why hormone receptors are sometimes called transcriptional machines. They control and coordinate the process of transcribing and translating information from the DNA so a set of target genes can be activated.

Every single cell in the body contains all the genetic instructions (the whole genome), but in an individual cell, only a small number of genes are ever expressed. For example, in your eyes you have the genes for every tissue in your body, but only the eye genes are turned on. You do not have skin genes turned on in your eyes. Conversely, in your skin, your eye genes (which are present there) are turned off, so you never have eyes growing out of the skin on your arm. (Although some frogs have been found with extra legs or eyes growing out of their stomachs. What does *that* say?) What this means is that some genes are always "on" or "off"; others are sometimes on and sometimes off. If it is always on, a gene will always be expressed.

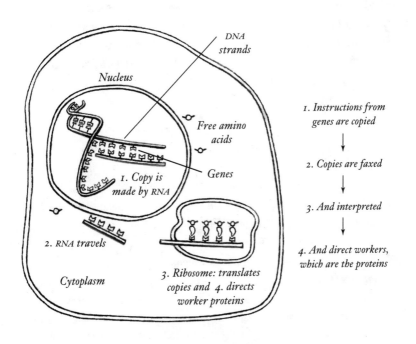

FIGURE 5.2 *Gene Expression Gets Your Body's Job Done*

Almost everything inside every organism is a product of gene expression, and gene expression is what can be altered by hormone disruption. Endocrine disruptors have the ability to turn genes off and on, not always appropriately.

Genetic expression is complicated and there are many opportunities for error, resulting in the wrong message being sent. Fetal exposure to hormones can program the way genes function for the rest of that being's life. Some genes are supposed to get turned on early in life, some later. If a fetus or developing child is exposed to a potent hormone disruptor during a specific window of vulnerability, the path his or her cells take in their development may be altered, possibly permanently. A girl may show signs of puberty at age five instead of during the early teen years. A boy's testicles may not descend. Intelligence may be affected. Sustained attention or response to stress may be altered. Or . . . nothing may happen. Individuals respond differently to these different signals.

For one reason or another, DNA is sometimes damaged and the genes are modified in a fundamental way. For example, when a woman has been exposed to excess ionizing radiation, genes in her eggs can get damaged to the point of mutation. Some DNA damage is a nondestructive alteration in the genetic code, such as changes that lead to a child growing taller than his or her parents. Other damage can be far more serious, such as passing along a genetically determined disease or deformity.

DES KARMA

Professor Risto Santti is a well-respected researcher in Finland who has spent his career studying the effects of DES on the male reproductive tract and prostate cancer. After his father's death in 1993, his mother was going through old letters and found records of which drugs she had taken while pregnant. She sent them to Dr. Santti. He was astonished to find that he himself was a DES son. Dr. Santti's recent research suggests a condition in males in which voiding becomes an inappropriately slow process, which he calls urethral dyssynergia. He feels this is a result of exposure to estrogenic compounds in the womb.

A haunting question, as yet unanswered, is whether or not hormone disruptors can cause cellular damage at the level of DNA. Most scientists are adamant that endocrine disruptors do *not* cause direct damage to genes but rather damage the process through which genes are expressed. Even the maternal transfer of pollutants, such as the DES I absorbed in the womb, is considered to be fetal exposure itself and not DNA damage to the parent that has been passed along to the child.

But never say never, especially in science. Some research is finding that some xenohormones can damage DNA directly and indirectly or can be metabolized into "damaging" metabolites. Fortunately, our bodies have repair mechanisms. We can therefore withstand a fair amount of DNA damage before mutation occurs. However, repair mechanisms are less vigilant in rapidly growing cells (where most cancers occur), such as colon, cervical, and breast duct cells. Also, repair capacities can get "maxed out," or be faulty in some people with underlying genetic glitches.

Timing Is Crucial

The sex hormones in adults primarily influence reproductive functions, such as sexual drive, the menstrual cycle, pregnancy, and sperm production, as well as affecting the immune and nervous systems. But in the womb, steroids also play an important role by steering the development of the reproductive organs as well as influencing the development of the thyroid gland, liver, immune system, and brain. This development has to happen according to a particular timed sequence of events. Even one very low dose of a hormone impostor at a specific point of embryonic development may cause permanent damage.

For example, on day fifty-six of human gestation, one particular hormone is required for the organs of the fetus to begin developing testicles or the fetus will not develop as a male. If the timed sequence of hormone signals is disrupted, development of the male reproductive organs can be skewed, resulting in undescended testicles or other problems. This has been demonstrated in animal studies. Pregnant rats fed one meal containing dioxin on day fifteen of their gestation (when sexual differentiation occurs in rats) produced male offspring that had smaller sex organs, a 75 percent reduction in sperm counts, and feminized sexual behavior. In females, the changes that turn the glands into ovaries begin in the third to fourth month of fetal life and are essential for normal functioning of the ovaries in later life.

Timing appears to be as important with exposure to phytoestrogens as it is with chemical hormone disruptors. A Basque from Spain told the USDA that one-eyed sheep were being born. The USDA discovered that if the sheep, on day thirteen of pregnancy, were allowed to graze on one side of the island where there were specific phytoestrogenic plants, sheep offspring would be born with only one eye. If the sheep were taken to graze on the other side of the island on that particular day, the baby sheep were born with two eyes.

The systems in our bodies are most sensitive when they are growing, before protective mechanisms are developed. Richard Hajek and colleagues from their experimental gynecology-endocrinology laboratory treated female mice neonatally (one to five days after birth) with a weaker form of estrogen than estradiol and found changes in vaginal tissue, smaller sex organs, and excessive uncontrolled growth of the cervical/vaginal area in nearly 100 percent of the animals. One-quarter of the mice developed tumors in their reproductive organs. The researchers stated, "These results strengthen the concerns put forth by McLachlan and colleagues that weak environmental estrogenic compounds . . . may demonstrate potent estrogenic effects in developing perinatal tissues."

ENVIRONMENTAL INJUSTICE

Increased exposure to environmental toxins, including endocrine-disrupting chemicals, may be contributing to some unnerving statistics on African Americans. Numerous general population surveys show that residues of chemicals such as DDT and its major metabolite DDE are found in greater levels in African Americans than in whites. African Americans have more exposure to chemicals in general because of where they live and work. Many also consume diets quite high in processed foods. One study revealed that half of tested African-American women had more than six parts per million of DDE in breast milk while only 5 percent of the Caucasian mothers reached this level.

Check the Environmental Justice website at www.es.epa.gov/oeca/oejbut.

BREASTFEEDING AND HORMONE DISRUPTORS

What happens when our precious newborn enters the world—at the very top of the food chain—and is fed the most perfect of all foods: mother's breast milk?

We know that through the process of bioaccumulation, even low dosages of ecohormones can become more concentrated higher up in the food chain. We also know how hormone disruptors and their breakdown products are fat soluble and are stored in fatty tissue, like breast tissue. (Those willing to spend money for the tests will find a minimum of a dozen chemical contaminants in their body fat, regardless of where they live.) Mother's milk is 3 percent fat. The chemicals stored in the mother's fat are not released in significant amounts except during breastfeeding.

Therefore, one result of breastfeeding is that it considerably lessens the mother's body burden of toxic chemicals, which may be one reason why women who breastfeed have lower rates of breast cancer. This implies, of course, that breastfeeding substantially increases the child's exposure, especially for the firstborn. The chemical levels in mother's milk become lower during each individual feeding, are lower after a three- to six-month period of breastfeeding, and are also lower for subsequent children. And what we get in the first six months of breastfeeding makes up more than 10 percent of the cumulative body burden of chemicals up until the age of twenty.

If breast milk was regulated like infant formula, it would commonly violate FDA levels for poisonous substances in food. Breast milk is the food with the highest level of known contamination from chemicals such as PCBS and DDT and its metabolites. (These are the chemicals we've known how to study; others—like plastics and flame retardants—haven't yet been tested.) If you compare the levels of persistent chemicals in breast milk in 1970 with those in 1980 and in 1990, you would find they are dropping due to bans on chemicals like DDT. However, despite the fact that DDT was banned many years ago, it still shows up in breast milk today, along with other chemicals.

Of course, other factors are involved. Studies have found that first-time mothers and women who regularly drink alcohol had higher levels of PCBS, while African-American women, cigarette smokers, and women who consumed sport fish during pregnancy had higher levels of DDE. Older mothers, who have had many more years to accumulate toxins in their

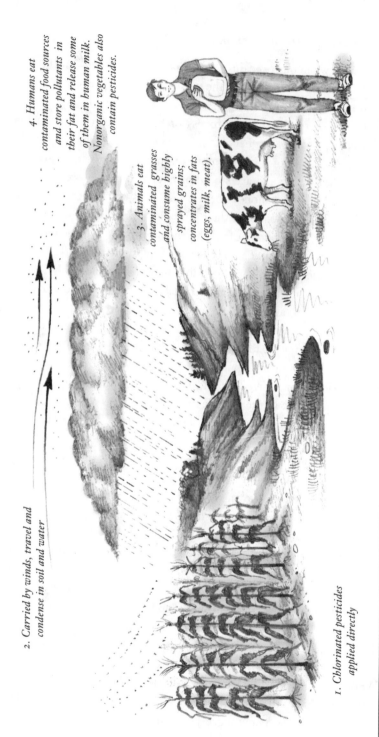

2. Carried by winds, travel and condense in soil and water

4. Humans eat contaminated food sources and store pollutants in their fat and release some of them in human milk. Nonorganic vegetables also contain pesticides.

3. Animals eat contaminated grasses and consume bigbly sprayed grains; concentrates in fats (eggs, milk, meat).

1. Chlorinated pesticides applied directly

FIGURE 5.3 Food Chain (Bioaccumulation)

bodies, have higher levels of chemicals in their breast milk (and more women are having babies for the first time at an older age).

A Mother's Ability to Breastfeed

Dr. Walter J. Rogan is an epidemiologist with the National Institute of Environmental Health Sciences (NIEHS). As part of a study of 700 children, Rogan and his colleagues looked at the children born to women in North Carolina from 1978 to 1982 and analyzed their exposure for total PCBs (polychlorinated biphenyls) and DDE (a metabolite of DDT). They measured these endocrine-disrupting pollutants in maternal blood, umbilical cord blood, and fetal blood so they had a very good idea about the children's exposure to PCBs and DDE while in the womb. They also analyzed the mothers' breast milk. Over the first six months of breastfeeding, they found that the maternal body burden of chemicals dropped due to some of these chemicals being transferred into the nursing infants. They also noted that the women with the highest exposure to DDE were able to breastfeed their infants for the shortest amount of time—an average of eleven weeks. The women with the lowest body burden of DDE were able to breastfeed for an average of thirty-three weeks. Studies on rats confirm this effect. Unborn rats exposed to the hormone disruptor dioxin in the womb developed altered mammary duct tissue, so when the rats became mothers, they produced less milk.

This data was so much like what they thought it would be that Rogan's team at first didn't trust their results. They asked the World Health Organization which countries had high exposures to DDE and found that China, India, and Mexico (where DDT is still manufactured and used) had the highest levels. Since Mexico was the closest, Rogan checked out an agricultural region in north central Mexico called Tiahuallo where cotton was heavily sprayed with DDT. This created high levels of the metabolite DDE in the butter, eggs, chickens, and dust of the area. The scientists tested almost 200 women and looked at the women with the highest levels of DDE. These women, in a completely different setting than the study in North Carolina, had a 40 percent decrease in the time they could breastfeed (a remarkable overlap with the results from North Carolina). In a third-world country, this is a deadly scenario. Without access to good water and money to buy formula, if you can't nurse your baby, the baby dies.

TABLE 5.1 BREASTFEEDING STUDIES

STUDIES ON LACTATION	EFFECTS
1978–1982, Walter Rogan and his coworkers at NIEHS looked at 700 children born to women in North Carolina; measured maternal blood, fetal blood, and cord blood for exposure to DDE and PCBS.	Women with the highest levels of DDE could breastfeed for an average of eleven weeks, compared to women with lower levels who breastfed for thirty-three weeks.
Rogan and cohorts did a second study on 200 women in Tiahuallo, Mexico, where cotton was heavily sprayed with DDT, creating high levels of the metabolite DDE in the butter, eggs, chickens, and dust.	The women with the highest dose ranges in utero of DDE had a 40 percent decrease in the time they could breastfeed (a remarkable overlap with the results from North Carolina).
Two German studies headed by Drexler and Drasch—one with 147 women and the other with seventy—demonstrated that the amount of mercury (an endocrine disruptor) in breast milk from the first week was statistically correlated to the number of dental amalgams in the mother's mouth, along with her level of fish consumption.	In both studies, after two months of breastfeeding the concentrations of mercury were lower in breast milk, and, in one study, even lower than in infant formula.
A study by Nagayama and coworkers of thirty-six breastfed Japanese children.	Background levels of chlorinated dioxins from breast milk significantly correlated with decreased levels of T3 and T4 (thyroid hormones) in the blood of the babies.

STUDIES ON LACTATION	EFFECTS
Korrick and coworkers measured breast milk levels of PCBS in 122 mother-infant pairs.	Four were found with exceptionally high PCBS and these were shown to live near PCB-contaminated waste sites in New Bedford Harbor and an estuary in southeastern Massachusetts.
Ayotte and Dewailley measured dioxinlike compounds in Inuit breast milk and *simulated* the effects of exposure from birth to seventy-five years of age by using a toxicokinetic model.	Their results suggested that breastfeeding strongly influences the body burden of dioxinlike compounds up to twenty years of age.
Rylander, et al., studied PCBS in the blood of Swedish women.	The longer the women lactated, the lower the levels of PCBS in the blood. They did not find high PCB concentrations associated with smoking and alcohol consumption, although two other studies did.

Children's Teeth and Hormone Disruptors in Breast Milk

In the late 1980s, Satu Alaluusua, a Finnish dentist from the University of Helsinki Institute of Dentistry, noticed that a fair number of her young patients had soft, discolored molars that were more prone to cavities. For something to affect molars (called structural effects), exposure had to have taken place early in life. Alaluusua and coworkers looked for the culprit and discovered that the children with defective molars had been exposed during lactation to dioxin from breast milk. Other epidemiologists around the world had also reported yellowish-brown discoloration in the teeth of children who had been exposed to high amounts of dioxin-like compounds.

Alaluusua and her coworkers tracked down children whose mothers' milk had been analyzed six years earlier as part of a World Health Organization study. She compared the finding of molar defects with the levels of hormone disruptors found in the mothers' milk. They found that breast milk with the highest levels of dioxins was linked with the children who had these permanent molar problems. Another study, published in the *Lancet* medical journal, shows that high background levels of dioxin from breast milk gave 17 of 102 children soft, mottled teeth that were permanently prone to cavities.

It was dioxins, not PCBS, that were associated with these dental problems. Linda Birnbaum, a toxicologist from the EPA in Research Triangle Park, North Carolina—a noted world expert in dioxins—emphasizes that the levels of dioxin (50–258 ppt) these Finnish researchers were finding in mothers' milk are within the normal range found in fat and breast milk in most Americans. Since most of the previous studies about mother's milk have been done in relation to PCBS and DDT (which are both banned), we don't yet know much about the effects of other endocrine-disrupting compounds.

What to Feed Your Infant

What's a mother to do? Does this mean we should stop breastfeeding our babies and give them cow's milk formula? Cows are vegetarian, so they don't eat fatty foods laced with hormone disruptors, and cows are milked daily so they are excreting their toxins on a regular basis. But what about the estrogenic growth hormones and antibiotics given to the cows? What happens when we heat up formula in plastic baby bottles? Are hormone disruptors leaching into the milk?

What about soy formula? Formulas based on soybeans can contain such large amounts of phytoestrogens that infants fed only soy formulas are being exposed to doses six to eleven times higher than doses known to alter a woman's menstrual cycle. Infant formulas contain at least tenfold (and possibly as much as one hundred times) the amount of phytoestrogens found in breast milk.

Infants seems to metabolize the phytoestrogens, but there are differing opinions on how these compounds act in their bodies. Even though phytoestrogens are far weaker than human estrogens, the blood levels of phytoestrogens in these infants can be 13,000–22,000 times higher than the infant's own estrogen levels. Researchers have concluded that there must be "some biological activity in the infant." Some believe the phytoestrogens can negatively affect development, while others believe there may be long-term benefits from exposing infants to the isoflavones in soy because this may confer some protection later in life against hormone-dependent diseases.

Soy-based formulas have been on the market for thirty years and have not been linked to any health problems. But has anyone looked for hormone disruption? No studies have been done to explore the effects of phytoestrogens in infants, including dose response, age of exposure, and length of exposure. As Dr. Sheehan says, "In the meantime, this large, uncontrolled, and basically unmonitored human infant experiment continues unabated."

All in all, breast milk is still considered by scientists and pediatricians to be the most ideal food for infants.

Breast milk has numerous redeeming nutritional factors that are missing from cow or soy milk—factors that help promote the infant's immune system and brain as well as factors that help seed the gastrointestinal tract to produce friendly bacteria needed for many aspects of health. And the intimate act of breastfeeding is known to increase many important factors, such as children's intelligence.

The present theory is that the higher rates of chemical exposure from breast milk are less significant than the smaller amounts that come from in utero exposure. In other words, even though more chemicals are transferred to the nursing infant, fetal exposure is considered more potentially disrupting. Dr. Joseph Jacobson found that it was the smaller exposures in utero that caused a decrease in IQ rather than the larger amounts of PCBS taken in by the infant during breastfeeding.

Scientists who have done studies on breast milk say that the benefits of breastfeeding far outweigh the risks. Don't stop breastfeeding! Rather, before and during pregnancy and breastfeeding, minimize chemical exposures as much as possible.

HOW TO MINIMIZE EXPOSURE

What should you do if you want to have a baby? What if you're pregnant or breastfeeding now?

- Eat lower on the food chain, preferably organic. Especially make sure high-fat foods like butter and cheese are organic. Eat a wide variety of colorful fruits and veggies throughout the week, such as orange carrots, red beets, leafy greens, and yellow squash.

- Eat organic meats. DES was identified in U.S. meat exports in late 1999, even though it's banned.

- Eat a diet low in detrimental fats (processed, hydrogenated, and animal fats), but include good fats (olive, sesame, walnut, and flaxseed oils) in your diet. Organic oils are the best choice.

- If you are thinking of getting pregnant, get tested to check your chemical levels and, if they are high, think about doing a detox

PACIFIERS, TEETHERS, AND BABY BOTTLES

PACIFIERS

Dispose of pacifier nipples that are manufactured from PVC plastic (vinyl) that is likely to contain phthalates.

Replace with latex pacifier nipples and silicone teethers, materials that do not contain phthalates. The good news is that most manufactured nipples on the market today already are made from latex and are labeled as such. (Note: some infants may be allergic to latex.)

TEETHERS

Dispose of all teethers and heavily mouthed toys made of soft plastic.

Replace with new items that manufacturers confirm are made from plastics that don't contain phthalates. Call toll-free numbers found on packaging. Gerber has withdrawn all phthalate-containing teethers from stores. Many major retailers (Kmart, Sears, Target, Toys "R" Us, and Wal-Mart) now stock only phthalate-free baby products.

BABY BOTTLES

Dispose of all clear, shiny plastic baby bottles, unless the manufacturers tell you they're not made of polycarbonate.

Replace with bottles made of glass or an opaque, less-shiny plastic (often colored) made from polyethylene or polypropylene. Evenflo has brought tempered glass bottles back on the market.

For more information contact *Mothers & Others for a Livable Planet* at 888/ECO-INFO or www. mothers.org/mothers.

WHAT THE SCIENTISTS SAY

- Dr. Bruce Blumberg (developmental and cell biologist at UC Irvine): "My daughter is two and has eaten organically since I read about the research on hormone disruption and, to tell the truth, I'm terrified."

- Dr. Peter Hauser (chief of psychiatry/veteran's affairs at University of Maryland): "I distill our own water at home and I and my pregnant wife try to eat organically, especially butter and cheese."

- Dr. Wade Welshons: "I don't have a daughter, but if I did and she were pregnant, I would definitely recommend that she not have her teeth filled and avoid any exposure to bisphenol A or any other potential estrogens, particularly during the first trimester. Based on the information we have, we can't say, 'Oh, don't worry because there's no effect.' We have information that there could be an effect, and there may very well be serious consequences."

- Dr. Susan Porterfield: "It's totally unnecessary to cause a hysterical panic. We have incredible adaptability. Even though endocrine disruptors are there, perhaps we have many adaptive mechanisms to protect ourselves from their potential harm."

- Dr. Tom Gasiewicz: "Pregnant women should eat mainly deep-sea fish and avoid sport fish and farm-raised fish. High levels of dioxins have been found in farm-raised fish because of the foods they're fed. Avoid fish caught in coastal regions close to big cities and polluted areas like Hudson Bay."

- Dr. Linda Birnbaum: "I think what they need to do is to eat healthy. If you eat a healthy heart diet, which is the recommendation of the Public Health Service, you're going to limit your intake of animal fat-soluble kinds of chemicals, which is where these persistent chemicals tend to reside. You're going to have more green and leafy vegetables."

- Dr. Dan Sheehan: "Well, I'm a developmental toxicologist, and I can tell you that in general it's wise for women to avoid any activities that may be associated with increased risk to their fetus. That includes such things as smoking, alcohol, and drug taking. But it also I think should include attention to exposure to chemicals. My position is, why take a chance?"

program for several weeks. Don't do a detox program while pregnant or breastfeeding, as it will release more chemicals into the breast milk.

- Discuss with your doctor the wisdom of consuming soy products during the first half of pregnancy. Soy has been suspected of contributing to an increase in hypospadias (penis defect) in boys born to vegetarian mothers.

- Don't have dental sealants (bisphenol A) applied during pregnancy. Frederick vom Saal exposed pregnant mice to 2 ng/g body weight of bisphenol A (the amount reported to be swallowed during the first hour after applying a dental sealant). At this level of exposure, there were permanent changes in size of part of the sex organs of males. At 20 ng/g dose of bisphenol A, the daily sperm production went down 20 percent. This work needs to be reproduced, but unless refuted it adds fuel to the need for precautionary measures.

  Try not to get any fillings, especially during the first trimester of pregnancy. Regular fillings contain mercury (a known hormone disruptor) and composite fillings contain bisphenol A (another hormone disruptor). If you have to have a filling, ask for a temporary made out of other materials. Two German studies found a strong relationship between the number of mercury dental fillings in the mother and the amount of mercury being transferred into breast milk and therefore into the body of the infant. They also found that during pregnancy some of the mercury from the mother's fillings crossed the placenta and entered the fetus in the womb.

- Don't handle or be around flea collars, flea bombs, pesticides, or lice shampoo. Don't use chemicals in the garden. There are natural alternatives.

- Avoid using spray chemicals (such as air fresheners and cleansers) and personal products (such as hairspray), especially in closed rooms without exhaust fans.

- Don't work with chemical solvents. Exposed women have more than twice the rate of miscarriages as unexposed women. Pregnant women who work with these types of chemicals and have poison symptoms heavily increase their risk of malformed fetuses.

- Avoid dry-cleaning establishments. Let someone else pick up the cleaning, and air it out for one week (after removing plastic) in the garage rather than in your closet.

- Avoid getting artificial nails and spending time in nail salons that have noxious chemical fumes. Many of the nail varnishes and glues contain hormone-disrupting chemicals.

- Don't microwave foods in plastic and try not to store foods in plastic or aluminum foil. Use glass containers.

- Avoid pumping gas, or if that is not practical, stand aside while the car's tank is filling to avoid the gasoline "smell" as much as possible.

- While breastfeeding, do not go on a diet to lose weight—a recommendation from the World Health Organization. (Don't worry about the weight that comes off naturally.) Losing weight can enhance the mobilization of some chemicals from fat and put more of your stored chemicals into the breast milk.

- Don't smoke and do avoid second-hand smoke. Dr. Erma Lawson, an assistant professor of medical sociology at the University of North Texas in Denton, connects mothers-to-be who smoke to a blood pressure monitor and a fetal heart monitor. Then she has them light up a cigarette and smoke so they can watch and listen as the developing baby tries to escape from the toxic smoke. The smoke itself constricts blood vessels, while tars, nicotine, and the chemicals in the tobacco go into the amniotic fluid and get absorbed by the baby.

- If you're pregnant while traveling in Mexico, China, or India and you start to spot, don't get a shot unless you know what's in it. Those countries still use injections of DES to prevent miscarriage, and the shots don't work!

- Remember, joy is an important factor throughout life and especially during pregnancy. Try not to get obsessive about this information, just do the best job you can.

Children

Once the software is misprogrammed . . . there's no way to fix it. Once the IQ potential is shaved off a child, you can't put it back in. That's the key to this. That's why endocrine disruption is so important to understand.

—Jim Ludwig, ecological researcher,
PBS documentary *Fooling with Nature*

I remember how proudly my friend Lena told me about her nine-year-old daughter being unusually wise for her age. In the next breath, she told me quietly how her daughter was also physically ahead of her age, already developing breasts. This disturbed Lena enough to take her daughter to a pediatrician, who consoled her with the fact that even though this would not have been normal a generation ago, today doctors are seeing eight-, nine-, and ten-year-olds with developing breasts and other signs of early puberty.

How could this be happening? Lena wanted to know. The physician told Lena her hypothesis: numerous chemicals in our environment, especially in our food, are mimicking estrogen hormones and thereby causing a more rapid maturation process. She explained that nowadays, during their first five years of life, children are exposed to the same level of endocrine disruptors that used to be considered safe lifetime exposures for seventy-year-old adults!

WHY ARE CHILDREN SO SUSCEPTIBLE TO HORMONE DISRUPTORS?

It seems that young children, up to the age of puberty, are more at risk for adverse affects from hormone disruptors. This is because:

- *Children's brains are still developing.* Some scientists suggest that the time in the womb is the most crucial period for the developing fetus's brain and cognitive ability, but exposure after birth while the child's brain is still growing (up to several years of age) seems equally important. Research at UCLA, the NIH, and McGill University in Montreal suggests that the gray matter of the brain is still actively growing and fine-tuning itself up through the mid-teen years.

Communication takes place in the brain when chemical messages leap across synapses—the connections between one nerve ending and another. During the first half of pregnancy, the total number of nerve cells is established. However, the interconnections—the pathways through which nerve cells communicate—continue to multiply during the first four years of life. Along with the increase in synapses, other steps in development build upon each other, much like making a tower out of blocks. If, during an early step, there is an alteration that results from an inappropriate hormonal signal, the neuro-network—the developing nerve communication in the brain—can go askew. The tower of blocks wobbles. This may result in decreased learning capabilities.

Postnatal brain growth, along with the continued development of the fatty protection around nerves called the myelin sheath (which takes seven years to develop fully), makes a child's brain very susceptible to toxic agents. Also, the blood/brain barrier, which prevents the penetration of toxins into the brain, does not develop fully until age one, leaving the infant vulnerable to ecohormones.

- *Children's bodies are still growing.* Shortly after birth, children have poorly developed systems for detoxifying chemicals, so the chemicals they are exposed to tend to stay in their bodies. Certain man-made chemicals may be particularly damaging right after birth because they may interfere with the hormones and other substances that send out the signals that normally control development. A child's vital bodily systems—such as the central nervous, immune, respiratory, and reproductive systems—are still dynamically developing, and each stage creates a new window of vulnerability to exposure. The highly complex hormone interactions that control the growth and development of our tissues, organs, reproductive functions, and so many aspects of our health can be urged in a different direction by a hormone disruptor.

- *Children, especially infants and toddlers, put more contaminants into their mouths.* Young children touch and ingest more contaminants than adults. Children, especially those one to three years old, have eating habits that increase their risk because they often have hand-to-food, hand-to-surface, and surface-to-food interactions. The way they handle food could contribute to 20–80 percent of their total dietary intake of pesticides. They also absorb chemicals through their skin, gastrointestinal tract, and lungs better than do adults. They crawl around on the floor where dust, especially in carpeting, has been shown by scientific data to be a serious route of exposure to chemical residues, many of which are tracked into the house on the bottom of our shoes.

- *Children are exposed to more toxic substances than adults.* Children inhale twenty-three times more air, drink three times as much water, and eat two to three times as much food per pound of body weight as do adults. They also have three times more surface area per pound than adults. These differences mean that children have greater rates of exposure to environmental chemicals than adults have. Fruits, vegetables, and juices are not necessarily safer than foods higher on the food chain since they are vehicles for pesticides, food additives, and colorings.

In a report released in November 1997, the Natural Resources Defense Council identified the five top environmental threats to children as lead, air pollution, environmental tobacco smoke, unsafe drinking water, and pesticides, all of which contain endocrine disruptors. Children are exposed to pesticides at home and school, in playgrounds, hospitals, and many public buildings and parks, in the water they drink, and in foods tainted with chemical residues. Total pesticide use in the United States is about 2.2 billion pounds of active ingredients in a typical year, or 8 pounds of pesticides per year for every man, woman, and child.

Government safety levels are finally being changed to take children into consideration. In August 1996, President Clinton signed into law an overhaul of the legislation that sets permissible levels for pesticide residues in foods, known as the Food Quality Protection Act. "Chemicals can go a long way in a small body," the president said in his weekly radio address. "If a pesticide poses a danger to our children, then it won't be in our food. . . . I like to think of it as the Peace of Mind Act. . . ."

It's a nice thought. Chemicals do go a long way in a small body. When the National Academy of Sciences studied pesticides and children's health in 1993, it concluded: "In the absence of data to the contrary, there should be a presumption of greater toxicity to infants and children."

CHILDHOOD DISEASES

Now that science has given us ways to avoid the usual childhood diseases, such as measles, and taken care of many of the epidemic diseases like typhoid, what is happening to the health of our children? Following are a few of the health problems that may be related to endocrine disruption:

- *Childhood cancer* has risen 10.8 percent in the last decade. Cancer is the number one cause of death from disease in the United States of children aged one to fourteen. Children regularly exposed to pesticides in the house have a 3.5 times greater incidence of *leukemia* than those not exposed.

- *Asthma* has doubled or tripled (depending on which statistics you read). Deaths from asthma among children increased by 118 percent between 1980 and 1993, and asthma is the number-one cause of hospitalization for children. DES has been linked to an increase in asthma and upper respiratory disease.

- *Middle ear infections* are a chronic problem for millions of children. One possible explanation is that PCBS and dioxins are structurally similar to thyroid hormones and thyroid disruption may affect the development of the auditory system in the fetus. This could be a contributing factor in the rise in childhood ear infections and the undetected hearing problems that play a role in certain learning disabilities.

- *Hypospadias*—an abnormality of development of the penis and urethra in young boys—has been increasing by at least 2 percent a year.

- *Birth defects, preterm births,* and *low birthweight babies* are increasing in number, according to data gathered by the Centers for

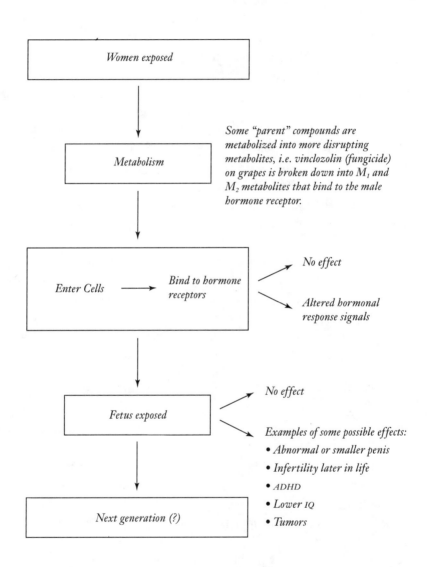

FIGURE 6.1 *What Can Happen Once Hormone Disruptors Get into the Body*

Disease Control from 1989 to 1996. Birth defects are the greatest cause of infant deaths in the first year of life. Premature birth rates were especially high among African-American women. Researchers believe that environmental factors, such as toxins in the air and water, may account for the rise.

Early Puberty

"Precocious puberty," as it is called, is a phenomenon documented in a study that found 27 percent of African-American and almost 7 percent of white girls had either breast or pubic hair development by age seven. Even more startling was the finding that 1 percent of white and 3 percent of African-American girls show these characteristics by age three. The data were collected from 17,077 patients seen by 225 physicians in suburban practices.

Although many scientists attribute this precocity to better nutrition, an increase in obesity in children, and lack of physical exercise, the authors of the study raised the question about environmental estrogens bringing on puberty at an earlier age. Xenoestrogens certainly could play a role, as they have been shown to bring on earlier puberty in rodents. Dr. William Kelce, from the EPA research center at Triangle Park, said they could manipulate the onset of puberty in offspring born to mice who had been exposed to methoxychlor, a widely used pesticide. If sexual development is occurring earlier, this may be an indication that other developmental changes are also happening, although they may not manifest for years or decades.

Puerto Rico has the highest known incidence of premature breast development ever reported, and for decades no one knew why. New research found significantly high levels of phthalates (which have been classified as endocrine disruptors) in almost 70 percent of girls with early breast growth.

From the mid-1800s to the present, girls in the United States and northern Europe are getting progressively bigger and fatter and are reaching puberty earlier. Is this connection really based on better nutrition? One part of Walter Rogan's North Carolina research was a puberty study on 302 girls and 267 boys who were followed for a twenty-year period. Once a year the children's height and weight were recorded, and they filled in pictures on a questionnaire to indicate their sexual development (the

BRAIN CANCER IN CHILDREN

A number of recent studies have found a strong association between some pesticides—especially sprays and foggers used to treat homes for fleas and ticks, pest strips, and termite pesticides—and brain cancers, the most common solid tumors in children. In preliminary studies, the Missouri State Health Department has shown that children got six times more cases of cancer if they were exposed to certain home and garden pesticides than children who did not have these exposures. This is a very strong association, stronger than most found in studying human populations. Studies continue to prove this association.

Families often aren't aware that many household products, such as pet shampoo and flea collars, contain active, toxic pesticides that are often not listed on the label. In the study, the likelihood that a child would develop brain cancer increased with the number of pets treated in the home. A survey run by the Missouri State Health Department found that 80 percent of polled women used some kind of pesticide while pregnant. One study found the risk of brain cancer was 2.9 times greater when the child was exposed through family use of a termite pesticide. Using fog bombs or roach control during pregnancy gave two times a higher risk of brain cancer. Children treated with anti-lice pesticide shampoo also had greater risk.

Look out for the ingredient *carbaryl* in flea/tick powders/dusts and in other household pesticides as it may be an important link to cancer risk.

Tanner Scale of secondary sexual characteristics). The researchers found that the higher the level of prenatal PCB exposure, the heavier the girls were at age fourteen, and their puberty was statistically earlier. Earlier onset of menstruation is a risk factor for estrogen-related illnesses such as breast and ovarian cancer. Boys with higher prenatal exposure to DDE also were fatter, but the age at which they entered puberty was not affected. More and more Americans are now overweight despite low-fat foods and diets. Could this be partially caused by prenatal exposure to endocrine disruptors?

Animal research supports this. Unborn mice exposed to bisphenol A in the womb, at levels comparable to what we humans get just by living our lives, caused the mice to go through puberty earlier and weigh 20 percent more than normal.

ANOTHER FACTOR IN SCHOOL VIOLENCE?

The timing of puberty is another factor to consider in adolescent behavior and possibly the rise we are seeing in school violence. Research on boys from the University of Edinburgh, Scotland, in 1999 is suggesting that "off-time maturers," those who go through puberty either too early or too late, have a higher level of crime, unruly behavior in school, and greater frequency of delinquent acts. Another study on girls, done at the Department of Pediatrics at the Albert Einstein College of Medicine/Montefiore Medicial Center, New York, in 1999 analyzed girls seen in doctors' offices. It documents that premature puberty can result in poor mental health, more behavior problems, and lower IQ when compared to children with normal age of puberty.

The Impact of Pesticides on Children

Elizabeth A. Guillette, research scientist at the University of Arizona and wife of Lou Guillette (who has done many studies on the impact of hormone disruptors on the alligators in Florida), is a nurse who became an anthropologist. Most anthropologists use high-tech methods, such as instrumentation, to test behavior and thought processes, but Dr. Guillette observes everyday life—play behaviors, daily activities, coordination—to evaluate the impact of contamination on children. She studied the Yakima Indians in the Sonora Yaqui Valley in Obregón, Mexico.

What made this a rare research opportunity into the impact of pesticides on children is that all factors between the two groups she examined were the same: they shopped at the same grocery store, bought the same products, had the same culture, played the same games, spoke the same language, and had the same family income. The only difference was that one part of the Yaqui population didn't want to use technological methods of farming or pesticides. Farmers who live in the valley apply pesticides 45 times per crop cycle and grow one or two crops per year. The families in the valley also use household bug sprays every day. The group that broke away to live in the foothills chose to swat the indoor bugs and not to use chemicals in their gardens. Their only major exposure to pesticides in the foothills came from government spraying of DDT to control malaria.

Previous research in the area showed that children in the Yaqui Valley are born with measurable amounts of pesticides in their blood and are exposed through breast milk as well. Guillette began a new study to screen preschoolers (thirty-three children from the valley and seventeen from the foothills) to see if these exposures were creating *behavioral* effects as well. First Guillette and her team made simple block formations that the four- and five-year-olds would copy. She tried to get them to stand on one foot, but culturally that was a no-no, so she had them jump up and down for as long as they could, catch balls, drop raisins into bottle caps, do memory drills, and draw pictures based on her suggestions.

In 1998 Guillette and her team reported that the valley preschoolers demonstrated cognitive, memory, and motor skill problems that were not seen in the foothill children. For example, the valley children had poor half-hour recall, had less stamina, and had poorer gross hand/eye coordination. The most obvious difference was visible in the children's drawings. The valley children could only do stick figures, while the foothills children had rounded figures with facial features.

When the children Guillette studied turned six and seven years old and were in school, she had follow-up conversations with their teachers. Teachers in the valley said that the children didn't remember what they were taught from one week to the next. Guillette didn't hear these complaints from the teachers in the foothills school. *She noted that the exposed children remained below their peers in mental and physical abilities.* New drawings established the most significant differences. The valley children were

---

SEEING IS BELIEVING

Those who observe children most closely know that something is wrong with their behavior and thought processes. Mothers in Mexico, Nairobi, and Venezuela and physicians in Northern India all report to anthropologists that something is going on in children who are exposed to environmental pollutants. Dr. Elizabeth Guillette said, "I'm not the only one who's scared about what's happening to our children as a result of contamination by these toxic chemicals or compounds. Contamination is now global. No one is safe. What is happening with wildlife *is* what's happening with people."

She says cows eat grass and all grass is contaminated with toxins such as dioxin. Mothers need to know that when they cut off the fat from meat, before they cook it, they are not just decreasing the intake of cholesterol, but they are also decreasing the intake of contamination and, thus, reducing exposure to their children.

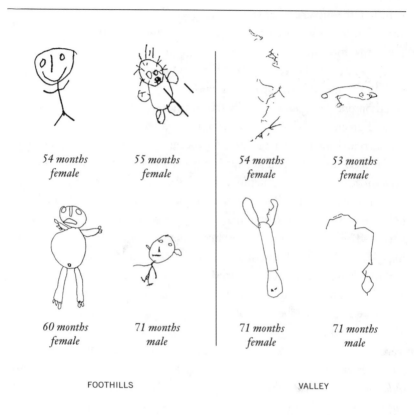

54 months *female*	*55 months* *female*	*54 months* *female*	*53 months* *female*
60 months *female*	*71 months* *male*	*71 months* *female*	*71 months* *male*
FOOTHILLS		VALLEY	

FIGURE 6.2 *Yakima Indian Children's Drawings of a Person*

drawing the way the foothills children had at ages four and five, whereas the foothills children were able to draw gender differences and add details such as buttons and sleeves to the women's dresses. Guillette calls what has happened to the valley children "integrative disruption." The children cannot take what they are seeing into themselves, assimilate it, and bring it back out again.

Guillette feels this is also relevant in America. She has interviewed farmers in U.S. agricultural communities where children play in the dirt, and where parents come home from the fields in their work clothes and hug the kids. There is ambient exposure as well as in food and dust. But it's not just children who live in rural agriculture areas who are exposed to pesticides. Half the pesticide use in the United States is in urban areas. For example, in New York (where pesticide sales have to be recorded), the borough of Manhattan has the largest pesticide sales in the whole state. *All* our children are getting exposed.

PESTICIDES IN INFANTS' AND CHILDREN'S FOOD

Pesticides are invasive in children's lives through the food they eat as well as through air, dust, and dirt. Nine out of every ten babies eat at least some commercial baby food. According to Gerber®, the average American baby eats 600 jars of baby food and fruit juices in his or her first year of life.

In 1995, the Environmental Working Group (EWG) put out a booklet called *Pesticides in Baby Food*. They had tested eight foods (applesauce, garden vegetables or pea and carrot blend, green beans, peaches, pears, plums, squash, and sweet potatoes) made by the three major babyfood producers—Gerber®, Heinz®, and Beech-Nut®—which account for 96 percent of all baby food sales. All samples were purchased at retail from grocery stores in Philadelphia, Denver, and San Francisco and tested for pesticides using the FDA's approved standard analytical methods. Sixteen pesticides were detected in the eight baby foods tested, including three probable human carcinogens, five possible human carcinogens, eight neurotoxins, five pesticides that disrupt the normal functioning of the hormone system, and five pesticides that are categorized as "oral toxicity category one" (the most toxic).

We need to factor the amount of pesticides children consume from food along with the amount they absorb from the environment. Children are exposed to various amounts and mixes of pesticides from lawns, parks, playgrounds, or carpets. And, as we have seen, children respond to these compounds in different ways and with greater magnitude than adults because so much of their development is still occurring in the central nervous system, including the brain, as well as in their reproductive and immune systems.

BEHAVIOR AND INTELLIGENCE

It used to be that the health risks that were looked at in relation to endocrine disruptors such as dioxins and PCBs were focused on cancer. Now the focus has expanded to include more subtle problems, such as the effects of toxicity on behavior and intelligence, which have become some of the biggest areas of concern about children's development. Dr. Philip

---

MARKETING PROBLEM?

In October 1997, Gerber (the industry leader) announced it was starting a line of organic baby food called Tender Harvest in competition with Heinz USA's Earth's Best. Gerber "faces an interesting marketing challenge: how to sell an upscale organic product without implying that its regular brand is riddled with farm chemicals and therefore less healthful." The announcement was taken to mean that organic foods have a growing appeal to mainstream shoppers, who have pushed annual sales of organic foods above the $4 billion mark. Other manufacturers have been waiting for organic shoppers to reach "critical mass," when organic products will become profitable.

Landrigan, a professor of pediatrics at Mount Sinai School of Medicine in New York and director of the new Center for Children's Health and the Environment at Mount Sinai, says, "About 3 percent of all Americans suffer from some type of neurodevelopmental disorder. Yet three-quarters of neurodevelopmental disorders have no known cause." He's talking about attention deficit/hyperactivity disorder (ADHD), aggression, delinquency, and certain learning disabilities.

New fields of study, called behavioral toxicology and teratology (the study of behavioral defects due to exposures during pregnancy), investigate how exposure to neurotoxicants such as heavy metals, solvents, and pesticides affect learning, memory, and behavior in humans and animals. If the neurons and neurotransmitters in the brain are seen as the hardware of the brain, then the software consists of our learning and memories, which have traditionally been the domain of psychiatrists and psychologists. A number of these new researchers are psychologists who are looking at the ways in which endocrine disruptors affect how our children think and act!

Research indicates a link between endocrine disruptors and intellectual function in children. Doctors Joseph and Sandra Jacobson, husband-and-wife psychologists at Wayne State University in Detroit, measured the PCBS in umbilical-cord blood of 212 children of mothers who had consumed moderate amounts of fish from the Great Lakes (a known source of dietary exposure to PCBS) while pregnant. Moderate consumption was considered to be an average of two to three fish meals a month for at least six years before the children were born. It turned out that the infants exposed to the highest levels of PCBs in the womb weighed less, were born earlier, and had smaller heads.

Most disturbing was the fact that the children in the Jacobson study who were exposed in utero to the highest levels of PCBs had lower IQ scores at the age of four; by age eleven, they had IQ scores that were 6.2 points lower than those of less-exposed children. The children at the high end of exposure were three times as likely to have IQ scores in the low average range and twice as likely to be at least one to two years behind in reading comprehension. They lagged behind on cognitive tests that measure short-term memory and planning ability and had difficulty in focusing attention, and their reading word comprehension averaged six months behind that of less-exposed eleven-year-old children. Jacobson said, "I thought that once the exposed children reached a structured school environment, whatever minor (PCB-induced) handicaps they had might be overcome. So I was quite surprised to find that, if anything, the effects were stronger and clearer at age eleven than they had been at age four."

Interestingly, the correlation was between their intelligence and their umbilical-cord levels of PCBs, not the levels of PCBs found in their blood at age eleven. This means that the exposure to PCBs they received from their mother's body was a significant factor in their decreased IQ, and this correlation was only detectable at birth blood levels, not at later ages.

The Jacobson team emphasizes that the levels of PCBs in the mothers they studied were similar to or slightly above the background levels of PCBs to which the general population in the United States is exposed. Background levels are the amount of chemicals we are all exposed to in our everyday lives. These middle-class mothers didn't eat PCB-laden fish every day and they did not live near toxic waste dumps. This is significant. This means that these effects are not limited just to women consuming Lake Michigan fish. Women who eat no fish may accumulate PCB compounds from dairy products, such as cheese and butter, and fatty meats, particularly beef and pork. In our interview Jacobson said, "You never know if the food you're eating is contaminated."

In another study on background PCB exposure, Rogan, Gladen, and colleagues followed 700 children in North Carolina from birth. In the first two years, the infants at the high end of exposure exhibited delayed *psychomotor* development—a general term used to refer to all voluntary movement, including fine motor functions such as writing or sewing and gross

ENDOCRINE DISRUPTION?

The Jacobson reports are being used as an indication of endocrine disruption affecting intelligence since PCB ingestion can affect hormonal signaling. However, when I spoke to Dr. Joseph Jacobson, who is a psychologist, he said he didn't know if the effects they were seeing had anything to do with endocrine disruption. "When the fetal brain is exposed to toxic agents, there are many aspects of that brain's development that can be affected by those agents. Hormones are one, but there are neurotransmitters, disruption of timing of neuronal migration, many factors that could explain why the PCBs that these babies get exposed to prenatally seem to disrupt brain development.

"We need to keep perspective here. I emphasize that the children are not mentally retarded, and even among those with the heaviest exposure, only some of the children were harmed. These are subtle deficits, things you would prefer not to have happen to your child, but they're not catastrophes. The levels in the environment are not at the level you might call poisoning. From my perspective, this is a societal-wide problem rather than something that individual parents should panic about."

---

motor functions such as walking or throwing a ball—but Rogan did not find an association between PCB exposure and smaller body weight and size or with mental/cognitive development. There is, however, the possibility that the North Carolina mothers had less exposure to PCBs than the mothers in the Jacobson study.

Even though Rogan and colleagues assessed school performance—through grades on school report cards—and found no effects pointing to a relationship between PCBs and intelligence, it has been pointed out that the Jacobsons tested the children directly themselves and did find PCB exposure associated with lower performance levels. Some scientists thought the design of the Jacobson study was flawed and doubted their results. In 1992 the EPA convened a group of experts to review the Jacobson study and decided that the relationship between in utero exposure to PCBs and memory problems *is* significant and not due to problems with how the study was designed.

What does a five-point shift downward in IQ really mean? Dr. Bernard Weiss, a neurotoxicologist and professor of environmental medicine and pediatrics at the University of Rochester Medical Center, said a five-point shift down the IQ scale in the U.S. population "could move nearly 2 million children who had been above an IQ of 130 to below 130, and push an equal number of children into the below-70 category." Scoring under 70 IQ means many school districts will have to have more mandated remedial education. Weiss said the social and financial consequences "could be stupendous. . . ." *The Bell Curve* (a book by Richard Herrnstein and Charles Murray) describes how IQ determines position in society. Data indicate that earnings, for example, are related to IQ. The authors of *The Bell Curve* conclude that lowering IQ by even three points would increase welfare dependency by 20 percent, increase the number of males in jail by 20 percent, and increase the number of children born out of wedlock by 15 to 20 percent.

IQ is a functional deficit—meaning it's not something you can see, as you might changes in physical shape or a clinical disease—and is certainly not as easily measured. Thus, many conventional studies on endocrine disruption do not take shifts in IQ into account.

A study conducted in the San Francisco Bay Area enrolled about 20,000 pregnant women during the 1960s and followed many of their children into adolescence. Dr. Irva Hertz-Picciotto, from the University of North Carolina, is presently analyzing data for several hundred children who were given cognitive examinations at five years of age as part of the study. She and her colleagues found that women pregnant in 1967 had children with substantially higher levels of PCBs than those pregnant in 1964, which may reflect the increasingly widespread use of these compounds during that time period. The older women were at the time of pregnancy, the higher the levels of the most highly chlorinated PCBs in their blood. Also, African-American women had 50 to 60 percent higher levels of DDT in their bodies compared to white women.

Even if your child's IQ is not affected, how about his or her ability to handle stress? Psychologist Helen Daly, while at the Department of Psychology at the State University of New York at Oswego (she passed away after a long battle with breast cancer), exposed pregnant rats to hormone disruptors by feeding them fish contaminated with PCBs from Lake Ontario. None of the offspring were fed fish directly at any point in their lives, yet Daly found behavioral changes in both the children and grandchildren of the rats fed contaminated fish. One of the main effects was their reaction to stress. The rat offspring were "hyperreactive" even to mildly negative situations.

AGGRESSIVE FEMALES

Dr. Frederick vom Saal is a key proponent of the idea that exposure to man-made chemicals, especially while a baby is in the womb, can affect what happens later in life. During his post-doctoral research in reproductive physiology, vom Saal noticed that one out of every six female mice was very aggressive toward other females. He then calculated that one out of every six females was positioned between two males in utero and thus was exposed to more male hormones. So he asked a question: would a random event—such as where the mouse was positioned in the uterus and who it was next to—create a variation in hormone levels that led to differences in behavior? The answer was a resounding *yes*. It turned out that not just behavior was affected by in utero positioning but also genital structure and at what point females would later go into puberty. Not only that, but if a female mouse developed between male fetuses, she produced litters with predominantly males in them. This has now been observed in mice and in gerbils and appears to be true in pigs.

In other words, vom Saal showed that development is determined by factors in the environment as well as by genes. He says, "If man-made chemicals get into a fetus's body during the time the cells are differentiating, and if they are chemicals that can interact with the natural hormone systems, we've got a real problem. We have extensive information from wildlife and laboratory studies that endocrine disruptors, at the levels at which animals are being exposed to them during development, permanently alter numerous organs, including the brain."

Because of this work with rats, Daly, Lonky, and others designed a similar study for humans; they used the same series of tests the Jacobsons used but also added tests for stress. The same hyperreaction to stressful events was found in human children. Dr. Lonky and others studied the children born to 243 mothers who had eaten varying amounts of fish from Lake Ontario. Even with low fish consumption, infants exposed to the highest levels of contaminants scored significantly more poorly on behavior tests than infants exposed to lower levels.

Studies are starting to show that chemical mixes have different effects on humans and animals than just the individual chemicals themselves. Researchers from the University of Wisconsin did a five-year study exposing mice to a mixture of a fertilizer (nitrate), an insecticide (aldicarb), and an herbicide (atrazine) at concentrations similar to those found in groundwater. They found evidence of altered thyroid hormones in young mice and increased aggression. The authors say children and fetuses are most at risk, and the study also showed that chemicals affect animals differently in different seasons of the year (more when animals have higher hormonal activity).

PCBs and Children's Brains

Since the prefrontal cortex (a part of the brain) does not mature until well after birth, it is shortsighted to say that just in utero exposure could cause damage in cognitive functioning. One researcher has shown that if mice are exposed to environmental agents such as DDT and PCBs during brain growth spurts it can lead to irreversible changes in adult brain function. Another scientist exposed baby monkeys from birth to twenty weeks of age to PCBs, at levels similar to those found in human mothers' milk, and found the monkeys were later impaired on cognitive tests.

THE STORY OF LEAD

Dr. Bernard Weiss believes brain development is the most important issue of endocrine disruption, and PCBs and dioxins, because they are everywhere, may exert more total damage than lead. Lead, which has been well studied, has been found to have very significant effects in children with only a one- to two-point downward shift in IQ. Dr. Weiss says that a 2.5 to 6.2 point downward shift in IQ (as shown in the Jacobson study) is huge. As a side note, preliminary study results show that bone lead levels are much higher among delinquents than non-delinquents.

"With lead," Weiss says, "we can trace a progression from the 1970s. At first, the Center for Disease Control thought that a level of 40 mcg percent of lead in the blood was the dividing line between problems caused by lead and none, or at least fewer problems. They went on to lower this level to 25 mcg percent of lead in the blood as the dividing line. Then they lowered it again to 10—a 'level of concern' by the EPA. Why did they lower the amount? Because of the shift in the IQ distribution that they found lead caused. The greater the level of lead, the lower the plotted IQ. This is a fact. So now we are turning our attention to endocrine disruptors rather than lead."

TABLE 6.1 HUMAN PCB STUDIES ON ENDOCRINE DISRUPTION

HUMAN STUDIES WITH PCB EXPOSURE IN MOTHERS	EFFECTS
In 1980–1981 the Jacobsons studied PCBS in umbilical-cord blood in 212 children whose mothers had moderate consumption of fish from Great Lakes—an average of two to three fish meals a month for at least six years before the children were born.	Infants • weighed less • were born earlier • had smaller heads Children • had lower IQs by age four • had still lower IQs by age eleven (not reflected in blood) • were three times as likely to have IQ scores in the low–average range • were two times as likely to be at least one to two years behind in reading comprehension • lagged behind on cognitive tests • had difficulty in focusing attention • had reading word comprehension that averaged six months behind that of less-exposed eleven-year-old children • were hyperereactive to stress
Daly and Lonky studied 243 mothers who ate an average of 40 pounds of Lake Ontario fish over their lifetime. First human study to document a wide range of effects on temperament from prenatal exposure to hormone disruptors.	Children with the highest exposure: • did poorly on behavioral tests • had same hyper response to stress as in the Daly animal studies • had shorter attention spans • had abnormal reflexes
In 1978–1982, Rogan and Gladen followed 700 children in North Carolina.	In the first two years the children had: • delayed psychomotor development but not smaller body weight or head size and no neurobehavioral deficits from six months to five years old

STUDIES	EFFECTS
1989, Dutch PCB/Dioxin Study of 395 children at forty-two months. Background levels of PCBS were equal to or slightly higher than those in the Jacobson and Jacobson study.	• Poor cognitive functioning in preschool children • Trouble with short- and long-term memory, verbal and numeric skills, and sequential problem solving
A review by Tilson of human studies and of animal studies on mice, rats, and monkeys.	All suggested that exposure to environmental toxicants can cause impairments in cognitive and psychomotor activity.

ACCIDENTAL EXPOSURES	EFFECTS
1968, PCB poisoning in Yusho, Japan, after 1,000 people ingested contaminated rice oil.	Follow-up studies on the children who had problems showed: • lack of physical coordination • apathy • IQS averaging about 70
1982–1983, Yu-Cheng, Taiwan—1,850 people were exposed to rice oil that was contaminated with PCBS. The offspring of exposed mothers exhibited very similar learning problems to those seen in the Jacobson study.	Babies had: • lower birth weight • developmental delays • lower IQS • behavioral effects • growth delays Children: • boys did not mature normally at puberty and had smaller-than-normal penises • higher incidence of behavioral problems that did not go away as the children aged • immunological problems • much higher incidence of infection and respiratory disease
A small follow-up study on mothers exposed to oil contaminated with dioxins used to keep road dust down in Times Beach, Missouri. U.S. government had to evacuate the town.	Abnormal EEGS of fourteen children born to exposed mothers. Altered immune system cells at the ages of nine to fourteen indicating long-term immune effects.

TABLE 6.2 THYROID, ADHD, AND ENDOCRINE DISRUPTION

THYROID STUDIES	EFFECTS
Dr. Hauser studied the children from a number of families that had a unique genetic disease of the thyroid receptor and compared them to children with normal thyroid function.	He found impairment of thyroid function caused by resistance to thyroid hormone resulted in 76 percent of the males and 50 percent of the females having ADHD and significantly lower IQs (though not mental retardation).
A German study on 671 children seven to ten years old who lived near a toxic waste incinerator	Children from four out of nine municipalities with higher exposure had statistically lower free T3 and T4 (thyroid hormones) compared to children with less exposure.
Sher and team	Strong suggestion that PCBS and dioxins interfere with thyroid metabolism, possibly altering the thyroid hormone milieu and thus altering the mitochondria's ability to generate ATP (energy).
Bonacci and coworkers	Showed estrogen signaling by PCBS may contribute to thyroid pathologies. Indicated that ". . . more than 200 different types of PCBS (congeners) show estrogenic effects, and estrogen receptors are present in human thyroid tissue."
ANIMAL STUDIES	
Porterfield	PCBS can act to promote, block, or partially block thyroid function depending on the type of PCBS. The development of the myelin sheath is regulated by thyroid. Because brain development occurs during very specific periods of time, not enough thyroid during these times can produce permanent damage.

Although they are banned, PCBs are still found in the environment and in the food chain, such as in the Great Lakes fish that are so often used as a source of PCBs in various studies. Even though there has been a massive clean-up of the Great Lakes, the levels of PCBs and other organochlorine chemicals have remained steady since 1985. A question remains about which of the chemicals are actually involved in hormone disruption since there are more than 2,800 different chemicals found in the Great Lakes.

PCBs are known hormone disruptors. Many of the issues about PCBs and other endocrine disruptors that researchers are now grappling with are the same as the ones that created controversy and spurred debate among researchers on lead, a heavy metal which is a potent endocrine disruptor. Joseph Jacobson told the *New York Times* that brain damage caused by low-level exposures to PCBs was comparable to the damage found in children exposed to low levels of lead. Experimental studies have shown that lead affects estrogenic signaling through various mechanisms. Like lead, PCBs have contaminated every human population. And the damage from PCBs is added to whatever brain damage has already been done by lead, mercury, pesticides, and other chlorinated hydrocarbons.

It certainly seems like PCBs and related dioxins are not good for the developing brain. In 1968 an outbreak of human PCB poisoning occurred in Yusho, Japan, after 1,000 people ingested contaminated rice oil. Follow-up studies on the children who were born to the mothers at the highest levels of exposure showed lack of physical coordination, apathy, and IQs averaging around 70.

Eleven years later, a mechanical accident in Yu-Cheng, Taiwan, also leaked PCBs into rice oil. Some 2,000 people were poisoned after eating the rice oil and suffered from stomach pain and horrifying skin eruptions. The offspring of the PCB-exposed Yu-Cheng mothers exhibited very similar learning problems to those seen in the Jacobson study. They were also developmentally delayed and had an IQ deficit. The boys did not mature normally at puberty and had smaller-than-normal penises. There was a higher incidence of behavioral problems that did not go away as the children aged. There were also immunological problems and a much higher incidence of infection and respiratory disease.

It is possible that the effects experienced by both the Yusho and Yu-Cheng populations may have been the result not only of the accidental PCB exposure, but also because dioxin-like compounds were degraded in the contaminated rice oil. So they may have received a double dose of endocrine disruptors plus their metabolites. Most people are not exposed to such large amounts of PCBS at once.

Not all ill effects come from accidental exposures. Even exposure to background levels of PCBS has produced developmental effects in animals, and the data we have on humans are consistent with the animal data.

A MISDIAGNOSIS ON PHTHALATES?

On June 22, 1999, a report was released by former U.S. Surgeon General C. Everett Koop (heading a review panel for the American Council on Science and Health—ACSH) saying, "Consumers can be confident that vinyl toys and medical devices are safe. There is no scientific evidence that they are harmful to children or adults."

The Council based part of their report on studies that suggested children clear certain pharmaceuticals out of their bodies faster than do adults. The Council said the same happens with xenobiotics and thus children had little danger from exposure. What a leap! We know from studies on women that they process some drugs faster and some slower than do men. How does this relate to how women handle xenobiotics? It seems—not at all. Italian studies over a twenty-year period demonstrate that women who were accidentally exposed to dioxin at Seveso held on to more dioxin and for longer periods of time compared to men. Women have smaller detox organs and thus can't clear xenobiotics as easily. Well, children have even smaller detox organs.

The National Environmental Trust (NET) has cautioned readers of the Council report (which was not peer-reviewed) not to rely on the makers of chemicals for unbiased information. ACSH is an organization that accepts 76 percent of its funding from corporations, including the largest makers of phthalates.

Health Care Without Harm, a nonprofit coalition of consumer, health, and environmental groups, had released its own report the previous week, which reviewed 100 studies on the phthalate DEHP (a known hormone-disrupting compound). They concluded the phthalate could harm multiple organs and interfere with sperm production.

Their findings were confirmed in December 1999, by the National Toxicology Program (a division of the NIEHS), which reviewed the data and found that oral exposure in animals to DEHP can cause miscarriage, birth defects, reduced fertility, abnormal sperm counts, and testicular damage. Most major toy makers—Disney, Mattel, Gerber, Warner Brothers, and Hasbro—are phasing phthalates out of toys that were intended for sucking or chewing. The European Union (EU) has banned the use of phthalates in PVC children's toys in fifteen countries.

Dutch children exposed to pre- and postnatal background levels of PCBS and dioxins were found to have significant delays in psychomotor development. In another Dutch study the background levels were equal to or slightly higher than those in the Jacobson and Jacobson study. They looked at 395 children under the age of two and found the children had trouble with short- and long-term memory, verbal and numeric skills, and sequential problem solving.

The Rogan study found adverse changes only up to twenty-four months of age; the effects went away as the children aged. This is different from the Jacobsons' work that found that developmental problems were still present at eleven years of age. The Netherlands study also found IQ deficits at age three-and-a-half. It is very important to point out that these early developmental problems, even in studies where they seem to go away, are occurring during important stages of brain development and we do not know if they herald difficulties that will occur much later in life.

According to Dr. Shanna Swan (chief of reproductive epidemiology at the California Department of Health Services), "We have a lot to learn about subtle effects of environmental contaminants and about serious childhood developmental disorders."

One idea of how PCB exposure may affect the way children's brains grow and develop is that when PCBS are metabolized in the body, some metabolites can inhibit a vital step in the metabolism of thyroid hormone. And PCBS aren't the only adversaries around. PAHS (polycyclic aromatic hydrocarbons) are toxic chemicals commonly produced from the incomplete combustion of petroleum products, wood, or tobacco. Studies indicate that persistent PAHS can also disrupt the thyroid system, which may have a profound impact on normal brain development in experimental animals, wildlife species, and human infants. If there is an underlying endocrine-system abnormality, such as a low-functioning thyroid, this may increase or decrease the effects of varied xenobiotics on the body.

What does this mean in simple English? Exposure to hormone disruptors in the womb and during infancy may keep some children from developing to their utmost potential.

ATTENTION DEFICIT HYPERACTIVITY DISORDER (ADHD) AND THYROID DISRUPTION

Some chemicals can bind to thyroid hormone receptors and disrupt thyroid signaling, especially in the developing brain in the fetus and young child. Hormone disruptors have been shown to alter both thyroid hormone secretion and thyroid functioning. Moderate to severe disruption of thyroid functioning in the developing fetus and child may have long-reaching effects. Some of these are:

- memory problems, learning disabilities, attention deficit hyperactivity disorder (ADHD)

- hearing loss

- brain myelination problems (the protective coating)

- problems of fine motor coordination, balance, growth, and motor dysfunction of varying severity (including cerebral palsy)

- seizures

- hydrocephalus, mental retardation, and other permanent neurological problems

Thyroid disruption may be contributing to some of the behavioral problems that appear to be increasing in children. According to Dr. Susan Schantz, a professor of environmental toxicology and psychology at the University of Illinois, it is likely that exposure to environmental contaminants such as PCBS and lead (and possibly bisphenol A) play a role in disorders such as learning disabilities, attention deficit hyperactivity disorder (ADHD), cerebral palsy, autism, and much of mental retardation that remains unexplained. Other scientists, such as Dr. Theo Colborn and her associates and Dr. Susan Porterfield, agree that thyroid dysfunction may developmentally play a role in ADHD.

Dr. Hauser, professor of psychiatry and internal medicine at the University of Maryland, speculates that in utero exposure to certain synthetic chemicals may cause central nervous abnormalities similar to those of RTH, a thyroid disease caused by mutations in the thyroid receptor gene, because the underlying mechanism may disrupt thyroid hormone action.

According to the surgeon general, close to 21 percent of children age nine and older have a mental disorder. These disorders include depression, attention deficit hyperactivity disorder, and bipolar disorder. Americans are also giving their children a huge amount of psychiatric drugs. The United States consumes 80 percent of the world's Ritalin (used to treat hyperactivity).

Another factor that could be affecting thyroid function itself is that exposure to background levels of dioxins and PCBS through breast milk may cause some effects on the status of the thyroid hormone in infants.

Yet Another Generation?

One of the biggest questions remaining about hormone disruptors in general is whether or not the sons and daughters who were exposed in utero will themselves pass along the damage to their offspring. In one study, DES-exposed female mice were mated to nonexposed males. Their female offspring (called DES-lineage mice) had significantly increased cases of uterine and ovarian cancer and adenomyosis (endometriosis inside the uterus). Spontaneous cancers of the uterus and ovaries are rarely found in mice.

Retha Newbold, who, along with Dr. John McLachlan, has been researching DES for longer than anyone else in the country, did research in which the granddaughters of DES-exposed mother mice had a striking increase in tumor formation, although they did not have reduced fertility. *These results suggest that the cascade of events that leads to tumors may begin well before birth.* There was also a transgenerational study that showed increased cancer susceptibility via males exposed to DES.

Some scientists have found that DES can have a multigenerational effect. The Society for the Advancement of Women's Health Research stated that "If DES results in inheritable changes to DNA, then a third generation of offspring also may be at risk. Further research is needed at the molecular level to clarify the range of DES effects and to apply this knowledge to the study of other environmental estrogens."

How we live and what we take into our bodies may leave its mark for generations to come.

Helpful Hints for Protecting Children

There are actions you can take to help minimize your child's exposure to hormone disruptors. Here are some ways to protect your children.

- Buy unfinished wood or natural fiber toys. Whenever possible, buy PVC-free plastic toys. There are a few toy manufacturers that don't use PVC plastic (vinyl) at all, so the toys they manufacture are free of phthalates: Early Start (distributed by International Playthings), Guidecraft, Lamaze Infant Development, and The Natural Baby Catalog.
- Don't let children chew on soft plastic toys. Since phthalates are added to soften PVC plastic toys, the stiffer and harder the PVC plastic toy feels, the fewer phthalates it is likely to contain. Be

especially cautious with soft plastic toys that are ripped or torn—phthalates can easily leach from them. Plastic toys also retain pesticides which are sprayed in the house for up to two weeks.

- Check with your dentist to see whether or not plastic-coating treatment for your children's teeth contains bisphenol A. Composite fillings contain bisphenol A. No research has been done comparing composite fillings to mercury amalgams, so we don't know which is worse. It would be nice to have a nontoxic alternative.

- Wash your hands and your children's hands frequently. Teach children to wash their hands often, not to lick their fingers or bite their nails. Since chemicals inevitably deposit on surfaces, frequent cleaning is preventative. Wash children's toys often.

- Avoid lindane and synthetic pyrethroid-based head lice and scabies shampoos. One study showed that lindane promoted tumor growth the same way that estrogen did. For head lice, use a fine-toothed comb with petroleum or plant-based jelly, followed by an antibacterial, nontoxic herbal shampoo. On the other hand, lice carry some of the worst diseases that have decimated humankind. Some scientists think it wiser to kill the lice and take the low risk from the pesticide in order to avoid any chance of some awful disease. Also, there is a new lindane-free shampoo put out by Lifekind called "Lice Out."

- Know and be able to detect lead poisoning symptoms:
    1. Common symptoms of severe lead poisoning include: fatigue, memory loss, balance problems, weakness in the fingers, chronic bowel troubles and visual difficulties; less visible symptoms may include: tantrums, short attention span, learning disabilities, or irritability.
    2. A simple blood test can detect high lead levels.
    3. If you suspect lead poisoning, take action immediately. Call the National Lead Information Center at 1-(800) LEADFYI for general information and for testing and treatment programs (which may include diet changes, medication, or hospitalization) in your area.

Men's Reproductive Problems

Hell has no fury like a congressman who discovers he's not the man he thought he was.

—From a report linking chemical pollutants to shrinking penis size and falling sperm counts, *Newsweek*, March 21, 1994

Hormone disruptors started to get a lot of attention when studies began to indicate that men's sexual virility—even their basic masculinity—could be at risk.

Basically, the brain is the control center for the process of sexual development, directed by the sex steroid hormones. Evidence is piling up from animal studies and wildlife observation—in gulls, terns, fish, whales, porpoises, alligators, and turtles—that exposure to certain man-made chemicals can disturb steroid hormone production and activity. So what happens when endocrine disruptors alter the way in which hormones in the brain direct normal sexual development? In men's lives, we have seen some of the results of hormone disruption in DES sons, whose difficulties echo the reproductive problems which are on the increase in men today.

DES sons are at increased risk for:

- testicular cancer

- underdeveloped or undescended testicles

- small penis size

- hypospadias (abnormalities of penis)
- problems with fertility due to abnormal semen and lower sperm counts
- possibly prostatic disease. Since they are just entering middle age, we do not know if they will be at increased risk for diseases such as prostate cancer.
- noncancerous cysts on the back of the testicles (on the epididymis)
- major depressive disorder (MDD). One study suggested DES sons are almost twice as likely as non-DES-exposed men to have at least one episode and significantly more recurrent episodes.

Not all health problems associated with hormone disruption are related to the reproductive system. Studies that followed 31,000 people for twenty years after the Seveso dioxin accident in Italy in 1976 found men with the highest exposure had elevated lung and respiratory cancers, Hodgkin's disease, leukemia, and multiple myeloma. Males had a higher incidence of heart disease; an increase in heart disease has been seen in several dioxin-exposed populations. Both men and women had a 70 to 80 percent increase in lymphatic cancer. Ironically, women had a decreased incidence of breast cancer. However, the scientific eye has been looking mostly at problems of the reproductive system in the male, which is the focus of this chapter.

Gender-Bending

Exposure to endocrine disruptors can alter hormonal balance and create changes in the characteristics that define males and females. There are specific terms for what can happen.

- *Feminization*—an increase in female characteristics
- *Defeminization*—a decrease in female characteristics
- *Masculinization*—an increase in male characteristics
- *Demasculinization*—a decrease in male characteristics

During the course of normal male development, testosterone from the male testes is converted within certain regions of the brain to estrogen. Estrogen then interacts with receptors on nerves to produce the cellular events that lead to masculine development. Thus, men can't become men without estrogen. But too much estrogen (or not enough androgens) will have the opposite effect and cause demasculinization.

Possibly the most studied gender-bending case is that of the alligators in Lake Apopka, one of Florida's largest freshwater lakes. In some Florida lakes, 90 percent of eggs laid by female alligators hatch. At Lake Apopka, hatching barely reached 18 percent and half the baby gators died within the first 10 days. Dr. Lou Guillette showed that 75 percent of the alligator eggs in the lake were dead or infertile and the males were all demasculinized. In the mildest form of demasculinization, the alligators had normal penises and testes but produced some female hormones. In more severe cases, the alligators had no phallus at all, even though the gonads were testes-type. About 20 percent of turtles in the lake also showed intersex conditions—a combination of male and female characteristics.

About a decade earlier, the Tower Chemical Company on the shore of the lake had had a chemical spill. At the time, 90 percent of the alligator population disappeared, but even now that water samples show the lake is clean, the alligators are still suffering from reproductive problems. As we know, estrogenic chemicals are stored in fat, not water. Therefore, the chemical residue is probably in the fat of the animals in the lake, while the water itself is clean.

Researchers found the female alligators in the lake had about twice the amount of estrogen typical for a female, but the males had almost no testosterone. At first, scientists thought the small penises and reproductive problems of these alligators were caused by excess estrogen from the estrogenic chemicals in the lake. That turned out not to be the case. We now know that these reproductive problems were actually due to the fact that the chemicals were highly antiandrogenic. In other words, the chemicals were seriously blocking the male hormones so that the female hormones predominated. Numerous environmental estrogens have been found to possess such antiandrogenic activity.

Ecohormones can act either as agonists (meaning they promote hormonal signaling) or antagonists (they block the signals). Interestingly enough, there are no natural estrogen antagonists inside the body, only those that come into us from the environment. So far there are few recognized androgen agonists—chemicals that act to promote androgen (masculine) signaling, but there are chemicals that act as antiandrogens. And when the male hormones are blocked, there is more potential for feminizing effects.

Lately, Guillette has been looking at alligators in other lakes in Florida besides Apopka, such as Lake Orange, Lake Woodruff, Lake Griffin, and a reference lake with less contamination. In the more polluted lakes, male alligators are feminized, with their penis length being 20 percent smaller than those of alligators living in less polluted lakes. (And if you think it's easy to measure alligator penises, think again.) The female alligators are masculinized, having less estrogen and more testosterone.

Alligator gender normally is dependent on the temperature at which the eggs are hatched. At 33°C, the alligators come out of the eggs as males; at 30°C, the hatchlings are all female. When Guillette's team put eggs at 30 degrees and added extra estrogen, all the gators turned out male instead of female. Then the researchers added contaminants (DDE, etc. at 100 parts per trillion), hatched the eggs at 30 degrees, and also got sex reversals— the eggs all turned out male. Atrazine—a pesticide used on corn—also created the same situation. It's plain to see that chemicals definitely can cause sex reversal. Guillette said, "I'm always cautious about saying anything about humans. But to say that all of our animal evidence means nothing for implications for humans is the height of unreasonableness and arrogance. It's clear that we have data suggesting that we have a broad public health issue that is not just isolated to wildlife."

Gender bending isn't happening only in the United States. In England, male fish that lived near sewage outfall in British rivers were becoming hermaphrodites. Female fish make an egg-yolk protein called vitellogenin. In England, male fish exposed to estrogenic compounds in England's

---

NEXT TIME YOU TAKE A VACATION . . .

Lake Mead is one of the most popular vacation spots in the United States and a main source of drinking water for Southern California and Las Vegas, Nevada. Treated and untreated waste, including chemical waste and pesticides, gets dumped in certain regions of the lake, which shows clear evidence of being contaminated with hormone disruptors. Male carp there are making an egg protein that usually only females produce for their eggs. Lake Mead attracts 7 to 8 million vacationers a year, many of whom eat the fish they catch. Carp are not game fish, but bass and catfish, two of the favorite sport fish in this lake, might also be contaminated.

sewage effluent started making this female protein. The fish were changing sex. Instead of producing sperm, these trout thought they had ovaries
and were producing a yolk protein although they didn't have eggs. This
information was kept classified for two years because the government was
afraid of scaring people. Effluent accounts for half the water flow in rivers
in England during the summer, and 30 percent of drinking water is taken
from rivers. The British looked at possible causes for the estrogenic effects
in the effluent, including studying whether or not ethinyl estradiol (a
potent synthetic estrogen in birth control pills) was getting into the water
from women's urine. The drug itself was not detectable, so they continued their search for the source of the estrogen.

Back in the United States, Dr. Ana Soto and Dr. Carlos Sonnenschein,
at the Department of Cellular Biology at Tufts, were sleuthing out the
reason breast cancer cells in their lab were growing out of control in plastic flasks, even though the researchers hadn't added anything to the flasks.
They eventually discovered that this rampant growth of breast cancer cells
was the result of contamination by an estrogenic compound—nonylphenol (a hormone-disrupting chemical)—which was leaching from the plastic flasks. Nonylphenol is a chemical compound that has been in use for
more than forty years; it is present in everything from plastics and detergents to spermicidal foams.

At least 20,000 tons of nonylphenol are produced each year in England
alone. When the British tested nonylphenol on fish, it proved to be highly
estrogenic. The mystery was thought to be solved—nonylphenol (and its
cousin octylphenol) were present in the river water and the drinking water
in England and were the estrogenic sources affecting the fish. Later, data
showed that the normal estrogens in urine found in sewage are actually
causing the feminization of the fish. However, when the pesticide DDT gets
into fish eggs, it really can gender bend. Scientists injected DDT into male
fish, and *tada!* they turned the males into mothers who were able to lay
eggs that actually produced baby fish. The study also confirmed that fish
contaminated with DDT can pass toxins on to the next generation through
eggs, profoundly altering development.

Masculine and feminine behavior are also at risk. In some exposed wildlife, creatures whose genes should instruct them to be male have been
looking and acting like females, and females have been behaving like males.
In the early 1970s, a study at the Channel Islands in southern California

---

DR. ANA SOTO'S "ACCIDENT"

Dr. Ana Soto and fellow physician Carlos Sonnenschein, researchers in cellular biology at Tufts Medical School in Boston, had been working for several decades on why cells multiply—a vital question in solving the mystery of cancer. They were experimenting with human breast cancer cells that multiply in the presence of estrogen. Soto and Sonnenschein ran a clean lab. However, in 1987, they came into the lab one day and found that the breast cancer cells had suddenly begun multiplying like crazy. They assumed it had to be some sort of estrogen contamination because the only cells that were multiplying out of control were the estrogen-sensitive breast cancer cells.

It took them two years to track down the culprit—the "inert" plastic test tubes they had been using in their lab experiments. Corning, the manufacturer, had recently changed the plastic resin in order to make the tubes less brittle, so researchers at Tufts (and at other institutions) had been using different tubes without knowing it. Corning would not, however, disclose the chemical composition of the tubes since it was a trade secret. Soto and Sonnenschein set about isolating the compound in the plastic that had caused the estrogen-like effect, which turned out to be p-nonylphenol, a member of the alkylphenol family. Since the food-processing and packaging industries use PVCS that contain alkylphenols, and nonylphenol has been known to contaminate water that had passed through PVC pipes, they wondered: how much of this compound is leaching into our food and water?

Dr. Soto is especially concerned about the plastics used in containers which are heated in microwave ovens. Though she says we do not yet have definitive proof that these containers are made with estrogenic substances, she encourages people to take precautionary measures. "I no longer use any plastics in microwaves myself," she said in our phone conversation. "Glass will do just as well."

---

showed that female gulls were nesting with other females. This phenomenon, dubbed the "gay gulls," was again discovered in a Santa Barbara gull colony. Over the next two decades, female pairs were found nesting in populations of herring gulls in the Great Lakes and in Puget Sound, and in terns off the coast of Massachusetts. DDT was suspected, as the eggshells were also thinning.

Scientists at the University of Wisconsin–Madison have shown that toxic doses of TCDD (the most potent form of dioxin) can reduce concentrations of androgens in the blood of adult animals, which made them wonder about possible in utero effects. They gave a single oral dose of TCDD to female rats on day fifteen of their pregnancy (when the male fetuses are ready to produce androgens—the critical day for male sexual development). When they were born, the pups had smaller accessory sex organs, appeared to mature more slowly sexually, and exhibited behaviors that were distinctly less masculine and more feminine than normal. Their sperm counts were 50 percent lower than those of the control group. The team could not find a level of TCDD exposure at which there were *no* effects.

This leads to an interesting question: could exposure to endocrine disruptors in utero lead to homosexuality? Many sex-related characteristics are determined by hormones during the early stages of development, and they can be influenced by very small changes in hormonal balance. A controlled DES study run by a university showed a statistically significant (beyond chance) correlation between being a DES daughter and lesbianism. Evidence suggests that once sex-related characteristics are imprinted, they may be irreversible.

THERE ARE NEVER ENOUGH GOOD MEN

There is another worrisome aspect to gender bending that has been demonstrated in humans—a changing sex ratio at birth. After an accidental exposure to dioxins—the 1976 Seveso accident in Italy—there was a higher percentage of female children born in ratio to boys than was the norm. In

SINGING THE WRONG SONG

Birds may not be able to change their feathers, but they are changing the tune they sing. Dr. Michael Fry, a wildlife toxicologist at the University of California, Davis, and director of the Center for Avian Biology, has been investigating the effect of endocrine disruptors on birds for more than thirty years. His latest research examines what happens when parent birds bring food that has been sprayed with pesticides and other chemical residues to the chicks in the nest. He has found that female birds become masculinized and sing male mating calls; courtship and mating behaviors alter; the birds fail to breed successfully; and chicks that are hatched are only partially developed.

1977 researchers studied thirteen families in which both parents had been exposed during the accident. Nine of the couples with highest exposure had no male offspring at all. Then, eight years after the accident, 65 percent of newborns were female and the parents with the highest levels of dioxin in their blood had only female children during this time. After a period of time, the altered ratio started to normalize, which implies the problem had been related to the exposure.

Even without a chemical accident, a study of all live births in Canada from 1930 to 1990 showed that male births have gone down since 1970; to a lesser degree, the same decline has been seen in the United States, although there are still more males born than females. The authors of the Canadian study say: "The decrease in the sex ratio observed in our study, subtle as it was, portends a greater biological significance as a highly sensitive and unambiguous measure of the reproductive health of large populations."

In Denmark, the sex ratio of newborns from 1951 to 1995 was studied and it was found that the number of newborn males had declined significantly since the 1960s, at the same time that testicular cancer rates rose and sperm counts declined.

Dr. Devra Davis and her colleagues analyzed data on birth ratios and concluded the reduction in the proportion of males born may indicate that "some as yet unrecognized, environmental health hazards are affecting the sex ratio of births as well as other unexplained defects in male reproduction." (Heaven knows, many of us think there aren't enough men as it is.) It should be mentioned that one factor in the increased female to male sex ratio might be the use of fertility drugs, which are heavily estrogenic.

REPRODUCTIVE ABNORMALITIES IN THE MALE

Exposure to hormone disruptors, either in utero or during childhood, has definitely been shown to lead to disorders of the reproductive tract. Some of these abnormalities, like malformations of the penis, are apparent at birth. Others, such as lowered sperm count, infertility, and cancer of the testes don't manifest until after puberty. Deborah Cadbury wrote and directed a BBC documentary, *The Assault on the Male*, which showed how various reproductive problems in the male were finally grouped together and related to endocrine disruptors. She expanded the documentary into a book, *The Feminization of Nature* (Penguin U.K., 1998)—a fascinating peek at the human drama that leads to advances in scientific understanding.

According to Cadbury, Dr. Niels Skakkebaek was one of the first major players in this particular drama. He heads the Department of Growth and Reproduction at Copenhagen University Hospital in Denmark, whose team sees thousands of young patients each year, specializing in male infertility and hormone disorders affecting reproduction (including puberty problems and intersex conditions). Dr. Skakkebaek became concerned when he realized that even healthy males had at least 50 percent abnormal sperm—sperm with no tail, all tail, two tails, grossly deformed heads, necks enlarged with cytoplasm—and some sperm were hyperactive while others didn't move at all. This is what science calls a biomarker of reproductive dysfunction. Dr. Skakkebaek searched the archives and discovered that records had been kept on sperm counts since the 1930s. He checked more than sixty studies on more than 15,000 men and found there had been a 50 percent drop in sperm count over the last fifty years, and the volume of semen had also declined.

When Dr. Skakkebaek announced his findings at a conference, one of the people who heard him was Dr. Richard Sharpe, an expert in male fertility from England. Sharpe had been noting a rise in his own patients of a number of serious problems in male reproduction:

- **Testicular cancer**—the incidence of this cancer has tripled in the United Kingdom and the United States over the last thirty years to become the most common cancer in young men. The U.S. Department of Defense (these guys keep good records) found that the rate of testicular cancer among active duty personnel rose from 8.62 cases per 100,000 in 1988 to 15.38 cases per 100,000 in 1996—a rate that doubled within eight years. Denmark has 300 percent more testicular cancer than it had fifty years ago. Rates in Ontario, Canada, have risen 60 percent in the last thirty-five years and the victims are getting younger. Two to four percent increases in the disease are being seen in men under age fifty in the United States, England, Australia, New Zealand, Wales, Scotland, and Nordic and Baltic countries. Men with decreased sperm count and men with low fertility have twice the risk of testicular cancer. Other risk factors included age of the mother (over age forty there is a 22.5 percent increased risk) and birth order, with the first born child being more at risk perhaps because free estrogen is higher and the first child gets the largest percentage of the mother's accumulated body burden of endocrine disruptors.

• **Undescended testicles** (cryptorchidism)—incidence doubled or tripled in the past thirty to forty years. One study showed that cryptorchidism and hypospadias increased among sons of gardeners or farmers in Denmark. Undescended testicles is one of the only known risk factors for testicular cancer.

• **Hypospadias**—an abnormality of the urethra and penis in young boys in which the opening is on the underside of the penis rather than at the tip. It is increasing at the rate of 2 percent a year. In its milder form, there may be just a little cleft in the penis. In more severe cases, the boy may not be able to stand to urinate or the penis may be so hidden that it's hard to tell if the child is male or female. William Kelce studied vinclozolin, a popular fungicide, which we wind up eating because it can't be washed off plants. He dosed pregnant rats with the pesticide and found severe reproductive problems in the offspring, such as hypospadias.

As Sharpe was noting the increase of male reproductive problems, he wondered if they could be linked to something happening in the womb. Dr. Skakkebaek had already come to the conclusion that events in the womb might be freezing certain cells (called Sertoli cells) at the fetal stage. He thought the damaged Sertoli cells could very well be the precursors of testicular cancer in the adult male (a hypothesis that is now widely accepted), even though the disease does not develop until being stimulated by hormones during puberty. By chance, Dr. Sharpe was asked to review an article by John McLachlan and Risto Santti describing their research on prostate cancer in DES-exposed rats, which showed that if hormonal activity was altered during fetal development, it would affect sperm count in adult life. The conclusion of the authors was that the most likely area of change was in the Sertoli cells in the testes, as the number of Sertoli cells determines how much sperm will be made in adult life.

The proverbial lightbulb lit up for Sharpe, who had never before considered the development of the Sertoli cells critical. He did an exhaustive search of the scientific literature on Sertoli cells during development and it became clear to him that all the reproductive problems he had been seeing—hypospadias, undescended testicles, and testicular cancer—could be tied together by the secretions of the Sertoli cells, which control all the other processes of development of the male. Later, data would also suggest that cryptorchidism, testicular cancer, and low sperm production are correlated in humans. What was the common factor that affected the Sertoli cells? Estrogen. Sertoli cells are very vulnerable in the womb and throughout childhood and puberty. Too much estrogen during fetal development could suppress other hormones and lower the number of Sertoli cells, and other agents that acted like estrogens could cross the placental barrier and disrupt development. Sharpe shared his new theory with Skakkebaek. They remembered the accidental human study with a synthetic estrogen—DES. When they looked up what had happened to the males born to DES-exposed mothers, they found an increased incidence in all the reproductive abnormalities, which backed up Dr. Sharpe's theory about male reproductive problems.

Back in America, Dr. John McLachlan (the scientific director at the National Institute of Environmental Health Sciences at the time) was worried about the incidence of prostate cancer doubling in recent decades. In his laboratory, McLachlan gave DES to pregnant mice on just two critical days during fetal development, which produced dramatic results:

- Male offspring had both male and female reproductive systems, side-by-side.

- The males were feminized at the molecular level, meaning their cells would actually express proteins that are normally expressed only in females.

- By age one, the mice showed signs of prostate disease.

Enlargement of the prostate gland afflicts 80 percent of men by the age of seventy in Western countries, and prostate cancer is now the most common cancer in American men, having increased 126 percent from 1973 to 1991. It is the second-leading cancer killer in older American men, with an expected death toll in 1998 of 39,200; some 184,500 cases were expected to be diagnosed in that year. Rat studies have found that long-term exposure to estrogen can induce prostate cancer. Dr. Frederick vom Saal showed that a tiny amount (1/10th of a trillionth of a gram per milliliter of blood) of circulating free estradiol in the fetus of a mouse can permanently alter the prostate. Even these minuscule increases in estrogen doubled the number of androgen receptors in the adult's prostate gland, which means the fetal exposure created a permanent increased sensitivity to hormones. This important research has recently been replicated. Other research has shown that prostate problems start in the womb when estrogen disrupts the communication lines between androgens and the developing tissue.

Next in the unfolding drama, Dr. Sharpe received a prepublication copy of *Our Stolen Future*, which described how Dr. Theo Colborn had found that exposure in utero to endocrine-disrupting compounds was causing problems in the offspring of various species. She examined wildlife studies and linked together the effects she had been seeing from pollutants in the Great Lakes, especially in the sixteen top predator species. The animals were all having developmental problems, from infertility to exploding thyroids. Adult bald eagles were having difficulty producing viable offspring after consuming fish from the Great Lakes for two or more years. In Florida, a large percentage of male panthers were being born with undescended testicles, which corresponded with what was being seen by Sharpe and Skakkebaek and McLachlan. Endocrine disruption was adding up.

DECREASED SPERM COUNT

One of the facets of men's reproductive problems—decreased sperm count—has been the focus of intense media coverage. Headlines blared in

---

SHOULD WE BE UPSET?

Dr. Lou Guillette, from the department of zoology at the University of Florida, says: "Imagine if for the last fifty years we had sprayed the whole earth with a nerve gas. Would you be upset? People would be screaming. Well, we've done that! We've released endocrine disruptors throughout the world that are having fundamental effects in the immune system, the reproductive system. We have good data that show that wildlife and humans are being affected. Should we be upset? Yes, we should be fundamentally upset. I think we should be screaming in the streets."

newspapers and magazines around the country: Silent Sperm; Downward Motility; Shooting Blanks; Down for the Count; It's Late in the Twentieth Century, Do You Know Where Your Sperm Went? In science, this is an area of hot debate.

Attention to sperm count began in 1992 with a study by Carlson and Skakkebaek that showed a significant decrease in semen quality (sperm concentration) from 1938 to 1990. This was supported by studies from a London fertility clinic and a Parisian sperm bank. However, a study of three U.S. sperm banks refuted these findings, and a reanalysis of the same data did not agree that the decline was worldwide.

Most studies (despite enormous differences in many of the study designs and methods) demonstrate that sperm density has declined from 113 million sperm per milliliter in 1938 to 66 million in 1990. In 1997 Shanna Swan and her colleagues reanalyzed the data from fifty-six studies on sperm and found "it was the rate of the decline, particularly in Western countries, that was most surprising. We observed a decrease of about 1.5 million sperm per milliliter per year in the United States, and a corresponding decrease of about 3 million sperm per year in Europe."

Even though there is no evidence so far that this alleged decline in sperm density has led to reduced fertility, there are important points to take into consideration, such as the following.

- *Sperm count may be a marker for other male reproductive problems.* For example, countries like Denmark, England, and the United States that have lower sperm counts have greater increases in incidence of testicular cancer, while Finland, where sperm counts are still high, has low rates of testicular cancer.

- *Lowered sperm counts may adversely affect couples with fertility problems.* One in every five or six couples now has trouble conceiving a child. Dr. Swan reminds everyone, however, that "Even though sperm counts have declined, even gone down to about 60 million sperm per milliliter, it's still 60 million. You only need one to make a baby."

An early indication of pesticides affecting sperm count came in 1949, when aviation crop dusters who handled DDT were found to have reduced sperm counts. Then, in the mid-1950s, a chemical called DBCP (dibromochloropropane) began to be used on bananas. Although its ability to kill off or disable sperm was discovered in the early 1960s in rats, nothing was done until workers in a DBCP plant in California noted there were very few children conceived by the men after they worked in the DBCP production area. Twenty-two men who worked in that part of the factory were tested and a high correlation was found between the duration of their exposure and a drastically lowered sperm count. Subsequent studies on factory workers in Mexico and field workers in Hawaii, Israel, and Costa Rica all showed similar results.

• *Regional differences do occur.* Most people agree that there are certain areas in the world where sperm counts are declining, but it's a hotly debated issue as to whether or not it's related to environmental pollution. While men from Northern California had typical sperm densities of 70 million per milliliter in the 1990s, compared to estimates taken before 1950 that revealed averages of 100 million per milliliter, there are areas where sperm counts are *not* lower. Seattle is one such bastion of functioning males. Dr. Alvin Paulsen, an endocrinologist and fertility expert at the University of Washington, published research that sperm counts in Seattle men have *not* decreased in two decades. Other studies, such as one by Fisch and associates, found that men who were donating sperm before vasectomies (in New York City, Roseville, Minnesota, and Los Angeles) did *not* have a decreased count. Men from these areas are known to have higher sperm counts than the average population, although no one knows why.

There was even a debate about whether or not briefs, as opposed to boxer shorts, were responsible for the decrease in sperm count—a theory

SO MANY SPERM

One of every five or six couples is infertile and approximately 40 percent of the time it is due to a problem in the male. The normal sperm count as recognized by the World Health Organization is 100 million per milliliter. A man's fertility is in question when his sperm count drops below 20 million per milliliter. Below 5 million, the man is often sterile. Why does it take so much sperm to impregnate a woman? Out of several hundred million sperm released in a single ejaculation, only several dozen finally make it up the woman's reproductive tract (the equivalent of a forty to fifty mile swim) in a hostile environment. If the count is too low and the quality of the sperm is impaired, it is less likely that one victor will finally penetrate the membrane of the egg and fertilize it.

that never bore fruit (of the loom). However, laboratory evidence shows that animals exposed prenatally to hormone-disrupting chemicals—at levels humans are exposed to on a daily basis through food, air, and water—have significantly decreased sperm counts. A number of animal studies have clearly shown that exposure to even low doses of EDCs in the womb cause decreased sperm counts in adult rats.

Dr. Paul Cook at the University of Illinois is looking at the number of sperm in the testes, which is another way of estimating sperm production. He is finding that fetal exposure to estrogens leads to testes with a lower apparent rate of production of sperm, which would correspond to what the sperm count data have shown. Several chemicals among the 12 persistent organic pollutants (called the "dirty dozen") identified for global phase-out by the United Nations have been found to decrease sperm count in animals and humans. Exposure to these chemicals has been declining since the 1970s and we may, according to Shanna Swan, now start to see a leveling off of this sperm decline.

Since the dirty dozen are only a handful of the thousands of chemicals out there, who knows what the trend in sperm count will be years down the road?

COULD CHEMICAL EXPOSURE LEAD TO VIAGRA?

A number of studies have shown that exposure to hormone disruptors can seriously affect men's ability to have a healthy sex life. Two decades later, workers at a plant that produced the insecticide kepone were reported to have lost their libido, become impotent, and had low sperm counts. Later experiments conducted in lab animals demonstrated that these pesticides were indeed estrogenic. In 1987 chemical production workers exposed to dioxins from New Jersey and Missouri plants participated in a medical evaluation. The exposed workers were found to have a lower level of testosterone than nonexposed control groups. Low levels of testosterone are associated with lowered libido and impotence. A study by the Occupational Safety and Health Administration (OSHA) in a large chemical plant that manufactured a stilbene derivative (a chemical with estrogenic effects) found that 36 percent of males who worked in that area had decreased libido (37 percent had decreased testosterone) and 21 percent were impotent.

Women's Health

> *Until rather recently, women's ailments were regarded simply as evidence of some design flaw or inherent weakness of women's constitution. . . . We now know that hormone balance is an important factor in a woman's overall health.*
>
> —John R. Lee, M.D., *What Your Doctor May Not Tell You About Menopause* (Warner Books, 1996)

This chapter looks at various women's health conditions that appear to have a connection to hormone disruption. Estrogen-dependent breast cancer and the use of synthetic hormones for menopause are examined in depth in Chapters 9 and 10.

WOMEN ARE DIFFERENT

Women are not just slightly smaller men. The sexes are biologically different. There are a number of reasons why hormone disruptors affect women differently:

- Women manufacture more of the natural hormone estrogen than do men, so additional estrogenic activity from ecoestrogens makes them even more susceptible to health problems caused by estrogen dominance.

- Women have more fat, with at least 21 percent body fat compared to 12–15 percent for men. More fat cells store more hormone-disrupting chemicals. Women's breasts and ovaries have high concentrations of fat, making these locations especially vulnerable. After menopause, when the amount of estrogen produced in a woman's body drops off significantly, women frequently gain an average of 8 to 10 pounds, adding yet more fat cells. Samples of fat cells located near tumors in breast and ovarian cancers have been shown to store environmental chemicals.

- In the normal course of how the body works, fat cells release about 5 percent of their content into the blood on a continual basis. In addition, women's weight tends to yo-yo more than that of men, and Dr. Robert Bixby, from the Indiana University School of Medicine, has shown that some of the chemical compounds that are stored in fat are released during weight loss.

- Women have been shown to retain higher levels of pollutants than do men. Landi and Bertazzi and coworkers at the University of Milan did a twenty-year follow-up study after the 1976 Seveso dioxin accident. They examined 30,000 blood samples taken within three months of the accident. Exposed women had statistically significant higher levels of dioxin in their bloodstream than did the exposed men.

- Women, generally being physically smaller than men, also have smaller organs. A smaller liver has less capacity for getting rid of toxins.

- Women spend more time at home, the place (according to the Total Exposure Assessment Methodology studies) that represents the highest personal exposure to Americans.

- Another way in which women differ from men is in how their bodies process pharmaceutical drugs. Some women can metabolize certain medicines up to 50 percent faster than men. One reason for this is hormones. Women's hormones fluctuate during their cycle, it affects the rate at which they metabolize drugs, with some women metabolizing drugs more slowly during ovulation, when eggs are released. Eggs have fat that can be "tainted."

- Certain stages in a woman's life—such as puberty, peri-menopause, and postmenopause—are all points at which women may be more susceptible to toxic exposures from the environment.

- Hormones, especially estrogen, affect the immune system. Women have more immune problems than men because these problems, such as lupus and certain thyroid illnesses, are driven by estrogen.

Even women in prime physical condition have problems male athletes don't encounter. A high-school female athlete who competed in cross-country and track experienced irregular menses, breakthrough bleeding, and flulike symptoms of fever, fatigue, sore throat, and aching muscles following meets. It was ultimately found that this only happened after meets at schools where certain herbicides had been used to kill grass along the fences to beautify the grounds. The young girl was getting estrogenic effects following exposure to these commonly used herbicides, which contained glycophosphate (the EPA confirmed it caused flulike symptoms). The principal banned use of the herbicide at the girl's school, but her symptoms continued when she competed at other places that used the herbicide. She went on to college, kept competing, and continued to experience breakthrough bleeding. One of her teammates reported vaginal bleeding after meets at golf courses (which are kept lush and green through heavy pesticide use).

WOMEN'S HEALTH CONDITIONS

There are a number of women's health conditions that we know are related to hormones and, therefore, by extension, are possibly related to hormone-disrupting chemicals in the body. Dr. John Lee has described a range of female disorders that arise (particularly in peri- and postmenopausal women) as a result of excess estrogenic signaling in relation to progesterone signaling when women are in their thirties and forties. The conditions that Dr. Lee associates with this excessive estrogen imbalance are:

- endometriosis
- uterine fibroids
- benign breast disease
- premenstrual syndrome (PMS)
- perimenopausal problems such as midcycle pain and spotting
- endometrial polyps
- ovarian cysts

- infertility

- possibly adenomyosis (endometriosis inside the uterus)

- increases in reproductive cancers such as of the breast and
ovaries

These conditions overlap with those seen in DES daughters. I have personally interviewed numerous DES daughters who have many of these problems. Much of what is known about the effects of DES exposure comes from the women who are being monitored as part of large cohorts. DES daughters could be:

- born with abnormalities of the genital tract, such as a misshapen or oddly sized vagina, cervix, or uterus.

- prone to reduced fertility and problems with pregnancy, such as ectopic pregnancies, miscarriages, and premature labor and delivery. A guesstimate from Pat Cody, the DES Action Program Director, is that 50 percent of DES daughters had problems with pregnancies. How ironic that a drug given to *enhance* pregnancy decreased healthy pregnancies in children exposed in utero to this drug.

- at risk for a rare form of vaginal or cervical cancer (clear cell adenocarcinoma, CCA) that previously was only seen in women in their sixties and seventies. CCA first appeared in DES daughters aged fifteen to twenty-two, but reports are being made of clear cell cancer in DES daughters in their forties. In other words, DES daughters are at increased risk of this cancer, not just in their twenties as was previously thought, but throughout their lives.

- at increased risk for menstrual irregularities and Fallopian tube, cervical, and uterine defects. Many animal studies suggest an increased risk of endometriosis, adenomyosis, cysts, and fibroids.

- at an increased risk for abnormal cell changes on the cervix and adenosis (abnormal cellular change) of the vagina.

- at increased risk for decreased thymus functioning (the thymus gland makes cells that act as the army of the immune system), lupus, arthritis, diabetes, asthma, chronic respiratory infections, and other diseases suggesting impaired immune function. Numerous animal and human studies show DES adversely affects the immune system, although some data do not support this conclusion.

- at greater risk for anorexia.

- at risk for problems with personality, intelligence, and mating habits, although this is controversial. Older studies suggested that exposure to DES in utero may have affected the personalities and levels of intelligence of DES children and may have predisposed them toward depression as well as anger, anxiety, low self-esteem, identity confusion, and guilt. Some of these studies couldn't be replicated.

- more likely to exhibit more masculine behavior, have less well-established sex-partner relationships, have less orientation to parenting, and experience more bisexuality and homosexuality. A well-controlled 1995 study comparing 117 DES daughters to matched non-DES daughters showed that DES daughters may have a trend toward lesbianism. The results of this study held up to statistical analysis.

- at increased risk for elevated levels of prolactin, a hormone that stimulates tumor growth factors (when not elevated due to breast-feeding). Increased prolactin may also indirectly elevate estrogen. High prolactin levels are suspected of playing a role in some breast cancers.

- at increased risk for indirect and/or irreversible genetic damage through various methods, such as demethylation (which makes leaks in the signaling system), that would lay the groundwork for cancers later in life.

- more prone to breast and ovarian cancer later in life. The oldest DES-exposed daughters are just now approaching the age range when the risk for developing these cancers is greatest. Even relatively slow-acting types of cancer may not act or behave the same in women who are DES daughters. Early animal studies of DES proved to be remarkably accurate forecasts of what would happen to DES-exposed humans. Some scientists who conduct animal studies have concluded that since their studies point to a link between DES and breast and ovarian cancer, the population of women with a history of in utero exposure to DES needs to be closely monitored for the development of gynecologic cancers.

It remains to be seen if DES daughters will have more problems with menopause.

Studies other than those on DES daughters are reporting similar findings in relation to other hormone disruptors. In 1992 German researchers published a study on the relationship of pollutant exposure to the exis-

TABLE 8.1 HORMONE DISRUPTORS AND HEALTH EFFECTS IN WOMEN

EXPOSURE TO	ASSOCIATED EFFECTS
Mercury	Hormonal disorders
	Alopecia (hair loss)
Cadmium	Thyroid dysfunction
	Habitual abortion
	Uterine fibroids

PESTICIDES (EFFECTS INCREASED WITH AGE)

DDT/DDE/DDD	Infertility
Pentachlorophenol (PCP)	Abortion
Alpha hexachlorocyclohexane (HCH)	Uterine fibroids
Polychlorinated biphenyls (PCBS)	Endometriosis
	Antithyroidal antibodies (the immune system starts attacking its own thyroid gland)

tence of fertility problems, hormonal disorders, abortions, and fetal malformations in a population of women. Their research shows that exposure to hormone disruptors was capable of affecting the female reproductive system. Table 8.1 lists the associations they uncovered.

BIRTH CONTROL AND FERTILITY

Fertility has become a growing problem. Between 1982 and 1995, there was a substantial increase in the number (1.6 million) and percent (21.4 percent) of women who had trouble with fertility, with the greatest increase seen in women under the age of twenty-five (41.9 percent). In Sweden, at the University of Lund, one study found that women who smoke cigarettes and eat fatty fish (salmon and herring) from the Baltic Sea take twice as long as normal to get pregnant. It seems that smoking makes the pollutants in fish more dangerous.

Women are frequently prescribed pharmaceutical drugs that act like hormones. In particular, oral contraceptives and fertility drugs are pharmaceutical hormones used to manipulate female reproduction—one to prevent conception, the other to facilitate it.

Birth-control pills have been both praised and blamed. When they first came into use in the 1960s, oral contraceptives were part of the societal changes deemed responsible for the era of free love. They are credited with allowing women to become more independent and in control of their life choices. However, there is a 7 percent annual failure rate for oral contraceptives, some of which is due to women not taking the pill as instructed while some is the result of actual medication failure. This means that, worldwide, almost 1 million women a year reportedly get pregnant while on the birth-control pill.

In the 1960s, women were promised that the birth-control pill was safe and then at least 500 deaths were found to be related to birth-control pills. Studies associate other significant risks to birth-control pills—allergies, migraines, alterations in blood sugar and fats, the lowering of key nutrient levels within the female body, and even rare cases of blood clots, strokes, and hemorrhages. Even though the scientific literature discusses these potential problems from ingesting birth-control pills, doctors rarely inform women about the risks or tell them how they might avoid these problems. Today's birth-control pills have much lower dosages of these hormones than the original pill.

Will a woman's birth-control pills affect an embryo?

Most women stop taking the pill before they become pregnant, so the fetus probably is not damaged. However, if a woman gets pregnant and doesn't stop taking the birth-control pill (perhaps because she may have some bleeding), the synthetic estrogen is available to bind with receptors in the fetus. What could that do? Studies on oral contraceptives have focused on seeing whether or not they caused birth defects, but the kinds

THE LEARNING CURVE

Dr. Wade Welshons: "The medical community right now doesn't think there are effects from ethinyl estradiol (the estrogen in birth-control pills). It's as though they didn't learn anything from DES."

of problems we're talking about with endocrine disruption are not detectable at birth. As far as we know, no one is keeping track of possible problems with the children of women who got pregnant while taking birth-control pills.

We do know that during pregnancy women have an elevated level of natural estrogen, and developing fetuses have high levels of binding proteins to protect themselves from getting too much of their mother's estrogen. Unlike natural estrogen, the synthetic estrogen in the pill—ethinyl estradiol—does not bind to protein in the blood, leaving it free to cross the placental barrier and enter the fetus, especially the developing brain. Ethinyl estradiol is far more active than natural estrogen and remains in the body for hours before it is excreted. Thus, it has more opportunity to affect estrogen signaling.

By age forty, 80 percent of women in the United States have used oral contraceptives at some point in their lives. This makes it difficult to run studies on the risks of birth-control pills since it's hard to find control groups of women who have not used them. But studies do suggest that women have an increased risk of getting premenopausal breast cancer if they used birth-control pills as teenagers, before first pregnancies (early on in life), or long-term at an early age. This trend reverses between the ages of forty-five and fifty-four when it appears that women who used birth-control pills early in life have a small protective effect from them. However, many women who first used oral contraceptives are just entering their high-risk years; much data still needs to be collected to form a clearer picture of what is really going on.

A side note: the estrogen from birth-control pills is still estrogenic (although in a less potent form) by the time it is excreted in a woman's urine. Sewage systems eventually channel some of this liquid back into the water supply, but water treatment plants are not equipped to filter out these estrogenic compounds. In other words, we could also be drinking estrogen metabolites from women on birth-control pills; from the normal estrogens in women's urine; and from the very high amounts of estrogen in pregnant women's urine. This is now a proposed area of study by the EPA.

Another form of birth control—injections of depoprovera (a synthetic progesterone at 150 mg/ml/shot)—is suspected of causing defects in the reproductive system of males exposed in utero, mostly irregularities like hypospadias (poorly developed penis). It has been shown that progestins can block the action of male hormones. Once used to prevent miscarriage, depoprovera is no longer prescribed for that purpose, but it is still prescribed for millions of women worldwide as a form of birth control. It has a failure rate of .03 percent, which means that an estimated three out of every thousand women become pregnant while using this drug, which adds up to many thousands of exposed fetuses.

What about fertility drugs?

Liz Tilberis, the late editor of *Harper's Bazaar* and former president of the Ovarian Cancer Research Fund, was convinced that the nine fertility treatments she had in the mid-seventies led to her ovarian cancer, even though no study has thus far shown a link. "I just feel that nowadays, however much money infertility clinics make, it is totally important to give a warning," she said.

And what about the babies born to the half million women who are treated for infertility each year with estrogenic drugs? Dr. Dolores J. Lamb, associate professor of urology and cell biology at Baylor College of Medicine, stated at the fourth Estrogen and the Environment Conference that the increase in some of the reproductive problems we are seeing, like abnormal penis and urethral formation in little boys, may be due to the excess estrogen received by babies born to women on fertility drugs. This would be endocrine disruption in action. Roughly 4.9 million women in the United States have trouble conceiving, of whom 43 percent seek treatment. About half of these women eventually conceive. These numbers are

---

FERTILITY DOESN'T ALWAYS REQUIRE MEDICATION

Dr. Chris Green, a physician in California, had a twenty-eight-year-old patient who had been on birth-control pills for several years but couldn't get pregnant after stopping the pills. Her follicle stimulating hormone (FSH) level was 70, an elevated level that normally would indicate she was in menopause. She had previously seen numerous experts who put her on fertility drugs, which failed. All the experts agreed she had less than a 5 percent chance of ever getting pregnant. But Dr. Green wanted to give nature a chance. She put the woman on a high-fat diet (because our bodies make hormones from fat) and prescribed a natural progesterone. The woman now has a healthy baby.

huge. It would seem prudent to monitor these mothers and their offspring for possible endocrine disruption effects.

There are indications that hormone disruptors, even those less powerful than DES, do affect the female reproductive system. In 1976, eighteen female monkeys were fed PCBS in foods (in levels equal to or half the concentration allowed in human food). Within two months, some females developed hair loss and acne; by six months all females had symptoms such as problems with menstruation and fertility; and infants born were smaller than normal.

The Women's Environment and Development Organization (WEDO) came out with a report in 1999 on the quality of women's health worldwide. Eighty-two percent of the countries surveyed—including the United States, Europe, Latin America, Asia, and nations in Africa—reported on occupational health hazards faced by women, including pesticide exposure. Forty-four percent of those countries indicated that these workplace exposures resulted in reproductive problems. In an animal study, ewes were exposed to two organochlorine pesticides—lindane and pentachlorophenol (PCP). Fertility was significantly decreased by the lindane, and in the PCP-treated ewes there was a decrease of thyroid hormone in the blood.

Cancer of the Reproductive Organs

Many studies in humans, in animals, and in the laboratory show that as a female's lifetime exposure to estrogens increases, so does her risk of getting cancers that grow in the presence of estrogen (this includes half of the cases of breast cancer as well as uterine cancer). An article from *Cancer Research* said that ovarian tumors are more deadly if they have more estrogen alpha receptors and less deadly if they have more beta receptors. At this time, alpha is associated with proliferation (growth); beta with control. Estrogens are considered cocarcinogens—chemicals that increase the ability of a cancer-causing substance to promote a tumor. In other words, estrogens can take a cell that is capable of becoming cancerous and increase the probability that it will do so.

In the last several decades, the number of cancers that grow faster in the presence of hormones has been increasing. Since the increasing incidence of hormone-dependent tumors overlaps the period of time in which synthetic compounds have become part of the environment, we must ask the question: is there a relationship between these tumors and endocrine disruptors? The next chapter discusses this question in detail.

PREECLAMPSIA IN PREGNANCY

Preeclampsia is a pregnancy problem in which toxemia occurs late in pregnancy, causing the expectant mom to develop complications like high blood pressure and severe fluid retention. One theory is that human retroviruses—part of our programming genes made by the body—go awry. According to researchers in Italy, endocrine-disrupting compounds may alter the normal genetic expression of human retroviruses and this may be one cause for preeclampsia as well as for a variety of other diseases.

ENDOMETRIOSIS

When I was in practice, one of the conditions I saw dramatically increase throughout the 1980s was endometriosis. Women would come into my office with long histories of severe pelvic pain, sometimes radiating down their legs, that often was not helped by medical treatment such as hormone therapy or surgery. Endometriosis can be mild, causing some pelvic pain and a feeling of fullness, or it can cause debilitating pain, complications, and even infertility. I have seen severe conditions in which the women developed problems with their pelvic lymph nodes, resulting in serious enlargement of their lower limbs that caused tremendous pain and made walking difficult.

Endometriosis is a very common gynecologic disease and is a major cause of chronic pelvic pain and infertility. In North America the National Institute of Child Health and Human Development estimates that endometriosis affects 10–20 percent of women of childbearing age in the United States, so this disease may be present in 6 million women in this country—meaning that approximately one-fourth to one-fifth of women may be affected—which translates into 300,000 new cases a year and requires 500,000 surgical procedures each year. Women in Japan are now getting more endometriosis, and some link the trend to endocrine disruptors.

Endometriosis is a disease that affects the endometrium—the part of the uterus that plumps up before menstruation and sheds during it. Endometriosis occurs when endometrial tissue grows in the wrong place;

it grows *outside* the uterus—anywhere in the pelvic cavity, on an ovary, or sometimes in other bizarre places. When it does occur within the uterus, as sometimes happens, it is called *adenomyosis*. Endometrial tissue, even though it's growing in an abnormal place, still fattens up before the period and bleeds during it, which causes local inflammation and scarring.

It's not easy for women to figure out if their gynecologic woes come from endometriosis. On the average it takes nine years for a woman to find out if she has this disease. The symptoms are varied and confusing, often mimicking pelvic inflammatory disease (inflammation within any number of female genital organs) or ectopic pregnancy (pregnancy in a fallopian tube). The most common symptoms are mild to debilitating lower abdominal pain, horrific cramps, severe fatigue, backache, painful sex, bloating, heavy bleeding, intestinal discomfort, and diarrhea. Approximately 40 percent of women with this disease grapple with infertility.

There is no way to test definitively for endometriosis except by "going into" a woman's pelvic area with an instrument and looking around (laparoscopy). Laparoscopies are abdominal surgery and are not without possible complications, such as scarring and adhesions, that often cause further pain and require more surgical intervention at a future time. All this contributes to a substantial cost as well as a decrease in quality of life, besides the fact that the recurrence rate is 40 percent within five years. Some endometrial spots are microscopic and can't be seen even with medical equipment. Unfortunately with endometriosis, it is often the smaller

---

IT'S 11 P.M: DO YOU KNOW WHERE YOUR PCBs ARE?

PCBs were first manufactured in 1929 by the Swan Corporation (which later became part of Monsanto). General Electric and Westinghouse also became major users of PCBS. Between 1929 and 1989, total world production of PCBS (excluding the Soviet Union) was 3.4 billion pounds, about 57 million pounds per year. Approximately 30 percent is in landfills, in storage, or in the sediments of lakes, rivers, and estuaries. Some 30 to 40 percent remain in use. About 1 percent has reached the oceans and is already causing major problems. Large birds and marine mammals (seals, sea lions, whales, and some dolphins) that eat contaminated fish lack the enzyme systems to detoxify PCBS. The whereabouts of 30 percent of all PCBS (roughly a billion pounds) remains *unknown*.

lesions that cause the most pain. Approximately 60 percent of women who go through laparoscopic intervention and its associated pain, recovery, and cost do not go into remission. As you can see, this uterine disease is common, serious, and debilitating.

TABLE 8.2 ENDOMETRIOSIS AND EDCs

STUDIES ON ENDOMETRIOSIS AND HORMONE DISRUPTORS

Dr. Mayani and team looked at one hundred women with chronic pelvic pain and identified those who had endometriosis. Blood tests found dioxin levels significantly higher in women with endometriosis than in women without this disease.

According to Gerhard, women with endometriosis had increased concentrations of PCBS in their blood.

Endometriosis appears to occur more in career women, which Koninck and coworkers from Gynecologic Endoscopic Surgery at the University Hospital Gasthuisberg say could be a consequence of urban exposure rather than lifestyle. Belgium breast milk has some of the highest dioxin levels in the world, reflecting that these women have high body-burdens of dioxin. Belgium has the world's highest incidence of endometriosis; 60 to 80 percent of Belgian women who are infertile or suffer with pelvic pain have been found to have the disease.

Osteen and associates have suggested that normal endometrial homeostasis depends on well-organized cell interactions regulated locally by a balance between cytokines and growth factors. This balance is under the influence of steroid hormonal signaling, which they suggest could come from endogenous hormones as well as environmental estrogens.

Sherry Rier and associates have demonstrated that chronic exposure to dioxin is directly correlated with the presence and severity of endometriosis in rhesus monkeys.

Cummings and research team studied mice and rats and found that exposing them to dioxin caused immune dysfunction in both and endometriosis in the rodents.

Exposure to dioxin in animals has been shown to increase the rate of abortion, alter the cycling of sexual receptivity, and cause endometriosis.

Lebel and team did *not* find an association in eighty-four women undergoing laparoscopies for chronic pelvic pain with exposure to organochlorines (chlorinated compounds).

One common theory as to what causes endometriosis is called retrograde menstruation. This is when a little of the blood flow during menses backs up into the Fallopian tubes. For most women, these little bits of endometrium simply follow their normal programming and die, but in some women the signal to die may be altered or inaudible. And this abnormal signaling of the endometrial cells may be provoked by environmental pollutants such as dioxins and PCBS. The incidence of endometriosis is higher in developed countries than in developing countries, overlapping with increased industrial production of PCBS and related dioxin pollution. Human and animal studies that have come out since the 1994 EPA Dioxin Reassessment have associated dioxin exposure with both causing and intensifying endometriosis. It also has been suggested that dioxin can block the protective effects of progesterone. Progesterone is one natural inhibitor of endometriosis, whereas estrogen and hormone disruptors like dioxin may promote diseases of the uterus.

It is also of note that endometriosis and adenomyosis are both associated with chronic inflammation and reduced T-cell activity and are considered autoimmune diseases. Dioxin is known to reduce the fighting cells of the immune system (T helper cells) and to alter other aspects of immunity. In studies based on the Endometriosis Association research registry, women with endometriosis also demonstrate other health problems, such as chronic allergies (to pollen, food, or even their own hormones), vaginal yeast infections, asthma, mononucleosis, eczema—all suggestive of decreased immune functioning. Thus, EDCs may be contributing to pelvic inflammation not just locally, but by immunosuppression that indirectly contributes to these diseases.

HERE, THERE, AND EVERYWHERE

"Until the United States Environmental Protection Agency released the draft of its latest reassessment on the health effects of dioxin [an endocrine disruptor] on September 13, 1994, I thought my move to Virginia had protected my children from further damage from dioxin. I didn't know we were feeding our children dioxin every time they drank milk or ate fish or meat. I didn't realize that the dioxin from a hazardous waste-burning aggregate kiln in Florida could end up in the milk of a cow or a new mother living in Michigan."

—Lois Marie Gibbs, *Dying From Dioxin* (South End Press, 1995)

Apparently, the endometrium is a prime place for dioxin to exert its toxic action. A team (from the Division of Environmental and Occupational Health at the University of Minnesota School of Public Health and the Tulane Center for Bioenvironmental Research) developed a human endometrial model to explore the interaction between dioxin and uterine tissue. They were the first to show that human endometrial cells contain the Ah receptor. Dioxin binds to the Ah receptor in the nucleus where it can regulate expression of certain genes. Normally, when the Ah receptor is turned on, three powerful enzymes go into action that help detoxify pollutants as well as maintain healthy levels of hormones such as estrogen by breaking them down. When high doses of estrogen are present in the body, the ability of these detoxifying enzymes to be helpful is reduced.

Certain foods such as broccoli, cabbage, and cauliflower may help maintain more optimal estrogen levels by binding in a healthy way to the Ah receptor and keeping the enzymes on their job for limited periods of time. This helps turn potentially "dangerous" estrogens into "safer" ones. When dioxin is present, however, these enzymes stay active longer. This inhibits estrogen from doing its normal job. The research team says that what goes on between the estrogen receptor and the Ah receptor is important in maintaining the proper balance of estrogens in the endometrium. When women are exposed to higher than normal estrogens, or to dioxins, this tightly regulated balance is upset, resulting in diseases of the uterus. They believe that their research provides a basis for understanding, preventing, and treating uterine disease.

FIBROIDS

Fibroids are benign tumors occurring in the smooth muscle layer of the uterus, scientifically called leiomyomas. Fifty to seventy percent of pre- and postmenopausal women have uterine fibroids, some of which can be felt and some of which can only be seen under a microscope. Five hundred and fifty thousand hysterectomies are performed each year. Fibroids are the major cause of these surgeries.

In her lab at the University of Texas, Dr. Cheryl S. Walker bred animals that spontaneously make fibroids. Dr. Walker discovered that in uterine fibroids, cell growth is increased while cell death is not. This causes fibroids. Interestingly enough, the layer of the uterus that gives rise to fibroids has a high concentration of estrogen receptor beta, which may participate in the balancing act between cell growth (proliferation) and

SUMMARY OF NATIONAL HEALTH INTERVIEW SURVEY FINDINGS

Condition	# reporting per 1,000	White Women	Black Women
Menstrual disorders	53.0	53.1	54.1
Uterine conditions	16.6	17.3	15.0
Fibroids	9.2	8.2	16.9

cell death (apoptosis). Dr. Walker found that lab animals whose ovaries had been removed formed no fibroids. She also studied fibroids in relationship to coumestrol and genestein (phytoestrogens), estradiol, the pesticides kepone and dieldrin, and DES. Almost every compound caused estrogenic action: cell proliferation, estrogen-receptor signaling, and turning on progesterone-receptor expression (which may, in the future, be used as a biomarker for fibroids). Leslie C. Hodge, a postdoctoral student of Dr. Walker's, found that every single organochlorine except dieldrin increased fibroid growth in low doses.

Kelly Morgan did an exhaustive review of fibroids and the environment while doing a fellowship at the Center for Bioenvironmental Research at Tulane and Xavier Universities. Morgan uncovered an observation made by researchers in India which indicated that DDT levels in the blood of women with uterine fibroids was three times higher than in women without fibroids. India's population has one of the highest body burdens of DDT residues in the world.

Endometriosis and fibroids together account for 750,000 surgical procedures annually performed on women in the United States. Fibroids and endometriosis are so common now, I have heard surgeons refer to them as "naturally occurring" rather than as signifying disease. In 1996 an analysis of data from the National Health Interview Survey, 1984 to 1992, demonstrated that fibroids were the third most common gynecological condition, reported by 9.2 out of every 1,000 women.

Fibroids are actively driven by estrogenic compounds. Risk factors for fibroids are unopposed estrogen, obesity, younger age at menarche, and race (incidence is higher in African-American women than Caucasian

---

ARE MODERN WOMEN MENSTRUATING THEMSELVES INTO HEALTH PROBLEMS?

Bleeding, anyone? It turns out western women now live so differently than women did °one hundred years ago that now women have many more menstrual periods during their lifetimes. When a woman ovulates, the egg bursts through the walls of her ovaries, which is a somewhat traumatic affair. To heal this, the cells need to divide and reproduce—cellular events which increase the risk of getting cancers. In 1986–89, Beverly Strassmann studied the menstrual life of African women in a village about 120 miles south of Timbuktu. These indigenous women go through puberty later (average age of sixteen), get pregnant earlier and more often (eight to nine times), and spend more time lactating (turning off ovulation for an average of twenty months, much longer than for western women). In total, the tribal women menstruate about 100 times during their lives, compared to the 350 and 400 times a contemporary western woman has her period. Incessant menstruation has been associated with increases in occurrences of abdominal pain, mood shifts, migraines, endometriosis, infertility, cancers, fibroids, and anemia. Environmental estrogens may be playing a role in some women having more periods.

---

women). Since certain hormonally active environmental pollutants can act as estrogens, antiprogestins, and antiandrogens (all of which enhance estrogenic signaling), and since these estrogenic compounds accumulate in body fat and tissues, the connection between hormone disruptors and fibroids needs more investigation.

VAGINAL YEAST INFECTIONS

Many women are plagued by vaginal yeast infections, and men and women both are reporting an increase in a condition called the Candida-related complex—health problems arising from intestinal yeast infections. It has been well established that estrogen stimulates the growth-promoting signals to these yeast organisms. It is possible that estrogenic compounds in the environment may be one of the factors responsible for the increasing incidence of this problem.

Breast Cancer

Hormone-disrupting chemicals are not classical poisons or typical carcinogens. They play by different rules. . . . Until we recognize this, we will be looking in the wrong places, asking the wrong questions, and talking at cross purposes.

—T. Colburn, D. Dumanoski, and J. P. Meyers,
Our Stolen Future (Dutton, 1996)

There is overwhelming evidence that estrogen levels are a critical determinant of breast cancer risk. This association is stronger than that between cholesterol levels and heart disease, suggesting that estrogen levels may serve as a clinical indicator of breast cancer risk (once we know more about which estrogens to test and how to test them correctly!). Data from a number of studies have added evidence to support an association between environmental estrogens and breast cancer.

The number of women getting breast cancer has been rising consistently over the past fifty years—a span of time that parallels the massive expansion of industry and our exposure to environmental pollutants (many of which are being investigated as estrogenic hormone disruptors), as well as major lifestyle changes, such as delayed parenting. Because elevated estrogen levels within the human body have been widely recognized as contributing to this disease, we must consider what role estrogenic hormone disruptors may play in breast cancer.

IT COULD HAPPEN TO ME—AND IT DID

After I was diagnosed with an estrogen-dependent breast cancer (grows in the presence of estrogen), people I had previously thought to be sane suddenly began spouting bizarre blame-the-victim rhetoric. One "friend" said, "Your thoughts create your body; just correct your thoughts and uncreate the cancer." Other comments I heard were that I needed to clear out my anger, eat less fat (dietary fat makes estrogen), work out less (muscles make estrogen), lose weight (fat makes estrogen), gain weight, get married, date less, and de-stress. A health-care professional I used to lecture with even said, "You gave yourself regular breast exams, didn't you? Well, maybe you find what you look for." (Those who knew how well I lived and ate and meditated joked that if cancer is a wake-up call to change, maybe I needed to switch to a diet of cheeseburgers and milk shakes.)

The main theme of all of these comments, well-meaning or just plain foolish, was that there was something I did or didn't do to bring this disease upon myself, and, therefore, there must be some way I could undo it. In other words, the cancer was *my* fault. On the other hand, I avoided telling my mother about my breast cancer until the very last day before this book came out—that's how terrified I was of relaying the news— because I didn't want her to feel that it was *her* fault. This may sound melodramatic to someone who doesn't understand the ramifications of being a DES daughter. One is never just a DES daughter or son but always a DES family.

When I was first diagnosed, I asked the surgeon if the breast cancer was possibly related to DES. "Absolutely not," he said. However, as I've looked deeply into the literature, it's very clear that mothers who were given DES during their pregnancies have a 30 to 50 percent increased risk for breast cancer (although the statistics from different studies vary in significance). Animal studies have long shown a connection between DES and mammary cancer. Not much is yet known about DES-exposed daughters getting breast cancer, but we're just entering our high-risk years. And not many doctors are asking women with breast cancer—or other estrogen-dependent diseases (such as ovarian cancer)—if they were exposed to DES in utero. Thus, no accurate report is being given to the DES tumor registry or to the cancer tumor registry in general. As a result, statistics do not reflect DES children and their rate of cancers (other than vaginal). However, beginning in 1994, more than 6,900 moms, 6,500 daughters, and 3,600 sons who had all been exposed to DES were sent questionnaires from the National Cancer Institute. Hopefully, when these data have been evaluated, we'll have a better idea of what's happening.

The predicament, though, is not just with DES daughters. We're *all* part of a unique experiment—we all have hormone-disrupting chemicals in our bodies.

BREAST CANCER: VITAL STATISTICS

In the Vietnam War, a total of 53,000 Americans were killed; in comparison, each year nearly 46,000 U.S. women are killed by breast cancer. It's the number-one cause of death in women thirty-two to fifty-two years old. Although heart disease kills far more women, breast cancer seems

---

DES AND CANCER

I asked many doctors if there was a relationship between my breast cancer and DES; they almost laughed at me as they said no. Dr. Herbst (who heads the Chicago DES project) said there was no data on DES and breast cancer in daughters, but I found a number of studies in animals that strongly indicate a link. Mammary and pituitary tumors have been induced in female rats by prenatal DES exposure. Other animal studies suggest that early DES exposure makes breast tissue increase in growth and more sensitive to chemical carcinogens—both implicated in breast cancer.

Dr. John McLachlan, a pioneer in the field of environmental estrogens, showed that animals given DES prenatally or neonatally are more sensitive to all kinds of hormones and hormone impostors. Other studies have also shown that DES-exposed animals are more sensitive to secondary exposures. This means that even though a hormone disruptor like DES may not, in itself, cause a serious endpoint like cancer, it may make the body more susceptible to carcinogens. I also spoke with Retha Newbold, a scientist who has been doing DES research for decades. She said it is very significant that a small percentage of DES-exposed daughter rodents are getting ovarian cancer in a strain of rodents that never get it. This association has been found in a number of other animal studies.

At the end of 1999, a DES research update report was released that stated for the first time that breast cancer was a suspected effect in DES daughters.

---

much scarier to many. According to Dr. Susan Love, "One out of three women dies of heart disease, and only one out of eight gets breast cancer. But most of the deaths due to heart disease occur when women are in their eighties or nineties. Below the age of seventy-six, however, there are more deaths from breast cancer than there are from heart disease. . . . Compared with some of the alternatives, dropping dead of a heart attack in my eighties might be just the way I want to go, thank you very much."

Fifty years ago, a woman ran a one-in-twenty risk of getting breast cancer; now it's one in eight. We are living longer and doing a better job of diagnosing this illness earlier, but the numbers still point to something in the environment contributing to this increased incidence. And not to be ignored, during this same time frame there has been an increase in DCIS, a precancerous breast condition that often requires radiation and surgery.

Breast cancer used to occur most commonly in women in their mid-sixties. Hester Hill, a social work supervisor at Beth Israel Deaconess Medical Center who runs breast cancer support groups, says, "I've been in this job for almost twenty years, and the increase in the number of women getting breast cancer in their thirties and forties—and not so rarely in their twenties—is appalling to me." It's possible that the early age of diagnosis is partially due to improved diagnostic methods, but premenopausal breast cancer may also be due to in utero exposure to hormone disruptors that program the breast to be particularly susceptible to breast cancer.

Breast cancer is a very complicated disease. Numerous human studies over the last thirty years have revealed a number of risk factors, which still account for only 20 to 25 percent of the cases of breast cancer. The most definitive risks are from ionizing radiation (x-rays, effects of radioactive substances, or the sun) and genetics, although heredity plays a smaller and more convoluted role than was originally thought. Only 5 to 10 percent of the total number of breast cancer cases are due to inherited genetic defects, and 40 percent of women who have these defective genes still don't get breast cancer. This points a finger at something in the environment.

The Steps of Cancer

To understand how estrogen, or estrogenic hormone disruptors, may play a role in you or your friends and relatives getting breast cancer, you first need to understand how a normal cell turns cancerous.

MY PERSONAL STORY WITH BREAST CANCER GENES

Mutations in the BRCA genes have been identified as altering a woman's susceptibility to breast cancer. I asked Dr. Generosa Grana, a breast oncologist from Cooper Hospital, about her experience with the BRCA gene and DES daughters. She said, "You're thinking your breast cancer is due to being a DES daughter. It's possible that it is due to your genes. We are now finding that some women of Ashkenazi Jewish descent have evidence of these genetic mutations without having a documented family history of breast or ovarian cancer. If you are a DES daughter *and* you have this BRCA gene mutation, we don't know what that would mean."

It took me two weeks to get genetic testing ordered anonymously. I was told by people in the medical field that if my insurance company found out I had a genetic contributing factor to this cancer, it could possibly affect my future insurability. After a tense week, I was pleased to learn I do not have mutated BRCA genes. This again suggested that, for me, in utero DES exposure played a role in the initiation of breast cancer.

A normal cell is sane and socialized, meaning it knows the rules—when to grow (divide), how fast to grow, how to repair mistakes (mutations in DNA), and when to die. A cancerous cell does not obey the rules. It is stark-raving mad and doesn't know that it should drop dead at a certain time. A cancer cell is fairly immortal (at least for as long as its host is alive). *Carcinogenesis* is the term for the origination of cancer—how and why some of the cells in the body suddenly start to run amok.

Here are the steps for the progression of cancer:

- *Initiation.* For cancer to occur, systems that regulate a cell to act normally must become disrupted. This can happen through a variety of means. Estrogens and estrogen metabolites, once thought only to promote growth in preexisting cancers, have now been shown to damage genes and thus play a role in initiating cancer. Human studies (plus laboratory and animal evidence), clearly illustrate that environmental pollutants acting like estrogens can in fact initiate breast cancer. This means that whatever causes cancer is more mysterious and frustrating than the straightforward identification of genes. On the other hand, cancers found to be due to excess estrogen or environmental chemicals that affect hormonal balance (or combinations of the environment and minor genetic abnormalities) may be more amenable to prevention in the first place.

• *Promotion.* Cells with damaged genes or damaged regulatory systems must then get the command to grow. Cells grow by division. It is well known that estrogen can make cancer cells grow by making breast cells divide faster. Research done by Drs. Ana Soto and Carlos Sonnenschein at Tufts showed that excess estrogen inhibits a protein in the blood that normally blocks cells from dividing and multiplying. More estrogen means the cells divide and multiply even if they are damaged. Much evidence supports the idea that as the rate of cell growth increases (proliferation), more can go wrong, which increases the risk of breast cancer.

Human studies clearly unveil the role of estrogen as a promoter of breast cancer. The Nurses' Health Study found that obese women had higher levels of estrogen in their bodies and more risk of getting breast cancer compared to lean women who have less estrogen. Heavier postmenopausal women, as shown in another study, suffer poorer survival rates once they get the disease. In the laboratory, animals exposed to higher than normal levels of estrogen developed larger mammary glands. The alterations in breast tissue set up the animals to develop mammary cancer later on in adulthood. These facts all point to estrogen as aggravating and worsening breast cancer conditions.

• *Progression.* Damaged cells form tumors, which then grow either slowly or rapidly depending on the type of cancer. *Metastasis* happens when the tumor cells spread from the point of origination to other parts of the body. This is how cancer kills. The crazed cells travel throughout the body, ultimately killing normal cells of various organs.

IMMATURE BREAST CELLS

When a female is born, her breast cells are immature. It is during the last month of a woman's first full-term pregnancy that a hormonal signal is sent to her breasts to get the cells ready for making milk. Only now are the breasts considered mature or differentiated. Although the process of breast maturation begins in puberty, it runs in a continuum: women who never have children have less mature breast cells than those who have had a child; having more children means even further maturation of the mother's breast cells. It is the undifferentiated or immature breast cells that are more responsive to estrogen and more easily stimulated to divide. More division means more growth; more growth means more potential problems. Errors in DNA repair or replication can occur, which can set the stage for cancer. In contrast, mature breast cells are less responsive to estrogen; they reproduce and divide more slowly, allowing time for DNA to repair any errors that occur.

Women who have their first child before the age of thirty have a decreased risk of breast cancer, and this protective effect is amplified if the first child is born before the mother is twenty. This may be because their breast cells mature at a young age. We know from studies that girls who get pregnant before the age of eighteen rarely (some say never) get breast cancer, and the breast cancer rate is very small for women who were pregnant at the ages of nineteen through twenty-one. (Also, after breast-feeding, levels of estrogen in the breast go down for several years.)

Thinking about the way undifferentiated breast cells are more vulnerable to breast cancer, Dr. Dimitrios Trichopoulos, an epidemiologist from the Harvard School of Public Health, decided to look back even further—to the immature breast cells of the fetus. If cellular immaturity affects vulnerability, he reasoned, than surely the fetus has the most immature and therefore the most vulnerable breast cells of all. Exposure to excess estrogen or estrogenic chemicals in the womb may program fetal breast cells, permanently imprinting the developing cells with traits that they would not otherwise have had (called estrogen imprinting by Dr. McLachlan and embryonic imprinting by Dr. vom Saal).

In other words, early exposure to environmental hormone disruptors or any form of excess estrogen may prime the body, especially breast tissue, for abnormalities and cancers later on in life. One essential idea to embrace is that the longer breast cells remain immature, the more vulnerable they are to cancer-causing substances. And exposure to hormone disruptors in the womb may lengthen this time of breast immaturity.

Work in Linda Birnbaum's laboratory at the EPA, headed by Sue Fenton, has shown that a woman's exposure to dioxin during pregnancy leads to altered development of the mammary gland of her unborn female, whose ducts will be less developed, more immature, and thus more susceptible to cancer. The ductal structures do eventually mature but never

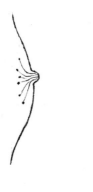

IMMATURE BREAST (BEFORE PUBERTY)

- *tiny ducts*
- *terminal end buds*
- *cells that are stimulated to grow and divide*
- *breasts are* undifferentiated *(aren't able to make milk)*

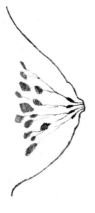

IN RESPONSE TO ESTROGEN (REPRODUCTIVE YEARS)

- *terminal end buds divide and multiply*
- *increase mass of breast*
- *each month estrogen surges*
- *causes more growth*
- *so more can go wrong*

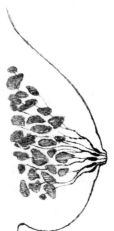

MATURE BREAST (PREGNANCY)

- *pregnancy stimulates terminal end buds to produce milk glands*
- *now breasts are* differentiated
- *more pregnancies, more breastfeeding causes more differentiation*
- *differentiated cells are* not *as responsive to estrogen and don't constantly divide*
- *less can go wrong*

FIGURE 9.1 *Breast Maturation*

TEENAGE SMOKING AND BREAST CANCER

Linda Birnbaum, head of experimental toxicology at the EPA, says: "I think that the increase in breast cancer is going to be associated with diet, lifestyle, and smoking. We know that if you smoke as an adult (even if you smoke for twenty years) and you stop smoking, after some years your risk of lung cancer has pretty much gone back to what it would have been if you'd never smoked. That's true for a number of kinds of smoking-related cancers. But for breast cancer, I believe that if you smoked as a teenager, when you were going through puberty, your risk never goes away because you permanently mutated or altered cells while they were differentiating and you basically set the stage for tumors to develop decades later. I'd like to see studies run to prove this."

Scientists at the Oak Ridge National Laboratory, chemical and analytical sciences division, have identified a number of compounds in cigarette smoke that are probably xenoestrogens.

"catch up." It is here in the ducts where most cancers of the breast, in humans, occur.

Other research, in 1998, revealed that exposing rats to dioxin during pregnancy caused their female offspring to have greater numbers of terminal end buds—the type of ductal cells most susceptible to cancer—in the breast tissue.

Results from both of these labs are weighty. They indicate that the critical window for people's exposure to dioxins, and other chemicals such as PCBS, is probably in their mothers' wombs. Pre-birth exposure to chemicals increases the amount of breast cells susceptible to cancer throughout their lifetime. So, no matter how many studies try to correlate breast cancer with exposure to hormone disruptors in adulthood, the results may be moot. Enhanced susceptibility may have been caused in the mother's womb, where no one was taking measurements.

ESTROGEN AND BREAST CANCER

It seems that exposure to excess estrogen is a consistent factor in many of the women (not all) who get breast cancer. Below is a list of findings based on studies that have found a correlation between women's exposure to estrogen and incidence of breast cancer. Numerous laboratory and animal studies support these findings.

- Asian women, who are at lower risk for breast cancer, have been consistently shown to have lower blood and urinary levels of estrogen than Caucasian women.

- Analysis of six studies showed that women with a 15 percent higher average concentration of estrogen (estradiol) levels had a higher risk of getting breast cancer.

ESTROGEN RECEPTORS AND BREAST CANCER

When a woman receives a diagnosis of breast cancer, certain biological "markers" give a general picture of the personality of the tumor and indicate what kind of prognosis and treatment the woman should have. One of the markers classically used by oncologists is to determine if the woman's cells are estrogen-receptor negative or positive.

- *Estrogen-receptor positive* (ER+) breast cancer means the cells still respond to estrogen.

- *Estrogen-receptor negative* (ER-) means the cells no longer respond to estrogen. (Some scientists feel that ER+ is an earlier stage of breast cancer and holds a slightly better diagnosis than ER-, which may be a later stage of the illness. Others don't agree because very tiny tumors may also be ER-.)

The discovery of estrogen receptor beta (see Chapter 3) may have special significance for a woman with breast cancer. It is possible that some women who are diagnosed as ER- for the alpha receptor are actually ER+ for the beta receptor. Up until recently, all research has been on the alpha receptor because no one knew other estrogen receptors existed. This new information may pave the way for more accurate markers and treatment.

Note: A highly publicized study in March 1998 showed that tamoxifen also helped to *prevent* breast cancer, although it had some dangerous side effects such as an increased risk for endometrial cancer or blood clots in the lungs. However, if blocking the ER sites helped prevent breast cancer because the women were getting less estrogen, what does that say about the risk of taking in *more* estrogen through hormone replacement therapy? And what happens to the fetus in the womb when it is exposed to excess estrogen from fertility drugs, oral contraceptives, or environmental estrogens?

- The Nurses' Heath Study correlated higher levels of estrogen in postmenopausal women with higher risk of getting breast cancer.

- A study of 130 women found a positive relationship between serum estradiol levels in postmenopausal women and the risk of breast cancer.

- Two studies on sixty-one women in Guernsey showed that women with the highest levels of estrogen in their blood had the highest risk of getting breast cancer.

Fifty to sixty percent of all breast cancers are estrogen sensitive, meaning the cancer grows faster in the presence of estrogen or estrogenic signaling. A normal cell has 20,000 to 50,000 estrogen receptors, but this number is three times higher in estrogen-dependent breast cancer cells—about 60,000 receptors per cell. Research suggests that the kinds of breast cancer and disease that are estrogen driven, as well as the number of estrogen receptors in women's breasts, may be increasing in the general population. Scientists from France and Texas worked together on a large-scale human study that analyzed 11,000 breast cancer tumors that had been collected from patients in hospitals across the United States from 1972 to 1993. They found a steady increase in the number of estrogen receptors over the last twenty years. Putting this human information together with what has been learned from animal studies, part of the reason there were more estrogen receptors in the breast cancer tumors could be due to higher levels of estrogen or estrogenic chemicals these women were exposed to in the womb.

Indirect support for the theory that in utero exposure to excess estrogen increases the risk of breast cancer comes from an English study of twins. Women pregnant with twins have higher concentrations of estrogen than women pregnant with only one child, and some research suggests that women with fraternal twins have even higher levels of estrogen. The study showed that if one twin under the age of forty-five gets breast cancer, her other twin has about eight times the average risk of also getting it—possibly due to genetics or exposure to the extra estrogen in the womb.

Scientists first wondered about estrogen's role in breast cancer when it was noted that nuns, who do not have children and thus are exposed to more ovulatory cycles and less estriol (the primary estrogen during pregnancy), get more breast cancer. Then scientists observed that surgically removing women's ovaries—the primary source of the female sex hor-

HIGH- AND LOW-RISK FACTORS FOR BREAST CANCER

HIGH RISK	LOW RISK
SIGNIFICANT RISK FOR BREAST CANCER—MORE EXPOSURE TO ESTROGEN	THE LOWEST RISK FOR BREAST CANCER—THE LEAST EXPOSURE TO ESTROGEN
Gender (women get more breast cancer than men)	Ovaries removed before thirty-five years old
Earlier menarche (onset before twelve years old), more menstrual cycles without ovulation (less progesterone, more unopposed estrogen)	Onset of menstruation after fourteen years old
Later menopause (for every one-year increase in age at menopause, the risk of breast cancer increases by approximately 3 percent)	Menopause before forty-five years old
Never had children	Women from developing countries have less risk and on the average have six or more pregnancies starting at earlier ages; in the United States, the average woman has two pregnancies at later ages
Having one child (evidence suggests that after the first pregnancy there is a brief one-time increase in breast cancer risk)	Have borne five or more children
Late age of pregnancy (greater risk than only one pregnancy)	Early pregnancies (giving birth before twenty years old; as far as I know, breast cancer has never been reported in a woman who had given birth at or before the age of eighteen)
Increased body weight and height; obese postmenopausal women (fat makes estrogen)	Lean postmenopausal women

HIGH RISK	LOW RISK
Alcohol consumption (a meta-analysis of six studies shows that drinking two to five alcoholic beverages a day increases a woman's risk of invasive breast cancer)	No alcohol use
Risk with higher blood concentrations of estrogenic dieldrin; modest exposure to triazine herbicides	Lower exposure
Ten years of HRT (HRT is estrogenic and inhibits the natural process of the aging breast becoming less dense)	Never used HRT
Current use of oral contraceptives, especially between the ages of thirty-five to forty-five and for thinner women (for premenopausal breast cancer)	Never used oral contraceptives
Fat consumption above 30 percent	Fat consumption 20–25 percent or less
Highest level of bone density (estrogen promotes bone density, the higher the bone density the higher the risk of breast cancer)—Framingham Study	Lower levels of bone density
Denser breast on mammograms	Less dense breast on mammograms

mones—and thereby reducing the number of times a woman menstruates, lowered the risk of breast cancer.

For centuries women gave birth to many children, starting in their early teens. Our lifestyles have changed dramatically in present-day westernized countries, with women giving birth to fewer children much later in life. This change, coupled with estrogenic signals coming in from the environment, has contributed to the increase in our lifetime exposure levels of estrogen, or unbalanced estrogen.

ARE HORMONE DISRUPTORS DISRUPTING OUR BREASTS?

Since excess estrogen appears to be related to many of the known risk factors, we need to explore the link between environmental estrogens and other xenobiotics and breast cancer. The association between xenoestrogens and breast cancer is controversial in the fields of cancer, toxicology, and epidemiology. Some human studies suggest that environmental estrogens at low doses may directly activate breast cancer cell growth and may be regarded as cocarcinogens in the genesis of breast cancer. Others disagree. (See chart in Appendix C for all the studies that do or do not show a significant correlation between xenoestrogens and breast cancer.)

What is known or suspected about the role of environmental estrogens in breast cancer is:

- They may influence when a woman hits puberty and begins to menstruate. Early menstruation (more years of estrogen cycling) is linked to an increased risk of breast cancer, so this may be one way in which hormone disruptors could increase breast cancer risk.

- A recognized fact from both cell and animal studies is that some EDCS—such as PCBS, DDT, some dyes, and certain ingredients in plastics—cause human breast cancer cells to grow. Plasticizers from food packaging materials exhibit estrogenic activity. Although the plastic component bisphenol A is FDA-approved, it is not broken down in the body as quickly as natural estrogen. When added to human breast can-

VEGETABLES AND BREAST CANCER

Most people believe that dioxin is not healthy. However, Dr. Stephen Safe from Texas A&M University believes dioxin or dioxin-like compounds from vegetables may have potential benefits for estrogen-dependent cancers, such as breast cancer, since these compounds act as antiestrogens and antitumorogenic agents in the breast. They do this by binding to the Ah receptor rather than blocking the estrogen receptor. Related dioxin compounds, such as the nontoxic ones from cruciferous vegetables, have been shown in animal experiments to inhibit mammary tumors and can turn carcinogens into nonactive, non-tumor–promoting metabolites.

cer cells in the laboratory, bisphenol A has been shown to cause cells to grow. It is still a debate as to whether or not bisphenol A actually has an effect on breast tissue in humans.

• DDT and a number of other pesticides now in use stimulate breast cancer cells to grow in ways similar to estradiol. It's of interest to note that one prospective study on 34,000 postmenopausal women from Iowa, which analyzed their food intake, showed a modest increase in breast cancer risk associated with apples, pears, peaches, and strawberries—the fruits that are sprayed with the most endocrine-disrupting pesticides.

• Another possibility, suggested by numerous animal studies, is that exposure to hormone disruptors in the womb may sensitize some women to the adverse effects of their own estrogen and carcinogens.

• In utero exposure to environmental estrogens may program genes in the fetal breast to be more susceptible to getting breast cancer in adulthood.

• In utero exposure to EDCs may increase the breast cells that are more vulnerable to developing breast cancer, as suggested by a 1998 animal study in which rats exposed in utero to dioxin had increased susceptibility to mammary cancer in adulthood.

• Environmental estrogens may play a role in unopposed estrogen, or progesterone resistance.

• They may promote "bad guy" estrogen metabolites that can induce tumor growth or further it along.

Some hormone-disrupting chemicals can damage DNA. Dr. Craig Dees, vice president of research and development at Photogen, Inc., a company doing breast cancer research, says that women who eat many processed foods might be consuming Red Dye No. 3 in quantities well above the levels shown to promote growth or damage DNA in laboratory tests. Our children, eating candies and fast foods, may be getting thirty times higher doses of Red Dye No. 3 than the level that causes genetic damage in the laboratory, especially at a time when developing breast tissue may be most susceptible to environmental hormones. As Dees says, "Red Dye No. 3 appears to have the means, motive, and opportunity to cause breast cancer. All we have to do now is catch it at the scene of the crime." It makes me wonder about red-dyed lipsticks that women wear and retouch all day long because some of these cosmetics contain Red Dye No. 3. If the chemical is applied to the skin, it is absorbed by the body—and this is a daily routine for many women.

Of course, we need to study what effects these substances have in women, not just on breast cells in the laboratory. A 1993 New York study showed that women with the highest blood concentrations of total PCBS and DDE had a four-times increased risk of breast cancer. Then a 1994 study in California found similar results in black women (and nonsignificant trends in white women). These two studies were followed in 1997 by a Harvard study, which could not confirm these results. An extensive review of women exposed to certain herbicides in 120 counties in Kentucky showed a significant increase in breast cancer risk with medium and high levels of exposure. These herbicides (atrazine, simazine, and cyanazine) have been used extensively throughout the United States (and have been for the past 35 years) to control weeds and grasses, mostly in corn production but also on citrus crops, sugarcane, nuts, sorghum, and cotton.

In 1998 a study from Copenhagen found a significant association between breast cancer risk and levels of dieldrin (an organochlorine pesticide, now banned) found in blood samples taken before the women were diagnosed, especially samples taken five years earlier. However, the previous year, Tom Brokaw announced on the Nightly News (NBC) that research had shown that the risk of breast cancer does not increase with exposure to the banned chemicals DDT and PCBS—"putting to rest" the question of whether or not pesticides can cause breast cancer. The Harvard study he was referring to, published in the *New England Journal of Medicine*, was accompanied by an editorial by Dr. Stephen Safe, a professor of toxicology at Texas A&M University, who said this should reassure the public and discourage "chemophobia," an unreasonable fear of chemicals. However, the blood samples in the Harvard study were collected only two years before the 240 women were diagnosed with breast cancer.

Dr. Frederick vom Saal, a biologist known for his work with hormone disruptors, immediately refuted the significance of the Harvard study, saying it is "lamppost science: you lose your keys and you look under the lamppost because that's where the light is." We know that the initiating factors for cancer often take place decades before the disease manifests. Yet studies frequently measure the levels of hormone disruptors in middle-aged women who already have the disease or measure their blood only a few years before they get the disease.

Referring to the 1997 Harvard study, biologist Sandra Steingraber, author of *Living Downstream*, said it well: "Maybe the lesson is that current blood levels of endocrine-disrupting chemicals are not necessarily related to cancer. Instead, the salient factor may be exposure many, many years ago. Chemicals came into our bodies, switched on and switched off certain genes, and had effects on certain hormones at that time. Those chemicals eventually went away, and then decades later you see effects. That is a really scary prospect because it means that you cannot uncover the connection by going in and measuring blood levels and measuring health outcomes and say, Aha! I see there's no connection." Dr. Coral Lamartiniere, a pharmacist at the University of Alabama at Birmingham, exposed pregnant rats to dioxin. This made the offspring more prone to mammary tumors once they became adults. This showed, again, that in utero exposure made the mammary cells more sensitive to carcinogens. That means the key time to measure PCBs and dioxins is in utero.

ASKING THE WRONG QUESTIONS

In other words, asking the wrong questions can guarantee getting the wrong answers. It is my belief that the studies we presently have do not accurately put to rest the association between hormone disruptors and breast cancer.

Dr. Nancy Krieger, associate professor of health and social behavior at Harvard, did a study that looked at women's blood levels thirty years before the onset of breast cancer. But even this may not be early enough. A number of scientific studies on children have measured umbilical-cord blood for hormone-disrupting chemicals and then followed the children for many years. These studies show that there is a distinct correlation between in utero exposure to chemicals and problems with behavior, cognition, and stress reaction. However, the measurable levels of chemicals in the blood did not continue. By the time the children were eleven years old, there was no correlation between the level of chemicals in their blood and the problems they were having. In other words, it is the exposure in the womb that mattered; the levels in the blood at older ages did not reflect the levels that had been present at birth. This means that testing blood levels of chemicals years after birth to see if there is a correlation to disease is missing the effects of in utero exposure.

Another reason studies that measure chemicals through blood levels may be inaccurate is that blood levels, although indicative of the body burden of chemicals, may not really reflect what's happening in the breast. Chemicals can concentrate in the fatty tissue of the breast at levels 200 to 300 times higher than in the blood. Some researchers suggest that breast tissue may be able to concentrate estrogenic compounds from plants many more times than the blood. If this is found to be true, it may be the same for hormone disruptors. Also, analyzing chemicals from blood that has been frozen for several decades may turn out to be unreliable.

It is most likely that hormone disruptors would initiate the deadly cancer scenario during the time in the womb and perhaps up to puberty, while the body is still developing and the breast cells are immature. Translating this hypothesis into a feasible study is not easy. In an ideal world, where plenty of money is available and scientists don't mind launching studies that may be ongoing long after their lifetime, we might be able to design appropriate research. Scientists would measure levels of pollutants in umbilical-cord blood, save this blood in blood banks, follow these children into adulthood, and see who gets cancer. Then the issue of whether pesticides and organochlorines cause cancer could be judged in a more exact light. Perhaps we cannot realistically do these kinds of studies, but studies should try to take into account some of these points.

OTHER CONSIDERATIONS

There are many factors that need to be taken into account before the association between xenoestrogens and breast cancer can be "put to rest." Some of these are as follows:

- Most scientists feel that cancer requires genetic predisposition, as well as initiation and promotion. It is possible that estrogenic chemicals may play a role in any or all three situations, especially through prenatal exposure, but may be more influential in genetically susceptible groups.

- The women in epidemiologic studies generally aren't asked whether or not they breastfed their children, which is one proven way of reducing a woman's body's burden of chemicals as well as decreasing her overall exposure to estrogen.

• Science needs to look at other chemicals besides the few tested to date. Most studies have examined only PCBS or DDT and its metabolite DDE. We haven't looked at many other potential endocrine disruptors, like flame retardants, plastics, and other pesticides. Widely used pesticides (such as atrazine on corn) consistently have been shown to cause mammary cancer in animals.

• Combinations of chemicals haven't been tested yet.

• The metabolism of estrogenic substances has to be taken into account. Chemicals can be metabolized from less to more active estrogens. This means that some metabolites may be more toxic than the original chemical, so just measuring the parent compound in the blood (to find correlations between that compound and disease) may not be accurate. However, some metabolites may be cleared from the body more quickly and thus be less toxic. Even if a chemical has been studied and shown to have no toxic effects, if the metabolites of that chemical aren't also examined, we won't have the whole picture. Estrogens also break down into metabolites. Devra Davis's team has shown that DDT and other chemicals can alter the metabolism of estrogen into more cancer-promoting metabolites.

• Epidemiologic studies have not yet taken into account the increased number of estrogen receptors in breast and tumor tissue, which may have been influenced by in utero exposure to hormone disruptors.

• Larger concentrations of chemicals may be found in the tumor tissue itself in contrast to blood. Most studies don't measure the amount of chemicals in the tumors themselves.

• New studies need to take into account the type of breast cancer and whether it is estrogen-sensitive or not, which may give more accurate information.

• It is possible that xenoestrogens may interact with what our moms ate while we were in the womb. Researchers at Michigan State University took mice known for developing tumors of the reproductive tract and, just to make sure they would in fact develop tumors, half of the mice were given DES. Then the pregnant mice were fed low-fat, high-fat, and no-fat diets. When the daughters were checked, tumors appeared in only 10 percent of the mice who had no DES in utero exposure and were on no- or low-fat diets, whereas 50 percent of the daughters on high-fat diets without the DES exposure got tumors, a fivefold increase. A whopping 68 percent of the mice born to mothers on the high-fat diet plus DES exposure got tumors. Clearly, fat might be altering our sensitivity to hormones later in life and sensitivity to hormone disruptors in utero. This may help explain why the role of fat in breast cancer appears to be so inconsistent—we may be looking in the daughter's supermarket basket when we should be examining the mother's.

• And what about the synthetic hormones used in birth-control pills? In a study on women in New Zealand who took progestin-only birth-control pills, there was an increased risk of breast cancer in recent users. In studies on monkeys given oral contraceptives, those given progestins alone or progestins in combination with estrogen caused the most severe abnormal markers in the breast (atypias) as well as cancer itself. Another study found that thin women between the ages of thirty-five and forty-five, and recent users of birth-control pills during that age, had a modest increase in risk of breast cancer. An analysis of fifty-four studies showed that current users of birth-control pills or those who have used them within the past five years are at higher risk. The analysis suggests birth-control pills may be enhancing growth of preexisting tumors, not necessarily causing breast cancer. The most remarkable finding of this huge analysis—which looked at 50,000 breast cancer cases and more than 100,000 control subjects—is that the breast cancer among birth-control users was significantly more localized rather than spread throughout the body. Once again, more research is warranted.

No Hormone Is an Island

Although we have been focusing on estrogen, endocrine disruptors may mimic or alter a number of the hormones involved in breast tissue biology, such as thyroxine, prolactin, insulin, growth hormones, glucocorticoids, and progesterone.

Thyroxine: Made by the thyroid gland, this hormone influences the response of breast tissues to estrogen. One study examined 102 breast cancer patients and found a prevalence of thyroid diseases. Dr. Susan Porterfield, an endocrine physiologist, explained that thyroid hormone receptors and estrogen receptors are similar. She said, "I believe that low thyroid functioning may make breast tissue and perhaps other tissues more sensitive to xenobiotics." Some xenoestrogens block normal thyroid functioning.

Prolactin: During pregnancy, this hormone elevates to urge the breast to produce milk. At other times, abnormally elevated levels of prolactin have been associated with a number of female problems such as menstrual abnormalities and infertility. Prolactin has been shown to increase the number of estrogen receptors and to affect tumor growth in response to estrogen. Some breast cancer cells can be stimulated to grow in the presence of prolactin, and, in the future, we'll probably be running prolactin breast tumor markers to assist in diagnosis and treatment. In utero exposure to hormone disruptors may set the scene for the body to make more prolactin, as some DES daughters have been shown to have higher levels of prolactin. Human estrogen and bisphenol A were both shown to stimulate elevated releases of prolactin in animal and laboratory studies.

And how about this idea? According to Dr. Timothy Murrell, emeritus professor in community medicine from the University of Adelaide in South Australia, excess prolactin causes free radicals that damage breast cells. He says nipple stimulation produces *oxytocin*—a hormone released during orgasm that causes contractions—which should flush the breast of free radicals and carcinogens. Dr. Murrell published studies which showed that implants of oxytocin caused regression of breast tumors in mice. He recommends "holistic nipple care," which is similar to massage techniques taught by lactation groups.

Insulin: This hormone is important for maintaining normal blood-sugar levels. Elevated levels of insulin and insulin-like growth factors have been implicated in increasing breast cancer risk and have been associated indirectly with elevated levels zof estrogen as well as with amplifying the signal that estrogen sends to the receptors. According to the molecular work of Dr. Craig Dees, insulin-like growth factors may make xenoestrogens more potent. Obese people are known to have more growth factors. Obese and some normal-weight women with elevated levels of growth factors may be more susceptible to xenoestrogens. And some environmental chemicals may bind to insulin receptors and contribute to insulin resistance and increased levels of insulin-like growth factor.

Aromatase: Dr. Tudor Oprea, an M.D. and Ph.D. in molecular physiology, says that hormones, like cars, are put together from various pieces. Part of the estrogen assembly line is performed by an enzyme called aromatase (which helps makes estrogen out of other hormones). It seems logical that aromatase itself may become a target for endocrine disrupters, and recent data suggest just that.

Progesterone: One study showed that women with progesterone deficiency had 5.4 times the risk of premenopausal breast cancer and a tenfold increase in death from the disease. Many doctors now believe that progesterone can also act as a protective agent during breast cancer surgery.

IN THE END

Breast cancer is caused by any number of different factors. It is my belief that hormone disruptors will be found to play a role, and their impact will probably be strongest in certain sensitive populations—such as the fetus, or in those with underactive thyroids, or those with diets low in indole-3 carbinol or B vitamins, or in women who abuse alcohol, or women with lipid (fat) problems, or women who have genetically reduced levels of the proteins that protect against DNA damage. This will all be affected by genetic predisposition, which probably comes in all kinds—from BRCA genes to other genes not yet found. It will also be affected by a person's balance of tumor suppressor and growth factors and the levels of other hormones, such as prolactin and melatonin. As we said at the beginning of this chapter, breast cancer is a complex disease.

Even though more conclusive studies are needed to demonstrate whether or not there is an association between estrogenic chemicals and breast cancer, it certainly makes sense to think in terms of *preventative action*, such as minimizing exposure to chemicals that may disrupt hormone balance and functioning.

Synthetic Hormones and Menopause

> *Members of the "baby-boom" generation have learned to expect medical solutions to "problems" like menopause. Growing up with birth-control pills, our generation is the first in human history with the option of spending the entire fertile life span taking hormones to control reproductive function. Why should post-reproductive, "menopausal" life be any different?*
>
> —Jonathan Wright, M.D., and John Morgenthaler,
> *Natural Hormone Replacement* (Smart Publications, 1997)

Janice, a lawyer, had been irritable, fatigued, and not sleeping well. But it wasn't until she was out on her first date since her divorce, trying to be flirtatious while a convoy of sweat drops slid down her nose and plopped loudly into her coffee, that she finally got the idea: she was going through *the Change.*

Her physician gave her a prescription for hormone replacement therapy (HRT). It relieved her menopausal symptoms, but she had a history of cystic breasts and taking estrogen made her breasts hurt. Janice also worried about increasing her risk of reproductive cancers from too much estrogen. Plus, she'd heard that HRT increased her risk of getting asthma.

On the other hand, she was afraid to go off the synthetic hormones. They were supposed to protect her against heart problems, colon cancer, and Alzheimer's disease. Hormone replacement therapy was also supposed to save women from the dreaded fate of osteoporosis, which ran in Janice's family. Her doctor not only strongly recommended HRT for her bones, he actually implied that if Janice didn't take hormone therapy, one day she'd walk out her front door and *poof* . . . there suddenly would be nothing left but a mere puddle of clothes, shoes, a purse, and keys—a calcium-deficient, boneless mass of what once had been a strong independent woman.

"I'm not stupid," sighed Janice, "but what is a woman to do?"

If you are confused about hormone replacement therapy, you're not alone. Should women be taking pharmaceutical hormones for most of their lives—birth-control pills and/or fertility drugs, followed by HRT? Will they make us younger, healthier, and happier, or are we playing a game of hormonal roulette? In light of information on endocrine disruptors, we must look anew at any hormones we take in from anywhere outside our body.

Most physicians honestly think that the average, healthy, menopausal woman *should* take hormone replacement therapy. Physicians have been taught that the advantages of HRT—a decreased risk for osteoporosis, heart disease, and colon cancer—outweigh the risks, such as breast cancer. A closer examination of scientific studies on the safety and effectiveness of HRT reveals an extremely controversial story. Many of the claims about the potential benefits of HRT may be misleading. Alternative methods do exist and are effective for some women (see Appendix B for natural remedies for menopausal symptoms).

MENOPAUSE

Menopause is defined as the cessation of the menstrual period for one year. Usually in her late forties or early fifties, a woman reaches the end of her menstrual cycling—a natural and inevitable transition from one stage of life to another. For some women, it happens earlier. Today, with our hormones so frequently out of balance, early menopause is becoming almost as common as early puberty. And the earlier the age at which a woman goes into menopause, the more symptoms she is likely to experience. Does this mean that our lifetime exposure to hormone disruptors will aggravate symptoms of menopause?

The pattern of hormone secretions actually starts to change years before a woman has her last period. *Perimenopause* is the segment of time when the hormones start to go out of balance, which can happen any time from a woman's mid-thirties to her forties—anywhere from one to fifteen

---

A NATION OF OLDER WOMEN

For some, menopause is a relief; for others, it leads to the depressing thought: "I'm not young any more." Well, a lot of women aren't young anymore. By the year 2000, 50 million American women were over the age of fifty. It is estimated that by the year 2015, half the women in the United States will be in their menopausal and post-menopausal years. One-third of their lives will be lived in this phase of womanhood. Needless to say, this is a large market for drug companies.

---

years prior to the onset of menopause. Because estrogens and progesterone have profound consequences throughout a woman's body, perimenopause can be marked by a variety of unpleasant effects that reflect the body's response to its changing hormonal milieu.

For some, symptoms that were experienced at a younger age may come back, such as sore breasts or menstrual cramps. Some women become much more uncomfortable than do others. Symptoms can include hot flashes (the only "documented" symptom), chills, insomnia, weight gain, irritability, poor stress-coping skills, a dry vagina, irregular and heavy bleeding, a shortened menstrual cycle, mood swings, depression, low self-esteem, anxiety, maldigestion, fatigue, short-term memory and concentration problems, loss of libido, increased dental and periodontal problems, wrinkles, and a lack of muscle tone in the urethra and supporting pelvic muscles, which can cause incontinence. Women may also experience low thyroid hormone levels or poor cellular response to thyroid hormone, which can create thinner and drier hair and skin, hoarse voice, constipation, getting cold easily (especially in the extremeties), water retention, facial puffiness in the morning, thickening and scaling skin, elevated cholesterol, and slowed speech and movements. All symptoms may be increased by emotional stress, cigarette smoking, alcohol consumption, and caffeine. What fun.

As if suffering with varying symptoms is not enough, after menopause there is a dramatic increase in the risk of serious cardiovascular disease—high blood pressure, heart attack, and stroke. The risk of osteoporosis increases. Heart disease, stroke, and four out of the five top cancers all appear to have a relationship to the hormone levels in our bodies. Another unwanted possibility is loss of memory or a decrease in mental acuity. It's no surprise that women are quite eager to alleviate their unwanted symptoms and reduce the risks associated with menopause.

HORMONE REPLACEMENT THERAPY

The major medical solution to menopause for the last three decades has been the use of synthetic hormones. If a lack of estrogen is making life miserable, why not just replace the estrogen? Estrogen has been shown to be helpful with many aspects of menopause and postmenopausal life. Estrogen can reduce the risk of osteoporotic fractures by 50 percent, can elevate the good cholesterol (which has been shown to help protect against heart disease), and may reduce plaque build-up in the arteries. These are all good things. Doctors have been so convinced about the importance of replacing estrogen that in 1996 more than 22 million prescriptions were written for Premarin in the United States. That's nearly $370 million a year for its manufacturer, Wyeth-Ayerst Pharmaceuticals.

When estrogen replacement therapy came out, it was "replacing" only estrogen. After a type of uterine cancer called endometrial cancer significantly increased, physicians discovered that the risk of developing endometrial cancer due to estrogen replacement could be reduced by also replacing the hormone progesterone, which blocks or opposes estrogen's cancer-causing tendencies in the uterus. Note, however, that natural progesterone is not the same as progestins, which are synthetic compounds that bear some similarities to natural progesterone. Doctors today usually prescribe a synthetic progestin called Provera. It is this combination of Premarin and Provera (or similar products) that makes up standard hormone replacement therapy (HRT).

If a synthetic hormone reduces perimenopausal discomfort and prevents the consequences of hormone depletion after menopause, why not use it? Some women get truly distressing symptoms during menopause and upon taking HRT they feel much better—their quality of life is greatly improved. Others take HRT and develop side effects that can be far worse than their original problems. A Massachusetts Women's Health Study showed that by the end of the first year of using HRT, half the women had stopped because of side effects, such as:

- resumption of menstrual cycle
- spotting
- stomach upset and nausea

PREMARIN

Estrogen was first made in the 1920s from the urine of pregnant women. In 1943 a synthetic estrogen was made from the urine of pregnant mares. It was called conjugated equine estrogen and named Premarin (since it came from PREgnant MARes' urINe). Although Premarin exerts estrogenic effects in humans, horse estrogen is not the same as human estrogen and is not necessarily as safe or as effective.

Note for animal lovers: in order to collect horse urine on a profitable scale, as many as 75,000 to 80,000 pregnant mares must be confined in tiny stalls for most of their eleven-month pregnancy. They live on restricted fluids so as not to dilute the urine, are allowed no exercise, and may not even be allowed to lie down. The rubber cups attached to the mare's urethra to catch the urine cause sores and painful urinary tract infections. After giving birth, the mares are pastured with their foals for only a few months before they are reimpregnated. Many of these mares become crippled or die as a result of the stress to which they are subjected. Most of the foals are sent to slaughter and exported to foreign markets for human consumption. To protest the conditions of Pregnant Mares Urine (PMU) farms, write to Dr. Donna Shalala, Secretary of Health and Human Services, Dept. of Agriculture, 200 Independence Ave. S.W., Washington, DC 20201.

- fluid retention
- swollen breasts, mastitis (breast infections), nipple sensitivity
- vaginal pain
- skin pigmentation changes
- leg and uterine cramps
- harder-to-read mammograms
- weight gain
- asthma

As you have learned throughout this book, a man-made chemical can produce different effects than a natural chemical because of the way it interacts with the cells of our bodies. The enzymes in a woman's body that chemically change, neutralize, and/or dispose of natural hormones—allowing them to produce their desired effects in the right amount for just the right time and then quietly and quickly leave—may not necessarily process patentable hormone molecules in exactly the same way. Equilin (the estrogen in Premarin) produces estrogenic effects that are more potent and longer lasting than those produced by natural human estrogens. For example, equilin has a more powerful influence on the growth of uterine tissue than does natural estrogen.

Can Women Really Become Estrogen-Deficient?

Replacing estrogen might be a good idea, but contrary to popular belief, menopause is *not* simply an estrogen-deficiency syndrome. Rather, it is a time in a woman's life when numerous hormones start to decline. Progesterone, which used to be produced at ovulation, is now absent except for the small amount produced by the adrenal glands. Testosterone decreases anywhere from 50 to 60 percent. Thyroid and DHEA hormones can go out of balance. This is in addition to the fact that women lose about two-thirds of their estrogen production—the 17-beta estradiol made by the ovaries declines (bringing about postmenopausal changes) and the adrenal glands take over, producing certain androgens that are converted into estrone. Estrone now becomes the main estrogen in the body rather than estradiol.

The breast (as well as other tissues) manufactures an enzyme (aromatase) that produces estrogens locally in the breast. Emerging data suggest that aromatase itself may become a target for endocrine disrupters. The ovaries continue to produce small amounts of estrogens, which vary significantly from woman to woman. According to George M. Stancel, from the University of Texas, there was a wide variance among healthy women's estrogen blood levels.

The fact is that perimenopause and the onset of menopause is a time when a woman's hormones are all over the place. Sometimes a woman's estrogen levels are elevated or the ratios of the individual estrogens are altered from what they were when a woman was premenopausal. Some symptoms come from *high* estrogen—bloating, tender breasts, and heavy bleeding—whereas hot flashes, vaginal dryness, and acne are from low estrogen. Women who are more prone to periods of surging hormones than others may be more at risk of breast cancer or other estrogen-dependent problems from taking HRT.

Consider that many contemporary women have been estrogen domi-nant much of their reproductive years due to the fact that they have had many more ovulatory cycles than most other women in history. They have children later in life, have fewer children, or never give birth. They are entering into puberty earlier (which may be linked to hormone disrup-tors and/or better nutrition). All this adds up to greater lifetime exposure to natural estrogenic signaling.

What happens when a woman who already has a history of an increased lifetime exposure to estrogen is also exposed to environmental estrogens?

Millions of women who are approaching or have entered menopause were born and grew up in the decades after World War II. The 1950s and 1960s were the heyday of chemical complacency, the days when progress was indeed the most important product. They were the years with the highest exposures to DDT and PCBS, the years when 13 million tons of DES were dumped into animal feed annually. Chemicals of all kinds were being used at preregulatory levels. Since fetal exposure to endocrine-disrupting chemicals is being implicated as the most dangerous window of vulnera-bility, many of the women born in those decades may already have been

---

ESTROGENS

Estrogen is an umbrella term commonly used to denote the three main types of estro-gens—estrone, estradiol, and estriol—which usually fluctuate in a woman's body in the following approximate proportions:

- *estrone*—the predominant estrogen found in postmenopausal women, produced in the body fat tissue. This is the form of estrogen that many researchers think may be related to the higher risk of endometrial and breast cancer in obese older women.

- *17-beta estradiol*—the most biologically potent of the three estrogens and the most generally known

- *estriol*—considered the least potent and the least likely to cause cancer and there-fore one of the safest of all of the estrogens

It makes you wonder why HRT doesn't use estriol along with other estrogens. Natural hormone replacement (see Appendix B) uses a high proportion of estriol and smaller amounts of the other two estrogens in Tri-est formulations.

---

far more estrogenic during their reproductive years than their forebears, giving them imbalances between estrogen and their other hormones.

We have to remember, again and again, that it is the balance of hormones in our endocrine system that is important. Estrogen is just the tip of the iceberg. Endocrine disruptors have been implicated in affecting a variety of other hormone signals in addition to estrogen, such as thyroid, adrenal, and vitamins A and D. Low levels of vitamin D are associated with an increase of abnormal growth of breast cells. Lowered levels of vitamin A or altered vitamin A metabolism have been associated with menstrual irregularities. Thyroid malfunctions have been related to estrogen problems and are possible causal factors in breast cancer. Thus, giving the body more estradiol (and synthetic progestins) at the time of menopause may not be as prudent a course of action as common medical thought has believed. The same may hold true for natural estrogen and progesterone products. Dr. Alan Gaby, the renowned medical nutritionist and educator, says: "The most effective hormone-replacement regimen is likely to be that which replaces *all* deficient hormones."

HRT AND THE LIVER

Women with a history of active gall bladder or liver disease, migraine sufferers, smokers, or those with elevated triglycerides will do better with the skin patch rather than the oral route of delivery if they are taking synthetic estrogens. When any oral HRT is first swallowed, it goes straight from the intestines to the liver, where it has an estrogenic effect. Dr. Walter Elger, a researcher specializing in HRT, says, "Excessive estrogenic action in the liver is considered a high price to pay for the convenience of oral estrogen therapy."

HRT AND CORONARY HEART DISEASE (CHD)

One of the main reasons (besides rescuing our bones) that doctors have classically recommended HRT to women is to *prevent* heart disease—the leading cause of death for women after menopause. It has been drummed into us that, since more postmenopausal women die of heart disease than breast cancer, the benefits of HRT far outweigh the risks. But as of March 2000, this no longer seems to be true. At their annual meeting, the American College of Cardiology stated that HRT is of no benefit to postmenopausal women who already have heart disease. And three major studies imply that *all* women on HRT may be more at risk of adverse cardiac effects than women not taking hormones. In other words, the latest results bring into question whether or not HRT protects good hearts or prevents bad hearts from getting worse. Let's look at this new information together.

Results suggesting HRT does not help hearts were first brought forth in the preliminary PEPI study (the Postmenopausal Estrogen and Progestin Intervention trial from the National Heart, Lung, and Blood Institute, part of the NIH) on 875 healthy postmenopausal women. After three years, women receiving HRT had 20 percent lower "bad" LDL-cholesterol and much higher "good" HDL-cholesterol than women who were given a placebo. This report was widely covered by the media, which hailed the study as the first real proof that HRT prevents heart disease.

However, many drugs that have been shown to lower bad cholesterol still fail to prevent heart disease. In the PEPI study, five new cases of heart disease developed, *all* in the HRT group, while *none* occurred in women receiving a placebo. Also, ten women on HRT developed blood clots, while none on a placebo got them. Applying statistical analysis to these results yields a 71 percent probability that treating postmenopausal women with HRT actually *causes* heart disease.

The PEPI study was looking at healthy women. The Heart and Estrogen/Progestin Replacement Study (HERS), on the other hand, was the first large randomized clinical trial that examined the effect of hormone replacement therapy on 2,763 women who already had heart disease. This study showed that the use of estrogen plus progestin in women with heart disease did *not* prevent further heart attacks or death from coronary heart disease. This occurred despite the positive effect of treatment on blood fats. LDL (bad) cholesterol was reduced by 11 percent and HDL (good) cholesterol was increased by 10 percent. HRT also increased the risk of clots in the veins (a serious and potentially fatal condition called deep vein thrombosis) and lungs (pulmonary embolism), as well as the risk of gallbladder disease by 40 percent.

In the HERS study, they found that during the first year on HRT, women had a trend toward increased coronary "events" such as heart attacks. This trend was gone after four years, with the risk being equal to women not on HRT. The authors suggested that until more research is done, women with heart disease should *not* be given combined HRT to reduce the risk of heart attacks.

STATISTICS CAN BE MISLEADING

Studies that have been done on HRT have what is called a selection bias. It is well documented that women who take estrogen also tend to eat healthier food, exercise more often, go to the doctor more frequently for checkups, have higher IQ ratings, and generally take better care of themselves than do nonusers of estrogen. In other words, they tend to be better compliers with recommendations about how to improve their lives. Furthermore, only healthy women are given HRT in the first place, and women are taken off HRT when they get seriously ill. Women in high-isk groups—such as those with fibrocystic breasts, a history of breast or endometrial cancer, high blood pressure, or women at risk of stroke—tend not to be put on HRT.

The PEPI study also eliminated women who were obese or who had hypertension, abnormal mammograms, diabetes, hypothyroidism, or severe menopausal symptoms. Eliminating high-risk groups from the studies is a good way to get inaccurate data about how the women who are taking it are reducing their risk of getting disease. It is quite possible that the statistics showing a reduction in heart disease risk associated with HRT are due to one or more of these other factors and are not related to the hormone replacement therapy itself.

A third study, presented at the American College of Cardiology by Dr. David Harrington and investigators in the Estrogen and Atherosclerosis (ERA) trial, supported the HERS results.

As if that weren't enough, here is another new wrinkle. The build-up of plaque in the arteries, called atherosclerosis, is one hallmark of heart disease. This process begins with high cholesterol, but more adverse events (such as heart attacks) are caused by inflammation. Inflammation is measured in the blood by something called C reactive protein (CRP). The higher your C reactive protein, the more your risk of heart disease, even more so than with elevated cholesterol. It has been shown that when healthy postmenopausal women are put on HRT, inflammation increases in their bodies, as evidenced by elevated levels of CRP.

These results make HRT look less like the perfect heart panacea we thought it was. What's going on here? Have the studies not been going on long enough for us to get a clear picture? Is combination HRT not doing a good job protecting the heart, or are the progestins blocking the heart-protective effect of estrogens?

Kent Hermsmeyer heads a team at the Oregon Regional Primate Research Center in Beaverton. They gave estrogen every day to eighteen rhesus monkeys who'd had their ovaries removed to simulate menopause. Half got natural progesterone and the other half got the most widely prescribed synthetic progestin for women in the United States (medroxyprogesterone acetate, called MPA, the progestin used in Provera). After four weeks, the animals were injected with chemicals to simulate a heart attack. The animals on the MPA had such severe constriction of their blood vessels that without intervention they would have died. The animals on estrogen alone or in combination with the natural progesterone recovered quickly without any treatment. When the researchers reported their findings, Hermsmeyer said, "The big surprise is that MPA poses such a huge risk. This is a really dangerous drug."

At Wake Forest University's Bowman Gray School of Medicine, J. Loudy Williams was not surprised. His studies had been suggesting similar findings. His research team's results show that MPA can "obliterate the beneficial effect of estrogen therapy on the progression of coronary artery atherosclerosis."

All this means that one of the major supposed benefits of HRT—reducing the risk of heart disease—appears to go out the window when we add progestins to protect against estrogen's increased risk of endometrial cancer. This should give us pause about HRT.

HRT AND CANCER

Estrogens are growth-promoting hormones used by a woman's body to stimulate the growth of cells in the endometrial lining of the uterus and cells of the breast to prepare for pregnancy and lactation. Excess estrogens can turn on too much cell division and growth. They do this, according to the research team of Ana Soto and Carlos Sonnenschein, by turning off natural inhibitors of cell proliferation.

Breast Cancer

At the beginning of the year 2000, new research shook up a lot of women—and rightly so. Studies clearly indicated that women on combination HRT (synthetic estrogens plus progestins) are more likely to get breast cancer than women who receive estrogen alone or are not on HRT. In other words, progestins, originally added to lower the risk of uterine cancer, are now increasing the risk of breast cancer. Exasperating, yes, but this new can of worms has been confirmed by three studies.

First, investigators from the National Cancer Institute followed 46,355 women and tracked the 2,082 cases of postmenopausal breast cancer that occurred among them. It turned out that women on estrogen-only HRT had a 20 percent higher risk, whereas women on both hormones had a 40 percent increased risk. Ouch. A second study from UCLA found that women who received combined HRT for five to ten years were 51 percent more likely to develop breast cancer.

A WORD OF WARNING

A woman who develops cystic breasts (benign breast disease) for the first time when she starts taking HRT may be at an especially high risk of developing breast cancer if she continues taking estrogen.

These studies added to what had already reared its head in 1997, in the Nurses' Health Study. This sixteen-year project, following 121,700 registered nurses on HRT to determine its effects, reported that initially women on HRT live longer, having a 37 percent lower risk of death from any cause. But after ten years, the reduction in mortality went down to 20 percent, as the women on HRT started dying from breast cancer.

Why is this happening? Well, perhaps it's hormone disruption. The progestins, which repress estrogen receptors in the uterus, appear to be stimulating the receptors in the breast.

Normally during menopause breasts start to sag (I hate that word). This happens partially because cell growth is low due to decreased levels of estrogen. However, now it appears that progestins added to HRT enhance estrogen's ability to make breast cells grow. Evidence from mammograms taken of women on HRT confirm that breast cell growth is greater when estrogen is given along with progestins than by itself. Apparently, all this growth and commotion in the aging breast may not be safe.

One month after the above studies hit the news, the American College of Obstetricians and Gynecologists (ACOG) sent out recommendations to physicians to *not* alter current use of combined hormone replacement therapy. Some good news is that most studies show that four to five years after women quit HRT, the higher risks for breast cancer disappear.

Earlier analyses of HRT and breast cancer studies were done on women who took HRT only for short periods of time—mainly to get rid of hot flashes. Nowadays women routinely take these synthetic hormones for long periods of time to benefit their bones and heart. If these hormones increase the growth of both normal and abnormal breast cells, we need to look at them more carefully. Studies show that women who go on HRT are thinner and have more symptoms and less bone density—all signs of having lower estrogen and, thus, lower risk of breast cancer. For other women with more estrogen, adverse effects may have been underestimated.

Some evidence suggests that women who are currently taking HRT and get breast cancer have less aggressive forms and have better survival rates. Avrum Bluming, a California oncologist, started a study in 1992 in which 200 women with a history of breast cancer are taking HRT. Their rates of recurrence and death (at the time of writing this book) are equal to those women with breast cancer who are not on HRT. Personally, I would be afraid to take classical HRT with my history of ER+ breast cancer and being a DES daughter.

Putting all the studies in one big pot and stirring them gives us a trend—there is a modest increase in the risk of breast cancer with estrogen-only HRT and a larger risk on combined HRT. It appears that the most increased risk comes from long-term and current use and that this effect increases every year as the woman ages. Women who drink alcohol and take HRT heighten this risk more.

Ovarian Cancer

A seven-year study of 240,000 women in Atlanta, Georgia, indicated the risk of fatal ovarian cancer increased with the length of time the women had been using HRT. Women who had been using estrogen for six or more years and then stopped were found to be as much at risk as continuous users. This is an issue that is seldom addressed with synthetic HRT, but it is important, as ovarian cancer is extremely difficult to diagnose and cure. Several other studies that investigated the association between estrogen replacement therapy and ovarian cancer have given inconsistent results.

Uterine Cancer

Conventional estrogen replacement therapy is known to increase the risk of uterine cancer. To overcome that increased risk, doctors prescribe Provera or other progestins. Unfortunately, as mentioned previously, progestins have a number of side effects and risks of their own.

HRT AND OSTEOPOROSIS

One fear related to aging centers around osteoporosis. Bone is hardy, but it is still a living tissue that is constantly being broken down and rebuilt throughout life. In osteoporosis, the osteoclasts (cells that dissolve or resorb older bone) are outrunning the osteoblasts (cells that construct new bone tissue), which results in a loss of bone tissue. After menopause, bone loss accelerates, sometimes reaching a rate of 1 to 1.5 percent per year.

The studies to date on HRT suggest it can reduce fractures caused by osteoporosis by 50 percent. (However, the women who take HRT may be healthier to begin with, so the statistics may not be accurate for the general population.) Estrogen helps reduce fractures by preventing the increase of bone resorption that occurs with menopause, but estrogen cannot enhance new bone formation. Even natural estrogens do not stimulate the growth of new bone cells. Thus, any bone loss a woman already has experienced (and bone loss often starts in the mid-thirties) is not reversed. And once a woman is on HRT and then goes off it, the bone loss continues, sometimes at an accelerated pace. Therefore, if estrogen is used to treat or prevent osteoporosis, it has to be given before significant bone loss has occurred, and it has to be given continuously.

Another approach to making bones stronger during and after menopause is to use natural progesterone and possibly DHEA and testosterone. Natural progesterone has been shown to stimulate bone formation. Dr. Jonathan Wright has seen reversals of osteoporosis in several of his patients who had bone density scans performed at the University of Washington. These patients were on natural triple estrogens, DHEA, progesterone, and testosterone (if appropriate), as well as the diet mentioned in Dr. Alan Gaby's book *Preventing and Reversing Osteoporosis* (Prima, 1994).

According to Dr. John R. Lee, the pioneer in the study of natural progesterone in postmenopausal women, it is progesterone (and, to a lesser degree, progestins) that actually works to restore bone tissue. Most American women are experiencing some bone loss long before they reach menopause and long before their estrogen levels drop. Since the mid-1970s, when the link between unopposed estrogen and endometrial cancer was discovered, most women who take patentable estrogens also take a patentable progestin.

Some of Dr. Lee's patients increased the density of their lumbar vertebrae by 20 to 25 percent in the first year of using a natural progesterone replacement cream. Over three years, the mean increase in bone density in his study was 15.4 percent. If the women had not used natural progesterone, a 4 to 5 percent loss in bone density would have been expected. Even women over age seventy had the same gains as younger women. Dr. John Lee wondered, why was estrogen—and not progesterone—given credit for preventing osteoporosis?

There are now "designer estrogens" being marketed, which are targeted specifically for the prevention of osteoporosis. Drugs such as raloxifene (Evista)—called selective estrogen receptor modulators (SERMS)—are designed to increase bone mass with no increased risk of breast or uterine cancer. However, they have only been tested in studies of up to three years (as of 1999). When I heard an impassioned infommercial about this product at the Estrogen and Foods Conference, I asked the scientist who had helped synthesize this drug, "What happens to women after five years of use?" He had no answer.

ESTROGEN AND ADULT ASTHMA

Researchers from Harvard Medical School studied more than 23,000 women who participated in the Nurses' Health Study. They found that women taking postmenopausal hormones were 50 percent more likely to suffer adult-onset asthma—which is triggered and/or driven by hyperimmune responses—than women who had never taken the hormones. This could help to explain why adult-onset asthma affects more women than men (although childhood asthma strikes more boys than girls). The number of women with asthma soars at the onset of puberty, when the ovaries begin to produce large amounts of estrogen. There is twice the normal incidence of asthma among women who use HRT for ten or more years. Again, doctors believe that estrogen's benefits outweigh any risk of asthma for most women. Of course, if you already suffer with asthma, you must discuss this with your physician.

EACH WOMAN IS UNIQUE

The real issue is whether or not HRT is safe for an individual woman and what her alternatives might be. Not all women respond the same way to estrogen. A study by Dr. Walter Elger on postmenopausal women who were taking HRT showed a wide range of responses to the estrogen. In some women, it lasted for hours, while in others it was present for only several minutes. How quickly a woman's body processes the synthetic hormone depends on many factors, including her fat, liver function, and levels of other hormones and enzymes.

Part of the whole frustration of health care in general and hormone replacement therapies in particular is that there isn't one simple answer that applies equally for every woman: each woman must work in collaboration with her doctor(s) to find her optimal treatment. Medicine is not the exact science we all want it to be, which is why it is called both a science and an art. The art is in matching treatment alternatives to the individual. In order to make a decision, a woman must understand the pros and cons of what is available and what these options mean in relation to her lifelong exposure to her own natural hormones and to environmental estrogens, to her personal and family health history, as well as to her particular lifestyle choices.

What makes sense here? First evaluate your total hormonal picture through blood, saliva, and urine tests and a thorough personal and family history workup. With a doctor, evaluate your risk of breast and colon cancer, osteoporosis, and dementia. Run lipid profiles and bone-density studies to give you more information.

Next, it is prudent to use protocols that take into account the balance of all your hormones. Many women do well with natural hormones and easy, safe-to-take dietary and herbal alternatives. In fact, at a recent symposium on menopause for breast cancer patients, oncologists recommended nutrients and herbs as the protocol for high-risk groups.

However, not all women are helped by alternative methods. If you do not get relief of menopausal symptoms from natural methods, then try more conventional treatments. One important new study has shown that women can use lower doses of replacement hormones to prevent postmenopausal bone loss with reduced side effects if they take calcium and vitamin D along with the hormones. The lower dose may also reduce the risk of breast cancer, although that was not part of the study.

There is no easy answer, but it comes down to assessing risk versus benefit. For example, an older woman with high risk for colon cancer and no family history of breast or ovarian cancer may have little risk from any hormone replacement regime, synthetic or natural, compared to the benefit she will receive from it. On the other hand, someone like me—a DES daughter with a history of breast cancer—probably has a bigger risk compared to the benefits.

In choosing any hormone therapy, synthetic or natural, you and your health-care practitioner should discuss your heart disease risk profile.

Risk factors that are beyond your control:

- being age fifty-five or older
- having a family history of early heart disease (mother or sister diagnosed before age sixty-five or father or brother diagnosed before age fifty-five)
- high blood pressure
- asthma

Risk factors under your control:

- cigarette smoking
- high blood cholesterol
- diabetes (high blood sugar)
- obesity
- physical inactivity

Other factors:

- drinking alcohol (too much increases risk of high blood pressure)
- salt intake (too much increases risk of high blood pressure in salt-sensitive people; however this is a complex and controversial area of hypertension research)

Have your doctor run your lipid profiles and C reactive protein.

Heart disease has declined among men and women in the last 20 years. This is due to the fact that there are a number of well-defined lifestyle changes that lower the risk of heart disease: quit smoking, control high blood pressure and cholesterol levels, and get regular exercise. Taking a daily multiple vitamin reduces the risk of heart disease by 25 percent! Breast cancer prevention does not, on the other hand, offer easy what-to-

RISK FACTORS FOR HRT

HIGH-RISK GROUP

- close family history of breast cancer (a controversial issue)
- personal history of ER+ breast cancer (a controversial issue)
- personal history of endometrial (uterine) cancer
- active thrombophlebitis
- active gallbladder disease
- personal history of asthma

No one knows yet about DES daughters.

POSSIBLE HIGH RISK

- more distant family history of breast cancer
- personal history of hypertension (high blood pressure)
- personal history of heart disease
- personal history of benign breast disease—atypical markers or DCIS
- personal history of fibroids (particularly large or painful ones)
- personal history of endometriosis
- personal history of diabetes
- personal history of heart thrombosis, pulmonary embolism, and/or stroke

---

dos because it does not seem to be related so much to lifestyle as to lifetime exposure to estrogen, hormonal events, and genetics that are mostly beyond our control.

The more informed you are, the better decisions you can make for your body. See Appendix B to learn about natural hormone replacement and hormone potentiators. Don't listen to any single doctor. No doctor is infallible. And don't make your decisions based only on what worked for your friends.

Other Health Problems

> *Time and time again, we observed that various persistent pollutants can cause damage to living organisms: dioxin-like compounds can promote tumours, pollutants with oestrogenic effects can affect reproductive capacity, other substances can harm the central nervous system, and so on.*
>
> —Swedish Environmental Protection Agency, Claes Bernes, "Persistent Organic Pollutants: A Swedish View of an International Problem," *Monitor* 16 (trans. Martin Naylor)

When Albert Einstein was active as a professor, one of his students came to him and said: "The questions on this year's exam are the same as last year's!"

"True," Einstein said, "but this year all the answers are different."

And so it goes with hormone disruptors. Each new study brings up new answers to old questions—and frequently brings new questions. Some health conditions that occur in both men and women that have long been looked at from only one perspective must now be examined to see if they are related in any way to hormone disruption.

Our Body's Army: The Immune System

When most of us hear of problems with the immune system, we tend to think of AIDS or cancer. We don't usually think of illnesses like arthritis or lupus, let alone problems of the thyroid or the hormonal system, as being influenced by the immune system. However, no part of the human body is an island. All our systems are like back-fence gossips, constantly informing each other about what is going on everywhere else—and the immune system is an influential member of this coffee klatch.

The immune system is definitively linked to the endocrine system. Once again, DES is the model of this interrelatedness. Studies on the children of DES-exposed mothers have provided compelling evidence that in utero exposure can profoundly and permanently affect the immune system. DES daughters have increased cases of lupus, strep throat, rheumatic fever, and other rare hyperactive immune functioning, and both DES sons and daughters show increased cases of upper respiratory infections and rheumatoid arthritis (an immune-related arthritis).

Autoimmune conditions—where the body attacks some part of itself, as in lupus, Hashimoto's thyroiditis, Grave's disease, and Addison's disease—happen when the immune system isn't regulated properly and starts to attack itself. Autoimmune diseases can cause a significant decrease in quality of life. Approximately 8.5 million people in the United States suffer with autoimmune diseases, and 1.2 million new cases occur every five years. These numbers may be underestimated because they are infrequently studied. It is well accepted that females are more prone to autoimmune disease. (Sometimes life just isn't fair.)

Autoimmunity and immune deficiency are often linked. Dr. Allen Silverstone, in his laboratory at SUNY Health Science Center in New York, is doing research that might explain why autoimmunity happens frequently in DES sons and daughters. He has found that exposure to DES or dioxin in utero hampers the proper development of certain immune cells (called T-cells because they are made in the thymus), which are an important part of the immune system. When the T-cells get damaged, the immune system can become its own enemy, in addition to having trouble fighting off foreign invaders.

Silverstone says, "Immunity is very complicated, and people don't quite understand that autoimmunity and immune deficiency can be tightly linked. People can have immunodeficiencies, and because they do, their immune system isn't regulated properly, so they develop autoimmunities. This is one thing I have been studying: why immune problems and autoimmunity are at such a high level in DES sons and daughters, and why we should be worried about these things with chemicals in the environment that act like estrogens. We should be looking for immune problems, definitely, from these environmental estrogens."

This is beginning to happen. The United States EPA in October 1999 approved test guidelines to be used in assessing chemicals for immunosuppressive effects. The science regarding environmental agents and autoimmune disease is in the early stages of hazard identification.

In 1996 Robert Repetto and Sanjay Baliga conducted an exhaustive review of scientific literature on the impact of pesticides on immune system function, including both laboratory studies of animals and epidemiological studies of people. They said it is clear that pesticides do impair immune system function, sometimes severely, and this suppression of the immune system may make people, especially children, more vulnerable to infectious diseases. They found that children from the agricultural district of central Moldova (the Republic of Moldova is a sovereign state situated in southeastern Europe between Romania and Ukraine), where pesticides are used heavily, were three times more likely to have infectious diseases of the digestive tract and two to five times more likely to have infectious diseases of the respiratory tract, and 80 percent of these children, while apparently healthy, showed signs of suppressed immune function. Dr. Repetto commented: "New research may well show that the most widespread public health threat from pesticides is immuno-suppression that weakens the body's resistance to infectious diseases and to cancers."

Data from the National Cancer Institute indicate that the incidence of non-Hodgkin's lymphoma (NHL) has increased since the 1940s in the United States and the United Kingdom. One hypothesis is that NHL may be indirectly related to environmental compounds that suppress the immune system, such as PCBs. Much of this immune suppression from pesticides is through the mechanism of endocrine disruption.

Animals are not exempt from the effects of hormone disruptors on their immune systems. Monkeys have adverse changes in their white blood cells (the immune system's army) when exposed to dioxin, even at levels *below* normal background exposure. One single dose of dioxin to mice significantly decreased their resistance to the flu virus. Seals fed PCB- and dioxin-contaminated fish from the Baltic Sea had significantly lower killer–T-cell activity (cells to fight off illnesses like cancer) and other diminished immune responses when compared to seals fed less contaminated fish. It is also thought that contaminated fish were the cause of massive die-offs of seals in the North Sea, seals in the Baltic Sea, and dolphins along the Eastern U.S. seaboard, because the animals' immune systems were weakened by contamination and they couldn't fight off infection. Mice exposed prenatally to the insecticide chlordane develop lifelong immune suppression. These findings, along with human reports, suggest prenatal exposure to certain immunotoxicants may play a role in autoimmunity in adulthood.

Systemic lupus erythematosis (SLE) is a chronic autoimmune disease that can have many symptoms, such as arthritis, kidney failure, seizures, and neurologic complications. People with this disease (and their relatives) have been shown to have more of a particular metabolite of estradiol that hormone disruptors might promote. Unopposed estrogen is possibly one of the causes of SLE. In the Nurses' Health Study, the risk of SLE was slightly increased in women who had ever used oral contraceptives (older forms with more estrogen than what is used today), and there is a suspicion that fertility drugs also increased risk. The authors of this study say that endocrine disruptors should be investigated as one cause of lupus.

Thyroid and Adrenals

If your date shows up dressed in a tuxedo and a bow tie, you'll see exactly where the thyroid gland is located—right where the middle knot in the tie goes over the front of the throat. Most people think of the thyroid as the gland that controls metabolism. However, the influence of thyroid hormones is far-reaching, including the essential development of the unborn child—affecting gender as well as aspects of the brain such as intellect, memory, and other aspects of cognition. Thyroid hormones are pivotal for normal brain function throughout life. Thus, hormones secreted by this small knot at the base of our throat are necessary for normal behavioral, intellectual, and neurological development.

Like its cousin, the estrogen receptor, the thyroid receptor has a fair amount of "wobble"—and the more wobble a receptor has, the more likely it is to accommodate ecohormones and to facilitate the ensuing hormone disruption. According to the authors of a thyroid study, ". . . the thyroid gland is a direct link between the human body and its surroundings. Problems with thyroid functioning are increasing throughout the United States." In a related note, a research team studied eighty-two women with breast cancer and found one-fourth had thyroid disorder and another quarter of the women were candidates for thyroid disease.

Since a number of EDCs have been implicated as thyroid disruptors, this may be another manner in which hormone disruption plays an indirect role in unopposed estrogen. In a study of twenty-nine women, thyroid hormone actually stimulated the release of active progesterone from the luteal cells (where progesterone is made). In other words, thyroid hormone is necessary to get progesterone into the bloodstream. If thyroid hormone is inhibited, there is a greater chance for estrogen to be unopposed.

What is important to understand is that multiple environmental pollutants (and some of their metabolites) are similar in structure to thyroid hormones. In humans, thyroid hormones are almost completely bound as they travel through the blood. It is the unbound *free* fraction that is available for biological processes throughout the body. Since less than 0.1 percent of thyroid hormone is free, Mother Nature has constructed a situation in which only tiny amounts of thyroid hormone are available to bind to thyroid hormone receptors. If a hormone disruptor is free to bind to thyroid receptors or to thyroid-binding proteins, even small changes in thyroid signaling or available thyroid hormone levels may cause shifts with profound consequences. For example, thyroid is necessary for normal hearing development. If it's blocked, hearing loss can occur.

Dr. Susan Porterfield—an endocrine physiologist who has been working for years on how the developing fetal brain is affected by thyroid during pregnancy—has shown that PCB exposure in utero (in rats) decreases the level of one of the thyroid hormones in the blood, which then decreases the amount that gets into the developing brain. However, she emphasizes that thyroid hormone is so important for the brain that the brain has fail-safe mechanisms. Thus, when the level of thyroid hormone in the brain lowers, there is an elevation in a certain enzyme that helps produce more active thyroid. (Somewhat like having an ace hidden in the brain's back pocket.)

The body does have a certain amount of adaptability—mechanisms that act as back-up systems that come to our rescue when normal functioning is threatened. Whether these back-up systems will thoroughly protect against endocrine disruption or not remains to be seen. We do not know what it would take to overwhelm these protective buffering systems. Just how many assaults can they handle and still keep everything humming? Certain sensitive groups, such as the unborn and the elderly, often have fewer buffering mechanisms than healthy adults. And some people have better back-up systems in general than do others. Those at the lower end of buffering-system capacity may be more vulnerable to assaults.

Thyroid problems and PCB contamination are being linked in Slovakia (the eastern part of former Czechoslovakia). From a personal communication with Dr. Pavel Langer, I learned that heavy PCB pollution exists in Slovakia because under the former communist government it was illegal to even *speak* about pollution. Dr. Langer started to work in this field just after the bloodless revolution in 1989. He has published papers linking thyroid problems (especially thyroiditis, where the body starts to attack its own thyroid) with PCBs, both in individuals exposed on the job and the public at large. Iodine levels (insufficient iodine is frequently a cause of thyroid-related problems) have been monitored for 45 years and are sufficient, but there are still a lot of thyroid disorders—most probably related to long-term exposure to toxic substances that are altering immune function and thyroid antibodies.

Thyroid isn't alone in its vulnerability to hormone disruption. The *adrenal glands*, each located beneath a kidney at about waist level, also may be victims of endocrine disruption by chemicals. Animal studies are showing that various xenobiotics may be directly affecting the adrenal gland. A high prevalence of adrenal gland degeneration has been identified in stranded Beluga whales from the St. Lawrence River. Studies on dogs in the 1970s showed adrenal activity was suppressed by chlorinated hydrocarbons, such as breakdown products of DDT. DDT itself was given to some human patients with adrenal, mammary, and prostate cancer and was shown to shut down adrenal activity.

Diabetes

Since 1958, the number of Americans suffering with diabetes, an endocrine disease, has dramatically increased. The Centers for Disease Control and the World Health Organization estimate that 125 million people worldwide have diabetes, and that number is expected to double by 2025. Diabetes is increasing worldwide, especially in children. One reason is that people are carrying more weight, and obesity is known to increase the risk of diabetes. Heavier folks also have more growth factors that affect blood-sugar stability and more growth factor receptor sites that may be affected. But hormone disruptors may be another contributing cause of the increase in diabetes. For example, we know that Vietnam veterans exposed to endocrine disruptors such as Agent Orange (a potent mixture of several hormone-disrupting pesticides) have a higher incidence of diabetes, as well as abnormal glucose and insulin levels.

A follow-up study on the dioxin accident in Seveso, Italy, examined blood from 31,000 people within months of the accident and followed the

we look at ways to reduce our personal exposure in our most vulnerable habitat—our homes. But there is another place where we spend even more time—in our bodies.

A chemical can enter the body through three basic routes of exposure: *inhalation, ingestion,* and *skin penetration* (dermal exposure). Chemicals that circulate through indoor air may be inhaled into the lungs. We also swallow chemicals in food. For example, 90 percent of our exposure to PCBS and dioxins, two potent hormone disruptors, comes from the food we put in our mouths—especially dairy products, processed foods, and meat products—while the other 10 percent comes from water, air, and soil. Water may be ingested or inhaled through mist or steam, as in the shower. A chemical can penetrate the skin through direct contact, such as when spraying pesticides. Exposure through the skin can also occur as a result of contact with contaminants in air and water, as during bathing or swimming.

Some chemicals can enter through all three routes of exposure. Chloroform, for example, can be ingested from drinking water, enter the skin from the water in a shower, or be inhaled from the steam in the shower. A pesticide that is sprayed can be inhaled during use and penetrate through the skin during mixing and application. It can also be ingested through food if the hands aren't washed thoroughly before eating.

It is also the *rate of exposure* that is important. If the time between exposures is so short that some of the chemical remains from the first exposure, then a build-up of the chemical can lead to toxic levels in the body. Think of the way downing one-ounce alcoholic drinks one after another may cause inebriation, while drinking one ounce every few hours may not.

Another factor is *consistent exposure*. For example, phthalates and other chemicals used in plastic food packaging are fairly readily metabolized and don't last long in the body. However, all day long we consume foods that come in plastic wrappings or containers that frequently include phthalates. Even though the half-life of any given chemical may be short, there could be a real problem from the build-up of consistent exposure to various chemicals in our bodies.

In 1995 Dr. Sharpe and his colleagues in England found that three chemicals used in plastics—octyl phenol, bisphenol A, and butylbenzyl phthalate—had effects on the male offspring of rats (smaller testes and reduced sperm production) that were exposed to low amounts for short periods of time while pregnant. The researchers were shocked that such small amounts could have such adverse effects. They repeated the exper-

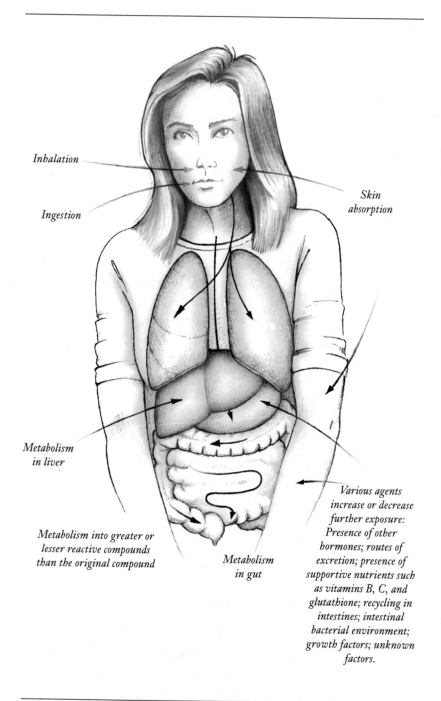

Inhalation

Ingestion

Skin
absorption

Metabolism
in liver

Metabolism into greater or
lesser reactive compounds
than the original compound

Metabolism
in gut

Various agents
increase or decrease
further exposure:
Presence of other
hormones; routes of
excretion; presence of
supportive nutrients such
as vitamins B, C, and
glutathione; recycling in
intestines; intestinal
bacterial environment;
growth factors; unknown
factors.

FIGURE III.1 *Routes of Exposure to Hormone Disruptors*

iments several times and got the same results. In another study on the off-spring of rats exposed to phthalates, the rats exposed during development showed reproductive/developmental problems and effects greater than the parents. They had decreased mating, pregnancy, and fertility as well as decreased sperm counts. The third generation was also affected, having lower weight levels.

RISK VERSUS BENEFIT

Some people say that we shouldn't use any new chemicals until we know all the possible consequences. That's a great idea, except that it would essentially halt human progress. No one can foresee all the potential problems that might arise with the use of any chemical. Not all plastics leach estrogenic chemicals and not all pesticides are estrogenic. Even totally natural approaches can create problems. For example, the animal wastes that the Mennonites were using as part of their sustainable agriculture were polluting Delaware Bay. It was too much natural all in one place.

It all comes down to *risk versus benefit*—the dangers presented by chemicals need to be evaluated in relation to the services they provide.

Take the case of chlorine. Some environmental groups believe that the use of all chlorinated compounds should be banned. It is true that when chlorine is added to drinking water it interacts with certain plant compounds and breaks down into metabolites that at high doses have been associated with liver cancer in rats. However, chlorine is an excellent disinfectant. It has kept untold numbers of people safe from infectious water-borne diseases like typhoid and cholera. These diseases have not disappeared; they are merely waiting for the opportunity to appear again. Alternative methods of disinfection (such as oxygenation) are less effective and prohibitively expensive to date.

The same is true with food preservatives. Although the food additives BHT and BHA may mimic the actions of the natural hormone estrogen, they also decrease the risk of illness from food spoilage. We must learn to evaluate chemicals not only on the basis of their hazards but also in relation to the good we reap from them.

In other words, don't panic. There are conservative measures that are sensible to take while science searches for the truth, such as avoiding unnecessary applications of pesticides in and around the home. Ben Franklin put it most succinctly: "An ounce of prevention is worth a pound of cure." Nowadays this is called the precautionary principle. We go into these precautionary measures in detail in this section of the book.

The next chapter tells you which foods are potentially highest in hormone-disrupting chemicals and how to reduce exposures through ingestion. Obviously we cannot completely eat or shop our way out of exposure to chemicals, but according to experts we can make a huge difference. Don't be discouraged. It is not that difficult to make certain lifestyle changes that can reduce your exposure to hormone disruptors.

This is not to say that we don't need *regulatory* change—new laws to protect us. We do. Based on the weight of evidence, the government can set and support research priorities on hormone disruption, a process they started with the establishment of EDSTAC and are continuing with EDSTP (the Endocrine Disruptor Screening and Testing Program). They can work toward reducing the use of chemical pesticides and regulate clean production practices. Industry can provide consumers with product and hazard information and can find ways to design products and industrial processes that don't rely on known hormone-disrupting compounds.

For the most part, in this book we are talking about *nonregulatory* action—the steps you can take individually that will make a difference for you and your family.

Food and Drink

> . . . if the people are properly informed, if they are educated, they will make intelligent choices to reduce their health risks. For most toxic environmental pollutants, the greatest reduction in public health risks can be achieved by reducing exposures at the personal level—by changing personal activities, habits, and lifestyles.
>
> —W. R. Ott and J. W. Roberts, "Everyday Exposures to Toxic Pollutants," *Scientific American*: 86–91 (Feb. 1998)

Corn chips with beans and cheese sounds good when you're hungry, but how does eating atrazine, bisphenol A, and butylated hydroxyanisole sound? All three of these chemicals (which can be present in corn, canned beans, and cheese) are implicated as hormone disruptors. More than 3,000 chemicals are deliberately added to food. Not all chemicals are hormone disruptors. However, most chemicals have not yet been tested to see whether or not they are endocrine disruptors, either by themselves or in combination with other chemicals. Therefore, it is currently a mystery as to which chemicals are hormone disruptors and which aren't.

What should you do? Reducing your overall exposure to chemical-laden food, and specifically to foods containing chemicals that are known endocrine disruptors, makes sense.

The Problems with Eating High on the Food Chain

Meat and dairy consistently have the highest levels of persistent hormone disruptors for a number of reasons.

1. Estrogenic hormones or "growth enhancers" are given to cattle (and pigs and poultry) so they grow bigger and fatter faster, and these growth hormones are given to dairy cows to up their production of milk. And recently DES has been identified in American beef!

2. Conventional animal feeds are among the most heavily sprayed crops. Most animal feed is laced with pesticides, herbicides, and fungicides, many of which are being investigated as hormone disruptors. Toxins, such as pesticides and drug residues, concentrate in animal fat. According to the EPA, 90 to 95 percent of all pesticide residues are found in meat and dairy products.

3. Most animal feed contains rendered fat (fat salvaged from fast-food restaurants and animal houses, often laced with melted plastic, etc.) and is a source of disrupting chemicals dissolved into the fat.

A survey of phthalate levels in fatty food samples (part of a Total Diet Survey in 1993 in England) found phthalates present in every sample of meat, fish, eggs, milk, and milk products (cheese had the highest concentration of phthalates). Richard Sharpe and John Sumpter are concerned about the fact that humans are eating amounts similar to the levels in their studies on pregnant rats, which caused male offspring to have smaller testes and fewer sperm. A diet high in fatty processed and packaged foods, along with generous portions of animal foods, adds up quickly.

Dairy

Milk and milk products (say pizza and ice cream) are a sacred cow in the United States, perhaps due to the fact that the United Dairy Industry Association spends more than $100 million a year on advertising, targeting women. Good consumers that we are, we proudly wear our milk mustaches, and along with the milk we unwittingly swallow bovine growth hormone (BGH), an estrogenic hormone given to cows. Although BGH may be good for dairy farmers because it increases milk production, it may not be good for humans. Why? Because BGH has been implicated as increasing the risk of breast cancer, although others say it is not a risk as it may not survive digestion.

BGH also contributes to the hormone-disruptor soup through another route. Although the FDA approved the drug, it admits that the use of this growth hormone often causes udder infections in cows. This leads to pus and bacteria getting into the milk. To prevent this, cows on BGH are given more antibiotics. According to some of the scientists I interviewed, certain subclasses of antibiotics are themselves estrogenic, or hormone disruptors.

Some of you may feel that milk is your major source of calcium and that eliminating or reducing your dairy intake will threaten your bone mass. This does not have to be the case. There are other available food sources of calcium, from sardines and almonds to garbanzo beans, kale, and tofu, all with far less fat than dairy and none of the hormones or antibiotics. There is also the question of whether or not dioxins and phthalates (chemicals found in plastics) are leaching into milk and milk products from their packaging in cardboard or plastic containers. Think about it.

There are ways to lessen your exposure to EDCs in dairy.

- *Eat less dairy, especially less cheese and butter, which are highly concentrated fats.* (Remember, EDCs are stored in fat.) Substitute low-fat cultured dairy products (such as yogurt and kefir) or nondairy foods.

- *Buy as much organic milk, butter, cheese, and other dairy products as you comfortably can.* For example, Horizon Organic Dairy (Boulder, Colorado) uses no pesticides, no antibiotics, and no hormones and treats their cows humanely, with access to clean water, organically grown feed, fresh air, and exercise. They know that cows are mothers too. Another company, Organic Cow, from Vermont and New Hampshire, also sells products in Whole Foods and Bread & Circus health-food supermarkets.

- *Remove cling wrap immediately from cheese or meat.* Most cling wraps used in supermarkets are made with a chemical called DEHA, which has been shown in animal studies to affect male reproductive function. (British manufacturers removed DEHA from cling wrap more than ten years ago. Some U.S. health-food chains, such as Whole Foods, make sure the brands they use don't contain DEHA.) You can remove most DEHA from hard cheeses by using a cheese slicer to take a thin section off the surface. When you use cling wrap at home over a bowl of food, don't let it touch the food. And even the plastic industry agrees you should *never* put food covered with cling wrap in the microwave.

Meat

Meat is a high source of hormone-disrupting chemicals for several reasons. One is that growth-promoting hormones are placed as pellets in the ears of cattle and are supposed to be removed five days before slaughter. It's possible that not all the hormone residues have left the cattle's body after only five days. Animals, like humans, don't all metabolize hormones in exactly the same manner or time frame. And the pellets may not always be removed (accidents do happen). Since estrogenic chemicals store in fat and meat is a high-fat food, just removing the pellets doesn't mean all the residues stored in the animal's fat will be gone.

Meat also has antibiotic residues. One-half of all antibiotics in the United States are used in livestock—25 million pounds a year. And antibiotics can contribute to hormone-disruptor exposure as well as contributing to antibiotic-resistant strains of bacteria. What to do?

Try to buy as much organic meat as possible for home use. When you go out to eat, don't fret. Simply enjoy your meal.

Poultry

Chickens and turkeys are not raised as they used to be. Chicken farms are highly effective industrial operations where the key incentive is to raise chickens *quickly*. In 1940 it took four months to grow a three-pound chicken; in 1990 it took six weeks. I spoke with a number of chicken growers. Commercial growers state that chickens now attain full size in six weeks due to genetic engineering, not hormones, with no bad side effects. Why then do organic farmers say that their chickens take ten weeks to

---

SOME SOURCES FOR NATURAL OR ORGANIC MEAT AND POULTRY

Shelton's (poultry)	909/623-4361
Nokomis Farms	414/642-9665
Organic Mail Order Directory Guide	916/756-8518
Pollo Real Ranch	505/838-0345
Roseland Farms	616/445-8987
Walnut Acres	800/433-3998
Welsh's Family Farms	319/535-7318

MEAT AND POULTRY: WHAT'S NATURAL? WHAT'S ORGANIC?

Commercial—With poultry, up to 80,000 birds may be packed into one warehouse and fed commercial feed, which contains numerous potential hormone-disrupting toxins (pesticides, herbicides, antibiotics, and drugs to combat the diseases that become prevalent when so many animals are housed together). The rendered fat in commercial feed contributes other toxins.

Natural—Legally, "natural" is a term that can be applied to any raw meat and refers only to foods not treated with chemicals during processing. So "natural" has different shades of meaning in different stores. Here are some examples:

- Animals may be given no hormones or additives such as nitrates, preservatives, or other chemicals.
- Animals are fed commercial feed.
- The "natural" chicken supplied to a commercial chain like Albertson's may be given antibiotics if deemed necessary.
- In health-food chains such as Wild Oats, the natural poultry never receive antibiotics.

Organic—Animals are fed a diet of organic whole grains with no added chemicals (this costs the farmer vastly more money and therefore the meat costs more for the consumer to buy). *Only meats and poultry labeled Certified Organic are guaranteed to be pesticide, herbicide, and drug free.*

Free-range—In the best case, free-range means the animals are allowed to roam on ground that has never been sprayed with chemicals and they are monitored from birth to make sure they have no chemical residues. Whereas organic farms may have 500 chickens to an acre, "free range" in some commercial lots may refer to an open pen of 50,000 birds in the same building with access to barren fenced yards. Too many birds in one space will fight, so they are debeaked. Without beaks they cannot eat whole grain and are fed only pellets of refined food which are often laced with rendered fat. And since birds (chickens and turkeys) fed this type of cheap feed are rather tasteless, more fat (such as coconut oil) is injected into the meat during processing. (Thus, poultry can end up being much higher in fat than is commonly assumed.)

grow to maturity? Raising chickens too quickly puts a strain on their internal organs, and the chickens then have to be treated with medications such as antibiotics (which are often masqueraded as vitamin mixes).

Try to buy organic chicken and turkey or natural free-range poultry at health food stores or co-ops. Eat more nonmeat proteins, such as tofu, tempeh, or beans.

Fish

Fish has always been considered a healthy alternative to eating meat. However, if you want to eat fish that you catch, follow sport-fish-consumption guidelines. Certain restrictions apply to various locations. This is especially important for fish such as salmon and trout, which have a high fat content and accumulate hormone disruptors and persistent organic pollutants (POPS). Canadian scientists have discovered that runoff of nonylphenols from pesticide spraying in Canadian forests has caused regional declines in Atlantic salmon. They suspect that any fish that migrates between fresh and salt water may be especially vulnerable to high concentrations of environmental estrogens because these fish must undergo major hormonal changes to adapt to salt water.

Top-predator fish, like pike and walleye, are likely to be the most contaminated with mercury, a heavy metal hormone disruptor. Shellfish tend to concentrate cadmium, another endocrine-disrupting heavy metal. Diets

---

HOW TO REDUCE YOUR EXPOSURE TO CHEMICALS IN FISH

FROM THE LAKE MICHIGAN FEDERATION

Choose younger, smaller fish to eat. Generally, larger, older fish have more contamination. For example, lake trout live for up to ten years, so they may contain more contaminants than chinook salmon, which only live three to four years.

Fish that eat other fish also build up more contaminants. Walleye and northern pike, for example, tend to have high levels of mercury. (Mercury cannot be removed from fish because it is in the flesh not the fat.)

Fish with more fatty flesh, such as carp and catfish, tend to have more PCBS because they are stored in fat.

high in adequate calcium, protein, iron, and zinc help protect against cadmium absorption.

Farm-raised fish are much better controlled. They are not fed for a few days before processing, so their empty bellies give them a firmer flesh with more consistent flavor and supposedly reduce bacterial contamination. A number of fish farms do expose fish one time in their life cycle to antibiotics. I have heard persistent rumors that farm-raised fish have more parasites and exposure to pesticides than fish in the wild, but I have not been able to substantiate this. I interviewed feed suppliers and discovered that farm-raised salmon and trout are fed diets high in fish meal and fish oils. Some suppliers add 5 percent poultry by-products and blood meal that contain rendered fats. Wheat is used as a binder in the food pellets. Those with serious wheat or gluten allergies may have trouble with farm-raised fish.

The best fish to eat are deep-sea fish, such as halibut, sardines, cod, and mackerel. Limit consumption of shellfish from coastal waters near contaminated coastlines, such as bay shrimp and bay scallops. Avoid eating big ocean fish, such as swordfish, marlin, and shark, as they are likely to be contaminated by hormone disruptors, and they may also be endangered.

THE CONVERSION FACTOR AS IT RELATES TO HORMONE DISRUPTORS

It takes sixty pounds of grain, feed, and hay to produce one pound of edible beef—a sixty to one conversion factor. Farm-raised fish have a conversion factor of one to one, meaning it only takes one pound of feed to produce one pound of edible fish. This is a very efficient conversion, which is much better for the environment. Thus, eating more fish (farmed and wild) means that a lot fewer hormone-disrupting chemicals get into our bodies via feed. Commercial feed for beef and poultry is highly sprayed and is a major contributing factor to the amount of hormone-disrupting chemicals in the environment.

By the way, the fish farmers I interviewed said they now have the technology to supply enough salmon to feed the world! (But this does include the use of antibiotics.)

PESTICIDES ON FRUITS AND VEGETABLES

If you eat in the United States or virtually any developed country, you eat pesticides, many of which are known hormone disruptors or have not yet been tested for hormone disruption. According to the Environmental Working Group, a nonprofit national research organization whose work has been generally accepted by the scientific community, "You eat small amounts of numerous pesticides, you quite likely eat them every day, and quite possibly in nearly every meal." Even pesticides that are now banned in this country, such as DDT, are still used in other countries and carried across global currents to our own soil or end up on our grocery shelves in foods imported from these countries. For example, DDT use in India is doubling every eleven years, and the chemicals used there and in Mexico and other developing countries will eventually get into our food supply.

In the last century, several hundred *billion* pounds of pesticides have been released into the global environment. As we enter the twenty-first century, an additional 5 to 6 billion pounds of insecticides, herbicides, fungicides, rodenticides, and other biocides are added to the world's environment every year—with almost one-quarter of this amount released or sold in the United States

We also need to be aware of the fact that fruit and vegetable growers in the United States, Mexico, Guatemala, Canada, and elsewhere commonly use illegal pesticides on crops that we eat every day. We even need to be cautious about foods we assume to be healthy. Ginseng, for example, used by many health-conscious people for its medicinal value, may not be as pure as one would hope. Most American ginseng is grown in Wisconsin, where state agriculture officials have uncovered widespread use of illegal pesticides on the crops of the 1,500 ginseng growers in the state.

In the EWG report *Forbidden Fruit: Illegal Pesticides in the U.S. Food Supply*, they found endosulfan—a chemical related to DDT that mimics estrogen in the human body—illegally on ten crops. There were at least sixty-six different illegal pesticides on the forty-two fruits and vegetables that EWG analyzed from local supermarkets. They say that a person eating the USDA's recommended five servings of fruits and vegetables per day will eat illegal pesticides at least seventy-five times per year.

Industry spokesman Dr. John McCarthy, the vice president for scientific and regulatory affairs for the Trade Association of Pesticides, said in

---

BEST AND WORST *NON*ORGANIC FRUITS AND VEGETABLES

This is excerpted from the 1995 EWG report *A Shopper's Guide to Pesticides in Produce*. This report and many others are available at http://www.ewg.org.

Have the most pesticides:

- strawberries (have the highest level of vinclozolin, a known endocrine disruptor)
- bell peppers (U.S./Mexico)
- spinach, cherries (U.S.)
- peaches
- cantaloupe (Mexico)

- celery
- apples
- apricots
- green beans
- grapes (Chile)
- cucumbers

Have the fewest pesticides:

- avocados
- corn
- onions
- sweet potatoes
- cauliflower
- brussels sprouts

- bananas
- plums
- green onions
- watermelon
- broccoli

The crops with the highest level of residue of endocrine disruptors and reproductive toxins from pesticides:

- strawberries
- spinach
- cabbage
- pineapples
- green beans
- asparagus
- apricots

- red raspberries
- cherries (U.S.)
- apples
- peaches
- grapes
- sweet peppers (U.S., Mexico)

our interview that companies do heavy testing with regard to food-use pesticides. According to McCarthy, "These tests range all the way from developmental tests of animals exposed in utero to multigeneration reproduction studies to chronic studies in animals in which they are tested in all phases of their lives. So that if products were to affect the endocrine system in any way, we would see the results in such tests."

Maybe industry just isn't seeing what others are. *Worst First*, published by Consumers Union, reports that exposure to insecticides (especially ops and carbamate insecticides) in foods must be reduced since it has clearly been shown that current levels are not safe enough for infants and children. *A child who eats three-quarters of an apple or a whole peach has a one-in-four chance of exceeding the safe daily intake for op insecticides just from that one food.*

To reduce risk, the EPA need not impose "draconian bans," although bans and severe restrictions on selected high-risk insecticides would not cripple agriculture as there are many alternatives for managing crop pests. *Worst First* identifies forty specific insecticides used on nine fruits and vegetables (apples, pears, peaches, grapes, oranges, green beans, peas, potatoes, and tomatoes) that account for a large portion of kids' overall dietary exposure and risk—the "Worst 40" that should be high-priority targets for EPA action under the Food Quality Protection Act.

If you eat nonorganic fruits and vegetables, peel and wash them (especially if waxed) with a mild solution of dish detergent or diluted vinegar. This removes some surface residues, although nothing can be done to remove pesticides that have been absorbed into the food. There are products that remove surface pesticides, chemicals, and dirt from fruits and vegetables, such as *Organiclean* (1-888/VEG-WASH or www.organiclean.com or *Healthy Harvest* Fruit & Vegetable Rinse, 203/245-2033).

Discard the outer leaves of leafy vegetables. Trim fat from meat and skin from poultry and fish (fat collects pesticide residues).

For more information on food and pesticides, contact www.epa.gov/pesticides/food or call 800/490-9198.

Another source of pesticides that we wind up ingesting comes from, believe it or not, cotton. Almost one-quarter of all pesticides used in the United States are applied to cotton, and every year half a million tons of cottonseed oil goes into processed salad dressing, baked goods, and snacks (like Fritos and Goldfish). Another 3 million tons of cottonseed is fed to beef and dairy cattle, as well as vast amounts of cotton by-products known as gin trash. Cottonseed oil is rarely tested for pesticides, and gin trash tests positive for toxic pesticides so often it was banned from use as livestock feed in California.

PHYTOESTROGENS

Not all estrogenic substances are bad for you. When you eat rye bread with raspberry jam or substitute a tofu burger for beef you are eating natural plant sources of estrogens called phytoestrogens. The term phyto-

---

PESTICIDES AND PESTS

David Pimentel, a professor of ecology and agricultural sciences at the College of Agriculture and Life Science at Cornell University, talked to me about our ability to reduce our dependence on pesticides by more than 50 percent without any reduction in yield and without any change in the cosmetic standard (blotches on fruit and vegetables).

Insecticide use in the United States has increased more than tenfold since 1945 with the new synthetic pesticides. Interestingly, says Pimentel, "crop losses to insects have gone from approximately 7 percent to 13 percent today." He explained: in 1945 there was zero insecticide use in corn production because all corn was grown in rotation after soybeans, wheat, oats, and so forth, which is gentler on the soil and produces healthier plants less prone to being attacked by critters. Corn losses at the time (according to USDA data) were 3.5 percent. Today less than half the corn is grown in rotation and corn is the largest user of insecticides in the nation, more than a thousandfold increase. Corn losses to insects are now at 12 percent.

He added, "I'm talking about pesticide use, not economics. In general, it is more profitable to grow corn continuously than in rotation with wheat or oats, even adding the cost of the pesticide. This is also not talking about the eight billion dollars spent annually for the health and environmental costs of using pesticides, which is not factored into the farmer's calculations." He finished by saying, "I've never said we shouldn't use any pesticides. What I favor is the *judicious* use of pesticides."

Dr. Pimental adds that 35 percent of all the foods we purchase in the supermarket have measurable pesticide residues, and 1 to 3 percent have residues *above* the tolerance level. He recommends eating a diverse diet, which reduces the chances of getting a high dosage of pesticides from any one food.

estrogens covers a wide family of compounds, including lignans, isoflavonoids, and flavonoids, which have mild estrogenic activity even though they are not steroid in structure like regular hormones.

PHYTOESTROGENIC COMPOUNDS

Isoflavones—the most famous of which are genistein and daidzein—are compounds found in high amounts in soy and mung bean sprouts. The highest to lowest amounts of phytoestrogens in soy are soybean flour, firm tofu, soft tofu, miso soup, soy drinks, and soy milk formula. A third isoflavone of soy, called glycitein, appears to be more estrogenic than the other two and much more absorbable by the body.

Lignans—compounds found in highest concentrations in flaxseeds (especially if ground immediately before consumption), rye bran, whole rye, barley bran, whole barley, and in moderate amounts in peanuts, whole berries, and some vegetables.

Whole-grain breads have more protective phytoestrogens than white breads because milling removes lignans and isoflavones. Fruits have very little phytoestrogens (except for berries, especially blueberries), but many vegetables have some. Pumpkin has the most, while zucchini, carrots, garlic, cabbage, turnips, red cabbage, broccoli, and cauliflower have a little. Green and black teas have high amounts of phytoestrogens. The phytoestrogens in food are not destroyed by cooking.

Phytoestrogens come from two sources: from plants themselves or from our intestinal tract as it metabolizes the precursors present in some of the food we eat. Intestinal production of phytoestrogens is very important. For example, if you take a round of antibiotics without rebuilding the intestinal milieu with friendly bacteria (by taking acidophilus supplements or cultured foods with added acidophilus), you can wipe out this beneficial metabolizing effect for months.

One benefit of phytoestrogens is they can protect us from excessive estrogenic estrogen. They do this by stimulating the liver to produce the hormone-binding proteins (SHBG) in our blood that prevent too much estrogen and some estrogenic substances from attaching to receptor sites. On the other hand, according to Dr. Herman Adlercreutz at the University of Helsinki, the typical Western high-fat diet may lower the production of these hormone-binding proteins. Another way in which phytoestrogens protect the body from too much estrogen is by binding with estrogen receptor sites and thereby blocking signaling from strong natural estrogens or EDCS.

The Soy Controversy

Phytoestrogens may protect our health at certain stages of our lives, yet they may not be so healthy at others. Presently, the protective or adverse effects of these naturally occurring plant estrogens are being debated.

Soy is famous for being the food with the most concentrated levels of isoflavones and, as a result, has been the subject of many studies. There is a lot of excitement about the potential beneficial effects of soy, but it is important to acknowledge that most of this information is speculative. We see in the lay literature and hear from professionals that soy reduces the incidence of breast cancer, but conclusions from six case-control studies do not clearly support this claim at this time. Personally, I found that even though I had an estrogen sensitive tumor, I felt much better when I ate soy products and decided to continue to do so, with my oncologist's blessing. Once again, all choices are based on your individual situation.

There's been very little data regarding the effects of phytoestrogens in men. In places where men eat more phytoestrogenic foods like soy, as in Asia, there are statistically lower rates of testicular cancer, prostatic cancer, and hypospadias. However, one Hawaiian study by the U.S. government suggests higher tofu consumption in Asian-Hawaiian men was associated with an increase in dementia.

Some studies do show that soy inhibits blood supply to tumors as well as putting the brakes on cancer traveling throughout the body. Major studies on women with terminal cancer are being done now to test high-soy protein beverages. Some studies show soy and its isoflavones protect against cancer, while other groups of studies demonstrate the opposite in women who already have cancer.

There are a number of reasons the data seem so confusing.

- Soy may act differently depending on the amount of estrogen a women already has in her body. It appears that if a woman is premenopausal or postmenopausal but taking HRT—in other words, situations where she has estrogen in her body—soy is probably protective. Once a woman has less estrogen in her body or has had diseases that are stimulated by estrogen—such as estrogen-positive breast cancer, cystic breasts, atypical breast cells, DCIS (precancerous breast cancer), or uterine diseases like endometriosis, fibroids, and cancer—whether soy helps or harms becomes a real question, as yet unanswered.

• Some tissues, such as ductile tissue in the breast, may concentrate phytoestrogens. This may differ from woman to woman, which means that soy's benefit or harm may vary.

• Studies on large groups of people have suggested that soy protects against cancer. It may be that soy protects against *getting* cancer, but once we *have* cancer it is a different story. Breast cancer is a multiple-stage disease. Thus the phytoestrogens in soy may act one way at one stage and differently at another stage.

• Soy may act differently in people who were exposed to soy in utero versus people who started eating soy foods as adults.

• A hefty portion of the research done on the "negative" effects of soy has been done on rodents. However, humans and mice may clear phytoestrogens out of their bodies in very different ways. Humans have a charming newly-discovered receptor (called SXR) that clears phyto-estrogens out of the body or breaks them down into beneficial products. Rodents don't have this receptor and don't clear phyto-estrogens as well as humans, thus more is left to interact with the estrogen receptor.

• Soy, being an endocrine modulator, has different effects at different dosages.

The bottom line is that just because something is a food does not necessarily mean it is safe. Dr. Claude Hughes, both a clinician and researcher, says, "Soy may be beneficial if given to the right person at the right time. And it may be adverse when given to the wrong person at the wrong time."

So do you avoid soy or use it as a medicine? It appears that women with estrogen-positive cancers, especially postmenopausal women, should be cautious about consuming soy and ask their doctors (who probably don't know what to say either). If soy is eaten, it should be consumed in large quantities. If a premenopausal woman has an estrogen-dependent cancer and eats soy, she should probably also consume large amounts. No one knows at this time. The conclusion is like the punch line at the end of every scientific debate: we need more research.

ORGANIC FOOD

You can find healthy food. It is more expensive but well worth it, especially if you plan to get pregnant, are pregnant, or have young growing children. Natural and organic foods are now the hottest items in food retailing. Sales of organic products, only $178 million in 1980, are now more than $4 billion a year, while the more widely defined "natural" products are selling $12 billion a year. One in four shoppers is now buying organic at least once a week.

What is organic food? Crops must be grown without the use of synthetic pesticides on land that has not had any synthetic chemicals applied to it during the previous three years. Farmers must maintain or improve soil quality. For processed and prepared foods to be labeled organic, at least 95 percent of the ingredients must be organic, with no artificial additives or preservatives. Cows and poultry must be fed only organic feed and be free of growth hormones and systematically applied antibiotics.

The USDA has drafted the first national standards that products must meet to be labeled organic. At the time I was writing this book, there was fear in the organic community that the proposed national standards were going to "relax" restrictions and allow four practices that would defeat the very idea of organic food. These are

- genetic engineering
- irradiation
- the use of toxic sludge
- the use of antibiotics

The standards also would allow dairy animals to be raised organically for only three months before selling their milk as "organic" and would allow 20 percent nonorganic feed for livestock.

What's really ironic is that it was the organic farmers themselves who asked Congress to write a law to regulate organic standards. The drafting process was a collaboration between lawmakers, consumers, environmentalists, and organic farmers. It was democracy at its best, until the USDA lawyers ignored the board's recommendations and wrote in large loopholes that would allow conventional agribusiness to cash in on the organic craze with only minimal changes in the way it operates. Fortunately, Congress was overwhelmed with more than 2 million responses from concerned consumers. We still don't know the final shape of this legislation, but it shows that we can make ourselves heard.

Europe seems to be charging ahead in the organic direction. In England, Prince Charles is an organic farmer. He gave the royal seal of approval to the British campaign against genetically engineered food. In Denmark, 25 percent of schoolchildren drink organic milk. Denmark's parliament has called for a switch to organic agriculture for the entire country by the year 2010.

Eating organically even part of the time helps. A study of male Danish organic farmers showed that those who ate organic food just 25 percent of the time had a 43 percent higher sperm count.

A review of the literature over the last fifty years looked at the benefits of organic versus conventional food crops. Thirty-four studies of the nutrient content of crops showed organic fertilization produces crops with higher levels of vitamin C, lower levels of nitrates, and better quality protein. Animal studies strongly showed superior reproduction and growth in animals fed organically grown feed compared to those who received conventionally grown feed.

EATING ORGANIC FOOD, EVEN AS JUST A PORTION OF YOUR DIET, CAN HAVE POSITIVE HEALTH EFFECTS

If you live in a small town or isolated area that does not have a health-food store, call Diamond Organics at 800/922-2396. They provide delivery nationwide of fruits and vegetables, teas and coffees, beans and grains, and some organic cotton clothing. Their website is http://www.diamond organics.com. Walnut Acres ships meats, cheeses, breads, soups, peanut butter, juices, canned fruits and vegetables, pastas, etc. (90 percent certified organic) through UPS or parcel post. Call 800/433-3998 or try their website at http://www.walnutacres.com. Or call a health-food store in your general area for local delivery services.

WHAT'S "FERTILIZING" YOUR FOOD?

Foods can be contaminated from fields spread with sewage sludge. Municipal sewage systems collect and treat 11.6 billion pounds of waste materials every year. Up to 36 percent of this sludge is spread on crops.

Oh, they don't really use sludge on fields, do they? Why not? Look at what else gets used.

The Associated Press broke a story that toxic heavy metals (cadmium and lead, which are known hormone disruptors, and arsenic), chemicals (such as dioxins), and even radioactive wastes are being dumped into fertilizer products and then spread over farmers' fields across the nation. In Gore, Oklahoma, for example, a uranium-processing plant gets rid of low-level radioactive waste by licensing it as a liquid fertilizer that gets sprayed over 9,000 acres of grazing land.

Many industrialized nations regulate fertilizers, but the United States doesn't. There are no laws to prevent wastes from the incineration of medical and municipal wastes and from heavy industries to be mixed with fertilizers. Nearly 30 percent (80 million pounds) of the toxic wastes sent to farm and fertilizer companies come from the steel industry. Some wastes contain nitrogen and magnesium, which can help crops grow, but these are often accompanied by toxic compounds. Federal and state governments encourage the recycling, which saves money for industry and conserves space in hazardous waste landfills.

Ask your local grocer to stock organic foods or foods certified as having "no detected" pesticide residues. If your grocer thinks you're being slightly hysterical, shop elsewhere.

FOOD ADDITIVES

Food by itself is fragile. It is prone to rot and is easily injured. Bugs infest it, bacteria invades it, mold assaults it, and the air makes it rancid. Something has to be added to food to protect it. Thus, technology has brought us food additives. In 1958 Congress passed the Food Additives Amendment to the Federal Food, Drug, and Cosmetic Act to ensure the safety of additives (colorings were added to the list in 1960). Additives are tested by being fed in large doses over time to at least two kinds of animals. This kind of testing does not show hormone disruption, which can occur at low dosages.

The additives everyone should avoid (because of their known toxicity or because of insufficient testing) include:

- acesulfame K (acesulfame potassium)
- artificial colorings (Blue 1, Blue 2, Green 3, Red 3, Yellow 6)
- olestra (olean)
- potassium bromate
- saccharin
- sodium nitrate, sodium nitrite

Try eating fewer processed foods and more whole foods. For example, look for nitrite-free hot dogs and sandwich meats.

Two food additives that are very commonly used have been shown to be slightly estrogenic. Butylated hydroxyanisole (BHA) is a food antioxidant—check the list of ingredients in the cereals you buy for the kids—which is slightly estrogenic. BHT, the chemical cousin of BHA, has also been shown to be estrogenic in laboratory tests. BHT is in chewing gum and dry active yeast, in processed foods and food-packaging materials. (Only 5 percent of BHT is used in our food; the other 95 percent is used in rubber and plastics as an antioxidant, and it's in liquid petroleum products like gasoline and motor oil. Sounds yummy.)

A food coloring, Red Dye No. 3, has been shown to be estrogenic and to make breast cancer cells grow.

Another several hundred substances that are added to foods are grouped under the term GRAS, an acronym for substances "generally recognized as safe" based on a history of safe use before 1958 or on published scientific evidence. Many spices and herbs, salt, sugar, and vitamins are included in this category. The third category of additives is "prior-sanctioned" substances—ingredients that had been approved by the FDA or the U.S. Department of Agriculture before the 1958 amendment. So nitrites, for example, can be used in meats because they were sanctioned for that use before 1958, but they cannot be used on vegetables.

Substances that leach from food packaging are indirect additives. Since they can end up in food, the FDA requires that they be evaluated.

Altogether, the food-additive industry generates approximately $10 billion a year in business. Fortunately, the concept of what is a safe additive is changing.

The Tin Can Question

Many food processors coat cans so the food inside doesn't react with the cans and thereby cause changes to the flavor or cause metal poisoning. Approximately 85 percent of the food cans in the United States are lined with plastic (compared to 40 percent in Spain). A report on bisphenol A (BPA, a constituent of plastic) from the society of the plastics industry showed that the average can gives off six to seven micrograms of bisphenol A into the food. BPA can leach from plastic when subjected to high temperatures. The degree of leaching depends on how the can is treated (not all are sterilized at high heat, called *autoclaving*) and what's inside the can. When I called numerous cola companies to find out if they had tested for BPA leakage, I got the royal runaround and never received any information.

Canned peas are the worst offenders (leaching 23 micrograms of BPA per can). Fatty foods (such as tuna packed in oil) and acidic foods (such as colas) may leach BPA into the food. Even distilled water added to empty cans, put under pressure, and heated leached BPA in the water. The liquids that contained bisphenol A from cans were shown to promote the growth of human breast cancer cells in tests. Seventy percent of the cans tested in one study showed estrogenic activity.

Avoid or limit use of foods packaged in tin cans to avoid lead and BPA. Also think about putting fresh fruits and vegetables in a paper or string bag at the supermarket rather than in the thin plastic bags that are provided. The more flexible the plastic, the more plasticizer is in it. At least, as a number of scientists I interviewed suggest, take the food out of the bags once you get home.

Water, Water Everywhere

There is nothing more basic to life than water (except air). Our bodies are made largely of water. Fruits and vegetables are mostly water. We should drink a good quantity of water each day. We bathe in it, cook with it, and wash our food and clothes in it. Healthy water needs to be a top priority in our lives. Today there are more than 700 chemicals found in common drinking water.

In 1997 the Environmental Working Group (EWG) came out with a booklet called *Tough to Swallow: How Pesticide Companies Profit from Poisoning America's Tap Water.* They found that 104 communities of 3.3 million people across the corn belt drank tap water contaminated with five or more toxic weed killers, years after a number of water utilities had begun special treatment to clean pesticide levels out of the water. An earlier EWG study found that weed killers came right out of the tap in twenty-eight of

CORN-FED GOODNESS

How about drinking a popular pesticide?

Ciba-Geigy, the company that patented DDT, had been looking for a chemical that could do to weeds what DDT did to insects. They found it in atrazine, which kills the two main weeds that threaten corn without harming the corn itself. Before the introduction of atrazine in 1959, only one-fifth of the corn grown in the United States was sprayed with pesticides. By 1988, 96 percent of the annual corn crop (grown on 65 million acres of land in the United States) was sprayed. Atrazine is the best-selling pesticide in the nation (68–73 million pounds in 1995) and accounts for one-quarter of Ciba-Geigy's crop chemical business.

Atrazine eventually gets into ground water and mingles with drinking water. The U.S. Geological Survey found atrazine in 990 out of 1,604 water samples in midwestern streams, rivers, reservoirs, and aquifers from 1989 to 1994. Even rainwater contained atrazine. One recent study that evaluated ten hormone-disrupting pesticides showed that only DDT had as damaging an effect as atrazine in altering how the body metabolizes estrogen. Animal studies show liver, heart, and kidney damage, tumors in the uterus and breast, and hormone disruption.

Ciba-Geigy has spent more than $25 million, submitted 14,000 pages of defense in response to the EPA desire to tighten restrictions on atrazine, and launched a letter-writing campaign (the EPA has received more than 87,000 letters) in order to keep atrazine on the market.

the twenty-nine cities sampled at levels that routinely exceeded federal standards or health advisories.

In February 1998 preliminary results from a study of California chlorinated drinking water indicated that pregnant women in their first trimester who drank five or more glasses of cold tap water a day might be at higher risk of miscarriage.

The problem with chlorinated water is not the chlorine, which is an excellent disinfectant that has helped stomp out epidemics of waterborne disease. But just because it comes out of the faucet in your home does not mean that chlorinated water is safe (and unless your water comes from a private well, it *is* chlorinated). The problem is that elemental chlorine reacts with organic compounds already present in water (such as dead leaves and algae), and their organochlorine offspring, known as disinfection by-products, can be toxic. When chlorine reacts with decomposing plant material, it forms trihalomethanes. By the time water gets into your sinks, showers, or washing machines, unless it has been filtered, the water usually contains these contaminating compounds.

Even though only 2 percent of the women in the California study had a high enough exposure to these chemicals to increase their risk of miscarriage, the EPA is planning to lower the allowable limits of trihalomethanes by 20 percent. In the meantime, health officials advised pregnant women to boil tap water for a minute and put it in the refrigerator or to leave carbon-filtered tap water standing in the refrigerator for several hours. Dr. Shanna Swan, one of the researchers on the study, said women should not switch to bottled water, which is not regulated as closely as tap water. "I don't think anyone would consider stopping chlorinating water," she said. "Chlorination has saved untold illnesses and lives."

Another study on the water from the central valley of California found estrogenic chemicals in both sediment and water samples, most likely having moved there from the fields through agricultural drain canals. It found that chemicals can survive the transport process while still maintaining their activity and persist for several weeks to several months (up to seven months) after the last spraying.

What is your child drinking? Children drink three times as much water as adults. Tap water is used as drinking water and in infant formula and reconstituted juices, comprising 30 to 40 percent of the infant and child diet by weight. More than 85 percent of infant formula sales are of concentrate or powder that is mixed with water in the home. So, what can you do? Here are some suggestions.

- Have your water tested. Know what you are ingesting. You inhale and absorb through the skin more of the contaminants from water in your house than you drink. Is the water heavily chlorinated? Full of trihalomethanes? To get your water tested, contact a reputable water treatment company that deals with a good laboratory. You could contact a lab directly, but a water treatment company will help you interpret the results.

- Know what your water pipes are made from. Copper/lead? Pvc plastic? If your water has a high pH (more alkaline) and is hard, copper piping is best. If you live on the East Coast or your water

GOOD WATER

Since exposure to many disinfection by-products comes mainly from inhalation from showers, washing machines, sinks, and toilets, I asked a number of scientists involved in home pollution if water filters at the main source of entry of the home would help. They all said no—that the gallons of water running through a house each day would overtax any filter within just one day. So I called up Greg Friedman at the Good Water Company in Santa Fe. He is a local water genius of sorts and very committed to helping people have safe water. After he interviewed many different specialists on water filters and spent long hours on research, he custom-designed a water filter for my home. After the filter had been in use for three months, he came out to my house and took samples of the city water versus the water out of the filter, which were tested by a laboratory in Ohio. The city water had trihalomethanes in it (the very chemicals that may be associated with adverse health effects—chloroform being one example). The filtered water had no detectable levels of trihalomethanes. He insists this four-foot-tall filter will clear at least 300,000 gallons of water, which should last approximately five years. We tested six months later, and it was still working. We shall continue testing to prove or disprove this, but the filter already has gone way beyond the expectations of the scientists I originally conferred with.

You can contact the Good Water Company at 505/471-9036. (This is not an advertisement, and I paid for the water filter.)

has a low pH (more acidic), hard plastic pipes are better because the acidity can leach copper, which may kill off the good bacteria in your body, leading to vaginal yeast infections.

- Filter the water supply in your house. Unfortunately, most filters are made from plastic. We don't know what chemicals are used in the plastic and if they leach out into the water.

- Buy bottled water if necessary, ideally in glass containers. But beware. An article in *Sierra* magazine states: "Yosemite brand water comes not from a bucolic mountain spring but from deep wells in the undeniably less-picturesque Los Angeles suburbs, and Everest sells water drawn from a municipal source in Corpus Christi, Texas—a far cry from the pristine glacial peaks suggested by its name. As long as producers meet the FDA's standards for 'distilled' or 'purified' water, they don't have to disclose the source."

- Use filtered water when making beverages such as juices from concentrates or other beverages. Two-thirds of the water we drink comes from these sources.

- When making foods that completely absorb water, such as oatmeal, use filtered water.

- Rinse pasta, such as spaghetti, before eating it. Unrinsed pasta retains more chemical byproducts from water treatment plants.

The only technology that can adequately remove pesticides once they have contaminated water supplies is Granular Activated Carbon. Not every water treatment facility uses this filtering system because it is expensive. And, when it is used, the cost is passed on to the water customers, not to the chemical companies. Since I live in New Mexico, where there is widespread contamination by naturally occurring radioactive particles, I use a reverse osmosis water system, the only treatment for removing these particular contaminants. Once you know what is in your water, you can work with a water specialist to clean it up.

WINE

Red wine may indeed be good for the heart because it contains resveratrol, which is a flavonoid with heart protecting qualities. Resveratrol, which protects grapes from fungal infections, acts like an estrogen by binding to the estrogen receptor. So even though it may help hearts, will it help breasts? While numerous studies suggest resveratrol protects against getting cancers, what will it do for women who have already had breast cancer? Some research has shown that this estrogen-like factor does make breast cancer cells grow. What to do? Personally, I'm still enjoying a glass of red wine occasionally.

COFFEE

Let's wake up and smell the coffee. Drinking two cups of coffee each day means buying some eighteen pounds of beans each year—the total annual yield of twelve coffee trees. To keep those dozen trees productive, coffee farmers will apply twelve pounds of fertilizer each year, as well as pesticides. When the fruits ripen, they are handpicked and fed into a diesel-powered crusher that extracts the beans inside. For each pound of beans, two pounds of the pulp wastes will be dumped into a nearby river. Pesticide residues will enter the food chain. Suddenly organic coffee doesn't seem so expensive.

Detoxification and Dietary Suggestions

*Work on the unpolluting of man must catch up
and pass the polluting of man.*

> —Dr. David Schnare, From the essay "The Unpolluing of
> Man," Foundation for Advancements in Science and
> Education

Human exposure to environmental contaminants, including hormone disruptors, is inevitable. We can minimize our exposure, but we cannot completely prevent it. This is true despite our best efforts to avoid exposure through environmental laws and personal lifestyle changes.

Once a chemical enters the body, it is absorbed into the bloodstream and can move throughout the body (a process called distribution). Then it can have several different fates. Often the chemical is metabolized and rapidly removed via the body's waste products. However, certain chemicals—like many hormone disruptors—are resistant to metabolism, yet they readily dissolve in fat, so they tend to be stored in the body's fat cells for many years.

Scientists have identified more than 400 chemicals in various human tissues. These chemicals are not easily removed from the body. Fat samples taken several years apart, on the same person, have shown that there is no reduction in the levels of chemicals like PBBS and PCBS over time. They persist for years, often for the entire lifespan of the person who owns those fat cells. Some chemicals have been found in the tissues of animals (and humans) decades after their use has been banned!

It is amazing how much research, money, and debate goes into trying to determine how and if chemicals are affecting our health, yet so little time and effort have gone into investigating safe methods of removing these chemicals once they are lodged within our cells. One study did try to reduce levels of dioxin during breastfeeding by controlling the mothers' diet, but there was no reduction of dioxin in breast milk. This shows that the dioxin in the milk was coming from the life-long body burden of chemicals rather than from what the mothers were eating at the time of the study.

Since we live in a chemical soup, and since it may take decades for science to figure out how this mixture affects us, and since these chemicals do not easily get cleared from our bodies through natural processes, it seems reasonable that we need to find a verifiable manner in which to reduce our accumulated body burden of chemicals safely. The process of clearing chemicals out of the body without any adverse side effects is called *detoxification*. Detoxification is the goal of deliberate programs that try to enhance our body's elimination of chemicals. There are a small number of studies that have shown that body levels of toxic chemicals can be reduced through deliberate detoxification procedures. This area clearly needs more investigation.

How beneficial it would be to all future generations if women who wanted to get pregnant first were able to clear their bodies of harmful chemicals!

The Body's Natural System of Biotransformation

Detoxification methods are based on the body's natural means of clearing chemicals. The body is designed for housecleaning—ridding itself of many chemicals, drugs, and environmental pollutants through the process of biotransformation. In this process, chemicals that normally do not dissolve easily so they can be excreted are altered or transformed into new compounds that are water-soluble and easily removed from the body.

Biotransformation uses three major tools:

- phase 1 enzymes

- phase 2 enzymes

- local repair stations at different areas around the body

The liver produces most of the phase 1 and 2 enzymes, so it is the star of the biotransformational process. Other organs—such as the lungs, skin, and kidneys—also have phase 1 and 2 enzymes, as well as local repair systems. This is one of the reasons that deep breathing, sweating, and drinking lots of water are generally good for helping to keep the body clean.

Phase 1 starts the transformation of toxic compounds by taking the original chemical and turning it into water-soluble products called intermediate metabolites. This first step is accomplished through the natural chemical processes of reduction, oxidation, and hydrolyzation. The chemicals now have been partially metabolized.

Then phase 2 kicks in. Different enzymes take the intermediate metabolites and attach them onto other molecules—sulfates, amino acids, glutathione, glucuronide (a certain type of sugar), and others. This joining together of a chemical metabolite with another molecule to make a new compound is called conjugation. The conjugates formed are now completely biotransformed metabolites of the original parent chemical and can be excreted from the body through urine, feces, or sweat.

To understand how this process works, imagine you're driving almost on empty, so you pull into a gas station, pay the cashier, take the hose from the pump, put the nozzle into your gas tank, and begin filling up. Smell those fumes—benzene is entering your body. Benzene is a nonpolar, fat-soluble toxin. The biotransformation enzymes start doing their job. Phase 1 enzymes add oxygen and hydrogen (a hydroxyl group-OH) to the benzene molecule, transforming what was once benzene into phenol—an intermediate metabolite. The phase 2 enzymes now add a sulfate group to complete the biotransformation process. The final product, phenyl sulfate, is a water-soluble compound that can be readily excreted in the urine. What was once benzene can now be flushed away.

BIOACTIVATION

Sometimes the intermediate compound produced by phase 1 enzymes is *more* toxic than the original chemical, a process called bioactivation. Often these toxic intermediates are highly reactive compounds (such as free radicals) that can cause adverse chain reactions, which can eventually damage tissues. However, if phase 2 enzymes are doing their job, or enough antioxidants are around, or local repair stations are up to snuff, these reactive intermediates are squelched and tissue damage is averted. It becomes obvious that successful biotransformation needs all the body's systems to be working equally well and to back each other up.

Biotransformation can be curtailed or altered by:

- a diet too low in protein
- a diet loaded with excessive carbohydrates
- vitamin and mineral deficiencies
- certain diseases of the thyroid, liver, kidneys, lungs, or gastrointestinal tract—such as chronic constipation, emphysema, or cirrhosis of the liver—that may promote toxic bioactivation and reduce the body's ability to clear itself of chemicals

You Need Bile and Guts

The liver is the most important organ of biotransformation, containing numerous enzymes that perform phase 1 and 2 functions. Let's say you're eating a juicy steak dinner that contains some DDT or PCBS. You chew a hunk of meat and swallow; it goes down your esophagus and through your stomach to your small intestine, which is lined with blood vessels (splanchnic arteries). The chemicals enter these blood vessels and are transported directly to the tiny blood capillaries that lead into the portal vein going to the liver. The chemicals are leaked out into the liver cells that contain phase 1 and 2 enzymes, which go to work on transforming the chemicals. The products of this enzyme action are released into the bloodstream as bile or go to the kidneys to be eliminated as urine. When released into the bile, the chemicals can recirculate a second time around the body. Effective detoxification methods enhance urinary, fecal, lung, and skin routes to avoid reexposure.

The gut may get rid of chemically biotransformed products in the feces or may rerelease them back into the system. The ability to eliminate pollutants is a complex phenomenon that depends on the functioning of all the organs that contain high levels of detox enzymes. If the liver is working overtime to detoxify drugs or alcohol, it won't be fully efficient at removing natural or environmental estrogens and thus may contribute to an increased body burden of unopposed estrogen.

BIOINDIVIDUALITY

Some bodies naturally perform the function of biotransformation better than others. Each one of us has an individual makeup—called bioindividuality—comprised in part by our diets, genetics, how well our livers function, and how much stress we live with. If you buy a house on the perimeter of a golf course that is heavily sprayed with pesticides, and I buy one next door to you, one of us might get sick and the other might not. Our health is a continual balancing process.

At certain stages of our lives, we do not biotransform chemicals as well as at other stages. Babies in the womb cannot biotransform chemicals very well at all. This is a very important factor contributing to the fetus's extreme sensitivity to environmental insults. The fetus may build up toxicants from the mother's circulation even if the mother is successfully clearing herself. We know that the fetus in utero is exceptionally sensitive to contaminants that cross the placenta and even more so during the time that organs are being formed (organogenesis). The elderly also do not generally clear chemicals as well as most younger folks do.

DETOXIFICATION

When I asked various scientists how we could get dangerous chemicals out of our bodies, most of them said that would be too dangerous a process because releasing toxic chemicals would cause reexposure. They said that the chemicals are stored safely in the body's fat cells and therefore don't affect the organs. This is not true.

It's true that chemicals are predominantly stored in fat. However, fat is not inert. Approximately 5 percent of fat cells are always in flux with the rest of the body. Thus, if you take a blood test, you can detect levels of these chemicals because a small amount is always leaking slowly out of our fat cells into the rest of our tissues. Thus, there is equilibrium between what's in fat and what's in the rest of our body. Detoxification programs turn this slow leak into a running faucet by enhancing mobilization and also by supporting the biotransformation process with nutrients. Participants in deliberate detoxification programs experience a decrease of symptoms from chemical toxicity, indicating that even though more chemicals are released, they are safely being removed from the body.

Getting rid of chemicals stored in the fat cells of the body requires

- mobilization of chemicals stored in the fat cells
- nutritional support of the biotransformation process
- enhanced excretion of chemicals through all the body's detoxification routes (liver, kidneys, lungs, and gastrointestinal tract)

Looking at which organs are involved in clearing chemicals from the body, it makes sense that therapeutic detoxification programs should include exercise, breathing, skin brushing, and supplementation with nutrients that support phase 1 and phase 2 enzymes, herbs that enhance liver enzymatic systems, friendly intestinal bacteria, and high-fiber sources that hasten elimination out of the intestines.

DIETARY STRATEGIES FOR GETTING RID OF EDCS

What can you do to reduce your body burden of synthetic chemicals if you cannot jump on a plane and go to a detoxification clinic for a month or two? Based on common sense, one could enhance the body's mobilization and excretion pathways in a safe and gentle way by doing some simple lifestyle actions.

Here are some ways to help your body eliminate harmful chemicals:

- *Drink five to eight glasses of healthy fluids a day*, including filtered or spring water. Adding water (hydrolysis) is a major detoxification mechanism.

- *Exercise daily*, or enough to make you sweat for at least thirty minutes four to six times a week.

- *Eat high-fiber foods, low-fat proteins, and plenty of fresh organic fruits and vegetables*, especially garlic and the cabbage family of foods (cabbage, broccoli, cauliflower, bok choy, and brussels sprouts stimulate the liver enzymes involved in phase 2 action). The active component of garlic (allicin and its products) supports liver functions involved in detoxification.

- *Get enough vitamins and minerals* to support the functioning of important biotransformational enzymes. Eat plenty of fresh fruits and vitamins and take a daily vitamin/mineral supplement. Especially important for the enzymes of detoxification are vitamins A, C, E; carotene and related cartotenoids; bioflavonoids; and minerals such as selenium, copper, manganese, and sulfur (you can get sulfur from protein, onion, and garlic).

- *Avoid eating too many refined carbohydrates*, such as breads and bakery goods made with white flour and sugar, candies, and colas. Sugar has been shown to lower P-450 enzyme action—a large superfamily of enzymes that are among the most well-known for detoxification. Some people genetically make less P-450 and other detoxification enzymes and are called slow metabolizers. Most phase 1 enzymes are found in the liver, but P-450s are found all throughout the body, including part of the adrenal glands, lungs, kidneys, and even in testicles. The kinds of fats we eat may also play a role in optimal production of P-450 enzymes.

- *Consume foods that are high in antioxidants*, such as red, yellow, and green vegetables; raw seeds and nuts; and fish. Antioxidants (such as vitamins C and E) mate with free radicals to produce offspring that are relatively nonreactive and do not cause injury. Consider supplementation with coenzyme Q10 (ubiquinone), which helps support enzyme detoxification. It has known antioxidant effects in the energy centers of cells (mitochondria, where the P-450 enzyme system lives). Coenzyme Q10 is a nutritional supplement found in health-food stores and pharmacies.

- *Consume foods high in amino acids* found in animal products or in nuts, seeds, and beans. Two amino acids—cysteine and methionine—are converted into glutathione, which is an important detoxifier and antioxidant.

- *Eat several helpings of protein a day.* The reason adequate protein is important is that your body manufactures glutathione from amino acids found in protein foods. Vitamin C helps this process. A daily dose of 500 mg of vitamin C increases the levels of glutathione in the body—a good idea as most forms of food processing (except freezing) destroy glutathione.

- *Avoid excessive use of alcohol and/or acetaminophen* (Tylenol), two examples of the many drugs that rinse out the body's store of glutathione.

BROCCOLI SPROUTS

In 1992 researchers at Johns Hopkins Medical Institutions in Baltimore isolated sulforaphane, a compound in broccoli and its kin that turns on detoxifying phase 2 enzymes. They then tested broccoli throughout its life cycle and found that the seeds were high in phase 2 enzyme precursors, as were three-day-old sprouts. Even the sulforaphane precursor dramatically inhibits chemically induced cancers in rats. They are now developing a way to certify that any sprouts that get marketed contain sufficiently high quantities of the sulforaphane precursor. Eat sprouts raw for effectiveness.

- *Include bioflavonoids in your diet* to stimulate glutathione-S-transferases (GST), a detoxifying enzyme. Bioflavonoids are found in fruits and vegetables with darker colors (bright yellows to blues and purples) and in certain spices and teas. You can also purchase bioflavonoids in supplement form. Starvation and fasting quickly lower the body levels of GST, which quickly elevates after resuming the consumption of food.

- *Turmeric*, combined with isoflavonoids (soy), has been shown to inhibit estrogenic effects. Several times a week take turmeric in capsules, add on top of food (after food is cooked), or mix a teaspoonful with honey.

- *Do a safe and sensible program for liver and intestinal detoxification*, working with a holistic medical doctor, naturopathic doctor, or nutritionally oriented health practitioner who specializes in such programs. My book *Healthy Digestion the Natural Way* (Wiley, 2000) outlines self-help programs. Any program you follow should include the careful balancing of protein and carbohydrate intake to allow for optimal activation of the body's detoxification system and is best undertaken with a doctor's supervision. Supplement with beneficial intestinal bacteria (forms of *L. acidophilus*) and milk thistle (an herb called silybum marianum), a remedy that has been shown in numerous studies to be effective in protecting the liver against toxins while having no adverse side effects. You may want to consider being evaluated by a detoxification clinic.

- *Keep the liver healthy and functioning.* To contain adequate repair mechanisms, body organs need to be healthy. This makes sense when you consider that many toxic metabolites of phase 1 biotransformation must be locally repaired by these tissues to avoid toxicity. Liver disease, drugs that tax the liver, inadequate B vitamins, junk-food diets, and abuse of alcohol (the liver is the main organ of alcohol detoxification) all reduce the liver's role in biotransformation.

Note: Sometimes people feel worse when they are detoxing or on a cleansing program. One theoretical explanation is that they initiated phase 1, but there was a problem with the next steps—such as an increase in free radicals with inadequate antioxidants to squelch them, inadequate minerals to support phase 2 systems, or inadequate excretion.

My Detox

After I had finished my orthodox treatment of breast cancer, I was looking around for what other treatments might offer ongoing protection and health. Dr. Alan Gaby (a holistic physician/nutritionist and my friend) and my surgeon were both fairly convinced that environmental chemicals play a role in many cancers and indirectly put a constant strain on the immune system. Having gone through the death of his sister from cancer, Alan was planning on doing a midlife detoxification program at the Northwest Healing Arts Center, a clinic run by a brilliant and innovative colleague of his, Dr. Walter Crinnion. He wanted to know if I would join him.

I arrived at the clinic and had a thorough workup. Dr. Crinnion, who is a naturopathic physician and one of the foremost experts in the United States on detoxification methods, ran tests to measure my blood levels. These showed I had higher than average levels of many of the chemicals that are possibly associated with breast cancer—DDT, DDE, and PCBS, and average levels of lindane and chlordane—even though I had been living a healthy lifestyle and eating organically grown food for most of my adult years. However, throughout my childhood I had been exposed to these chemicals, as was everyone else in the 1950s. I remember running behind the trucks that frequently sprayed pesticides on the trees near my home and the truck that sprayed insecticides every day at camp to keep the bug count down.

At the clinic, I took herbs each evening to help excretion through the liver and intestines. The morning began with aerobic exercise and skin brushing to enhance mobilization. Alan and I sat in the sauna (with heat around 130 degrees, also for mobilization); drank lots of water; and took herbs, vitamin C, minerals, and nutrients to help the detoxification enzymes, such as zinc, manganese, selenium, and N-acetyl-cysteine. Every hour we had a ten-minute break, then did more skin brushing. After the sauna we had naturopathic hot and cold therapy along with electro-physiotherapy to heighten liver excretion and immune functioning.

Colonics were performed at the end of the day to help eliminate the chemicals out of the body. I wanted proof that this procedure actually worked. Dr. Crinnion had a nearby lab test random samples of the effluent that came out from my colonic. Sure enough, some of the samples tested positive for a number of the chemicals that had been seen in my blood. Even though this information was anecdotal—it was just done on myself and one other woman—Dr. Gaby and I felt it was fairly significant.

I did the program for four weeks. Dr. Crinnion recommends a six-week program, but I had other commitments. Dr. Crinnion said the body

---

JUST IN CASE

Dr. Gordon Gribble has been a professor of chemistry at Dartmouth College for the last thirty years, studying chlorines and organochlorines. When I asked Dr. Gribble if he takes any precautionary action based on his knowledge of chemicals, he said: "I drink regular water out of the tap and don't eat organic food. I think there is a great danger in *not* using properly applied pesticides. Foods without pesticides can contain higher amounts of mycogens and pathogens [fungal and contaminating organisms]." He says that vegetables that are readily attacked by insects make more natural carcinogens in their attempt to fight off these insects and these natural carcinogens (such as glycoalkaloids) are more of a risk to us than pesticides. "Our body is well equipped to adapt to carcinogens and all the natural carcinogens we are exposed to," says Dr. Gribble. "If we didn't have these natural defense mechanisms, why, we'd all get cancer before the age of four." He does, however, eat a balanced diet and take vitamins, especially vitamins C, A, and E, which science has clearly shown assist in detoxifying chemical carcinogens.

continues to excrete these chemicals for many months afterward. He said that running my blood levels twelve to eighteen months afterward should show significantly lower levels than on the first day of treatment. Seventeen months later I was tested again by the same lab. PCBs and lindane had gone below detectable levels (my total PCBs had been elevated 4.5 times above the norm before the detox), DDT was reduced, and DDE and chlordane were the same.

Do not try this detox on your own.

STUDIES ON DETOXIFICATION

Scientific studies show that chemicals that have entered the body can be flushed out. These studies have used various methods to strengthen the body's natural excretion of chemicals.

The Michigan Seven

By 1978, 97 percent of individuals of a cross-section of the population tested in Michigan had demonstrable levels of PBB (polybrominated bisphenyl) in their fat tissue from inadvertent exposure. PBB is the major constituent of fire retardant, and it accidentally had been added to cattle feed in 1973, contaminating milk and meat. Seven men were treated for twenty days with a detoxification method that consisted of dry sauna for several hours a day, vitamins and minerals, and polyunsaturated oil. This treatment is currently used in Sweden and the United States for a variety of contamination accidents and drug rehabilitation. Pretreatment levels of sixteen chemicals, including PBB, PCBs, and three common chlorinated insecticides were taken. At posttreatment tests, thirteen were lower, with seven being statistically lower (in other words, not due to chance). A second posttreatment set of chemical measurements was taken four months later. The chemicals had been reduced even further, and ten of these reductions were statistically significant.

Electrical Workers

Electrical workers are frequently exposed to toxic chemicals such as PCBs, HCB (hexachlorobenzene), and other persistent organochlorine-based chemicals. Dr. Schnare from the EPA and Dr. Robinson from the Foundation for Advancement in Science and Education studied five electrical workers who were treated for three weeks with a rigorous detox program versus five who were not. Sixteen chemicals were tested, all of which were lower after treatment, while eleven were higher in the control group. The important part of this study is that the reductions in chemicals occurred even though the men were still working at their jobs and getting reexposed. This means, according to the authors, that excretion pathways were being enhanced, and this appeared to be a useful way to clean out the body. Schnare reports that many studies have shown that clinical symptoms reduce as chemical levels decrease.

Yugoslavian Capacitor Workers

From the 1930s to the 1980s, PCBS were made in Slovenia (a part of former Yugoslavia). One factory that made condensers had dumped approximately seventy tons of PCBS, some through incineration (releasing toxic waste into the air) and the rest through inappropriate handling methods. Many people living around the factory developed symptoms of toxicity, such as rashes, anxiety, numbness, gastrointestinal complaints, sleep disturbances, and joint problems, along with liver problems. Medical treatment did not help.

Eleven workers took part in the Hubbard detoxification program in a medical facility. They used daily aerobic exercise, stress heat, B_1 vitamins and polyunsaturated oil, vitamins, and minerals. Thirteen other workers were followed as a control group. For those on the program, posttreatment levels of PCBS were reduced 42 percent in blood and 30 percent in fat tissue, and their symptoms had improved. Levels of PCBS in blood and fat remained elevated in the control group. Four months later the differences between the experimental group and controls remained. Serum levels of the PCBS did *not* elevate during treatment. This finding is consistent with previous work.

Taiwanese Study

This study clearly showed that if you enhance mobilization of chemicals but not excretion, the chemicals don't leave the body. Sixteen Taiwanese patients who had been exposed to PCB-contaminated rice oil were put on a fast from seven to ten days without exercise, heat, nutrients, etc. The fast did not enhance excretion; it just increased mobilization. At the end of the study the patients had higher blood levels of PCBS than before the study had begun, but it is impressive to note that they still had symptomatic improvement.

Cycling Weight Studies

These studies indicate that some fat-soluble chemicals are released by dieting, which may be one reason why women who yo-yo diet are at higher risk for certain hormonally dependent tumors. This does not mean that weight loss is bad, but it points to the fact that fat cell mobilization without enhanced excretion is not good. If you're going to get the chemicals out of your tissues, you have to make sure they are removed from your body. This is also demonstrated in data about police officers who experienced hallucinogenic flashbacks after they had been occupationally exposed to drugs. Their fat stores released the drug back into the bloodstream, but the drugs were not excreted out of their system.

Some studies have shown that reduced levels of body chemicals have resulted in subtle behavioral changes, such as improvement in mental abilities, memory (long-term), and personality. In fact, Schnare and Robinson felt that human behavioral changes might be seen as early and subtle indicators of chemical toxicity. Something to think about with all the increase of violence and behavioral problems in our modern industrial society.

Room-by-Room Tour

Many people these days feel so overwhelmed with the problems of the world that they succumb to despair and helplessness. Or they say that the problems are just too massive to confront—better to cultivate one's own garden, take care of one's own family. We can't expect everyone to become an environmental activist outside their personal sphere of activity. However, if people actually took care of their family, their garden, and especially their spirit the world would be a much better place to live.

—Gary Cohen, "Toward a Spirituality Based on Justice, and Ecology," *Social Policy* (1996)

It seems that the old saying "home is where the heart is" may now need an addendum—"Home is also where the pollution is." It turns out that our greatest source of environmental exposure usually occurs not next to a toxic waste site but in our own homes. Not that living near a Superfund site is healthy; we still need to clean up the environment. However, according to scientists who call themselves human exposure assessment experts or environmental toxicology specialists (one man I interviewed called himself the "world's expert on home dust"), our houses are waste dumps, often carrying higher levels of toxic exposure than what would be allowed at any occupational work site. Drain cleaner, spray paint, rubber cement, toilet bowl cleaner, spot remover, antifreeze, bug spray, fertilizer—the typical American home contains sixty-three hazardous chemical products.

According to EPA information, 75 percent of American households used at least one pesticide indoors in 1997, mostly as either an insecticide or a disinfectant. Eighty percent of most exposure to pesticides occurs inside the home. Up to a dozen pesticides have been measured in most homes.

The American Association of Poison Control Centers reported in 1990 that some 79,000 children experienced pesticide poisonings or exposures. The EPA reminds us that the "-cide" in pesticides means "to kill."

This may sound alarming, but if home is our greatest source of contamination, we are in a far better position to manage this exposure than that which is in the environment outside our homes.

Most of us do not want to hear this, preferring to maintain what Wayne Ott, who has a Ph.D. in civil and environmental engineering from Stanford University, calls a "conspiracy of ignorance." We do not want to hear that we have some responsibility in the contamination issue, that it is not *all* the fault of nasty industry or slack government. True, many of these pollutants begin with commercialization and industry. But if our greatest source of exposure to pollutants is in our kitchens, bathrooms, living rooms, and workshops, then we have a measure of control.

There *are* ways you can protect yourself and your family. Not all the chemicals we address in this chapter are necessarily known or suspected endocrine disruptors. Most chemicals have not been tested yet for their endocrine-disrupting potential. Until more research is done over the next number of decades, all chemicals that haven't been tested are possibly hormone disruptors. But toxic is toxic. Even if some of the chemicals we discuss here don't prove to be endocrine disruptors, the likelihood is that they are toxic in some other way. Thus, the sensible approach is to minimize exposure as much as possible. The general idea, from almost every scientist we talked to, is that we should try to decrease our environmental pollutant exposure to the best of our ability, and this will minimize our contact with endocrine-disrupting chemicals.

THE TEAM STUDIES

From 1980 to 1990, the EPA conducted a series of scientific tests called the Total Exposure Assessment Methodology (TEAM) studies. The TEAM studies looked at more than 3,000 people from different parts of the country who were chosen in a statistical manner to represent more than 3 million people from these various locales. Personal, indoor, and outdoor exposures to a list of pollutants were evaluated.

Personal exposure is the actual exposure of a person. If we are talking about air pollution, it is personal exposure to the air a person is breathing, wherever he or she might happen to be during the day. To estimate

---

MR. EXPOSURE

Wayne Ott is a man who really understands exposure. He has been with the U.S. Environmental Protection Agency (EPA) and its predecessor agencies for thirty years and is one of the leading proponents of a new science—*human exposure assessment*—which looks at the manner in which pollutants come into actual contact with the human body.

Dr. Ott explains that *environmental regulators* start at the source of pollution, such as waste sites or industry, and try to figure out whether or not the sources are reaching anybody. *Exposure scientists* start with people and measure what's actually reaching them and then find out where it's coming from. He says, "Exposure is contact. That's what it means. What is contacting the person, and at what level, what concentration? It's a simple axiom: if you're not exposed, you can't get sick. You can't change the way the body works, but you can change exposures. In fact, it's the only thing you can change."

Ott is quite adamant about the fact that it is in our own homes that we are the most exposed. "What the public doesn't understand," says Ott, "is that your house *is* the hazardous waste site. All the things you have in your house are made of the same chemicals that are on the hazardous lists. Once you start thinking, all the chemically based products in a hardware store, like cleaners and solvents, they have to be made of something. What do you think they're made of? They're made out of the same substances that someone is worried about in minuscule concentrations one hundred feet underground."

---

that exposure, assessors give the test subject an air-quality monitor that can be carried throughout her or his daily activities (indoors, outdoors, or in a vehicle). Indoor exposure is estimated by a fixed monitor set up in one room, such as the living room. Outdoor exposure is measured by a fixed monitor set up at an outdoor site.

The first seven-year study took place in northern New Jersey, an area that holds the greatest concentration of oil refineries and chemical plants in the United States. More than 350 people—divided into those living near industrial sites and participants residing farther away—were monitored for two consecutive twelve-hour periods, day and night. According to Dr. Wallace, "The results were an eye-opener. No difference in exposure was seen between residents who lived near the plants and those farther away. Moreover, the personal exposures were typically three times higher than the concurrent outdoor concentrations for all of the eleven volatile organic compounds (vocs) they measured. The vocs included a known human carcinogen (benzene) and a number of other compounds known to cause cancer in animals. At the higher percentiles, personal exposures soared to 10 to 70 times the outdoor levels. Even overnight, when the monitor was on the bedside table most of the time, the indoor exposures exceeded the outdoor concentrations."

What this means is striking: living close to an industrial source of con-tamination like a chemical plant is not more polluting than what any of us may be exposed to at home. However, we must remember that the TEAM studies were looking at personal exposure to important carcinogens, not at actual cases of cancer or other illnesses.

Another TEAM study looked at personal exposure to particles, as opposed to toxic gases, in Riverside, California. The most important find-ing of the Particle TEAM Study was that personal exposure (the concen-tration measured by the personal monitor) was about 50 percent higher than either the concentration from the indoor monitor or the concentra-tion as measured by the outdoor monitor. The results of these studies overturned standard ideas concerning sources of pollution. The results all shared a common theme: *the most important sources of pollution are close to the person.* Not even dust is innocent anymore.

Some people visualize this exposure as a kind of "personal cloud," rather like the cloud of particles surrounding the character known as Pig-pen in the *Peanuts* comic strip, so it's also commonly refered to as the Pig-pen effect.

TAKE IT ROOM-BY-ROOM

To demonstrate how we are exposed to multiple chemicals in our homes—in other words, how we create the Pigpen effect—let's take a tour of your house (or apartment or office), indicating where the potential hormone-disrupting compounds are and what can be done about reducing your exposure to them.

THE AIR IN THE HOUSE

How long can we live without food? Perhaps a month. How long can we live without water? Perhaps several days. But how long can we live with-

EDUCATING THE PUBLIC

Dr. Wayne Ott (who spent thirty years with the EPA) says, "I joined EPA's predecessor organization in 1966—a time when the public did not believe that outdoor air pollution was a problem at all. The New York–New Jersey power plants burned high sulfur coal that caused elevated sulfuric acid that coated the New York Stock Exchange on Wall Street, making the building look black.

"Despite the obvious effects of air pollution on their surroundings, the public did not feel that outdoor air pollution was particularly important. As a result, the Division of Air Pollution of the Public Health Service (at which I was a staff scientist) conducted one of the largest and most aggressive public information campaigns ever. Hollywood studios were commissioned by the federal government to make documentary films about outdoor air pollution. Community discussion groups were organized throughout the United States and Public Health Service specialists fanned out to tell the people the story. Millions of color pamphlets showed the horrors of outdoor air pollution. Radio public-health service announcements were taped and mailed to stations across the United States. Even cartoonists at U.S. newspapers were enlisted in the war to educate the public. CBS News (with the help of Public Health Services) created a one-hour documentary that was aired during prime time with many spectacular pictures of smokestacks spewing out plumes. The U.S. Surgeon General went on TV repeatedly to warn the public.

"These ambitious efforts had a major effect: the public changed from (a) knowing almost nothing about outdoor air pollution to (b) being highly concerned and motivated about controlling outdoor air pollution.

"When scientific discoveries concerning indoor air began to occur in the early 1980s, no massive campaign was mounted by EPA to make people aware of the findings of the TEAM studies. I believe that the public still is programmed to believe that outdoor air pollution is a critical problem—even though most of the pollutants of concern in 1970 have all but disappeared from the nation's outdoor air. Outdoor exposures to carbon monoxide, for example, have dropped by 50 percent every decade for thirty years to almost negligible levels, even though indoor carbon monoxide levels still remain a serious cause of death in the United States—the second largest cause of nonintentional poisoning in the United States after heroin."

out air? Several minutes at most. Our air is vital to us. We each consume approximately 35 pounds of air per day. The TEAM exposure studies to date reveal that *it is the air in our houses that exposes us to the most pollution.* Here are some ways you can cut down on air pollution in your home.

- *Ventilate. Ventilate. Ventilate.* Open windows and doors. (For those living in Los Angeles or other cities with heavily polluted air, it might be best to keep windows closed.) Consider using window fans or other means, such as a free-standing air-filtration system, to eliminate chemicals in the air.

- If your new carpet or carpet padding is to be attached to the floor, request that it be tacked down. If not, ask for a glue with low-emitting chemical fumes.

- When you use your clothes washing machine, open a nearby window for an hour or two.

- Even in winter, open windows a crack for an hour or two every several days. Newly constructed airtight houses contribute to moisture and the indoor chemical load, but opening a window helps. Remove or seal the surface of all particleboard in your home with nitrocellulose lacquer because particleboard emits fumes for a long time.

- Add houseplants to help neutralize toxic indoor air. They take up carbon dioxide and give off oxygen.

Breathing In Trouble

The following is only one example of endocrine disruption brought into our homes and lives through the air in our houses. From the 1950s through the 1980s, the pesticide chlordane was used to kill termites. In more than 30 million American homes, chlordane was poured into the soil before the foundational concrete slab was laid—hundreds of gallons of pesticide per 1,000 square feet per home. Many people living in homes built before April 1988 (when chlordane was banned) are breathing in chlordane on a daily basis. There are a number of illnesses that have been associated with chlordane exposure: upper-respiratory problems, ovarian/uterine disease, migraine, increased incidence of infections, and autoimmune problems. Some health problems may occur even at what are considered safe and acceptable levels of the chemical.

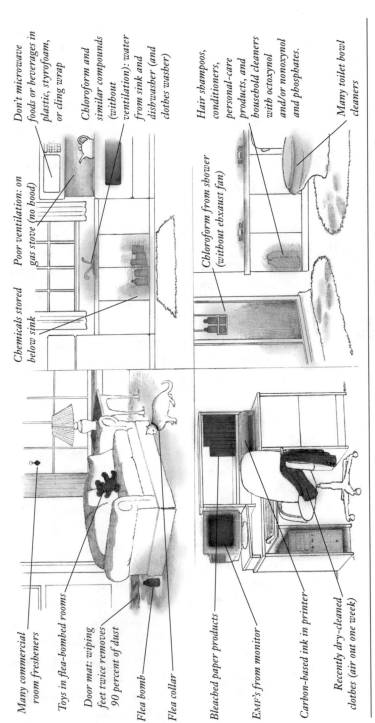

FIGURE 14.1 *Home Exposures*

Startling associations between chlordane and attention deficit disorder and other mental problems were uncovered by researchers at the University of Southern California School of Medicine. Two hundred and fifty adults and children had lived in an apartment complex in 1987 that had its outside walls treated with chlordane. In 1994 researchers showed that chlordane exposure in this group was linked to adverse effects on their mental functions, including problems with memory, attention deficit, tension, depression, anger, and fatigue. These same exposed adults had a significant increase in physical illnesses such as asthma, allergies, chronic bronchitis, headaches, and indigestion. The authors concluded that these problems seemed to be coming from indoor air exposure to chlordane, which they linked to "irreversible dysfunction of the brain." Chlordane has also been associated with childhood blood and brain cancers, infertility in mice, and even obesity. All these possible adverse health problems are in body systems that are affected by endocrine disruption.

Just as radon gas is now known to move into a home through the soil underneath a house, pesticide vapors can enter into a house the same way. The best method of dealing with this is by installing a system that reroutes the radon and pesticide vapors around your house by pressurizing the house or depressurizing the soil under the house and cement slab.

At the Front Door

As the front door to your home gets opened and closed, the dust that lines the indentations, carvings, and windows of the door gets blown into the house, carrying hormone disruptors like lead and pesticides along with it.

Dust also enters the home on our shoes. Studies have shown that dust tracked in on the bottom of shoes can contain high levels of pesticides and lead. Pesticides are sprayed by homeowners on or near patios, lawns, and the outside of the house. They are sprayed by town or city governments in parks and playgrounds and on trees lining the streets. Pesticide-laden dust drifts down onto pathways and roads, is picked up by car tires, lands on the driveway or front porch, and ends up on shoes. As we walk into our homes and onto the living room or bedroom carpet, the dust gets tamped down into the carpet pile, where babies crawl and kids play. If you live in an area with construction going on, the dust is also likely to contain a fair amount of lead contamination, most likely coming from disturbing the lead-laden soil from past years of auto emissions. Shoes worn outside the home are a major source of lead exposure in the home. Repainting and remodeling older houses generates lead dust that can be tracked into the home. Levels of organophosphate pesticides are much higher in house dust than in soil samples because house dust stays dry, keeping the pesticides in their original form for a much longer time.

There are ways to minimize the dust entering your home.

- Take off your shoes before entering your house. The Japanese have worn no outdoor shoes in the home for centuries. This may be one reason, other than all the soy they eat, that they have less incidence of illnesses like breast cancer.

- Wipe your feet twice on a good doormat. This may be 75 to 90 percent as effective as taking off your shoes. Large commercial doormats reduce exposure to the home, but these mats must be

---

THE KING OF DUST

John Roberts is a mechanical engineer and EPA consultant who hypothesized that house dust is a major source of exposure for infants and convinced the government to do a risk assessment. By 1990 he had helped develop a machine to study pollutants on surfaces, which was used in the TEAM studies. He says, "There are a number of compounds like the PCBS, DDT, PAHS (that come from incomplete combustion of cigarettes, coal, food, oil, and gasoline), and we find all those persistent compounds building up in house dust. The average kid is exposed to these compounds that we try to protect them from at Superfund sites. It's quite common to find lead in the middle of the yard at 100 parts per million and in the house at 1,000 parts per million."

He explained the mechanisms that enable these compounds to get into and stay in the house: "First is the preferential track-in of small particles, which stick to your feet better than big particles and have higher concentrations of pollutants. Next, whatever is in the air is deposited on the high outside surface areas of the house—the roof, the sides of the walls—and it collects around the foundation and walkways, then it's tracked in. Third, which is probably the most important, there's no sunlight inside. Sunlight is the major way in which organic pollutants like PCBS, PAHS, phthalates, and pesticides are broken down. The UV light breaks the carbon bonds and degrades many pollutants. Plus, there is more bacterial action outside in the soil. So pollutants that would degrade quickly outside may last for years in the carpet."

kept clean. There should be a sign above the mat to remind guests and family members to use it. It is easier to prevent dirt from being tracked into the house than it is to clean it up once it is inside. The first few steps we take on the carpet in the house remove 95 percent or more of the contaminated dust, so wiping your feet on a mat is really effective. A commercial-grade doormat should last a lifetime.

- Dust the front door weekly, just as you would the inside of the house.

- If you work with lead or in a lead-contaminated environment, change out of your work clothes before entering the house.

LIVING ROOM

Americans spend only 5 percent of their time outdoors, so indoor sources of pollution are a major contributor to human exposure. And where do we hang out? In the living room, where dusty rugs and fleecy surfaces provide a reservoir for hormone disruptors such as lead, pesticides, PAHs, and PCBs, especially in larger cities where high vehicle traffic contaminates the soil, which already harbors dust mites, molds, and bacteria. A combination of high-quality door mats, removing shoes at the door, and efficient vacuum cleaners can reduce dust levels by 99 percent. This is hopeful.

Rugs and carpets may contain 400 times as much house dust as bare wood or tile floors. The higher the pile of carpet, the more the dust can embed and get spread as children play and family members walk over the floors. Since house dust is the number-one cause of lead and a major source of pesticide exposure in the home, this is especially important if you have infants and toddlers who crawl and play on the rug, ingesting and breathing in the dust. They are more vulnerable to these pollutants than anyone else. Homes treated for termites showed residues of the pesticides chlordane and heptachlor—both endocrine disruptors—in carpet swatches placed on the floor in the homes.

A few weeks after installation, most carpets are considered low emitters of volatile organic compounds (vocs). It is how the carpet is maintained or contaminated with remodeling or with outside dust that mostly affects indoor air quality.

VACUUMING

Use a vacuum with a power head, high-efficiency bag, and HEPA filter. "Dirt finders," offered on vacuums by Hoover, Panasonic, and Sears, sense when dust is no longer coming into the vacuum and a green light goes on, telling you when the carpet is clean. It might take hours of vacuuming the first time to get that light to turn green everywhere on the carpet. These vacuum cleaners are "smart" and not expensive. If you can afford the very best, the Kirby vacuum is a marvel of "Micron Magic" filter efficiency combined with a powerful air flow that removes 99.9 percent of dust particles.

According to Roberts, "If a rug can be turned over and vacuumed from the other side, a series of three such flips with repeated vacuuming on each side has been shown to pick up as much as 55 percent of the total lead in the carpet." The less often street shoes are worn in the house, the less cleaning is required. Flipping old rugs can generate much toxic dust, especially if these rugs have not been flipped in years. Never do it with children or pregnant women around. It is best to do on a piece of clean plastic outside. Be kind to your lungs and immune system by wearing a good two-strap dust mask when you vacuum or flip rugs.

Here are some ways to minimize exposure in your living room

- Vacuum upholstered furniture regularly. Dust settles into fabric.
- Vacuum and/or wet wash the surfaces people touch once a month, such as furniture, woodwork, and window wells. Use a high phosphate detergent with a wet mop, sponge, or rag to wipe floors, baseboards, and window sills.
- Vacuum rugs and carpeting frequently (once a week or twice a week if you have a crawling child), using a high-efficiency particulate air (HEPA) vacuum cleaner. Normal vacuuming removes only 5 to 15 percent of house dust caught in the carpet or rug.
- Take extra care to clean up any ash on the carpet from fireplaces or wood stoves. Polycyclic aromatic hydrocarbons (PAHS) are toxic chemicals commonly produced from the incomplete combustion of petroleum products, wood, food, or tobacco.

- Lay out a clean sheet or blanket before you put a baby down on the carpet.

- Lead paint was banned from housing in 1978. If your home was built before 1979, have the house dust tested for lead. For information, call the National Center for Lead-Safe Housing at 410/992-0712.

Here are some tips for renovating and redecorating.

- Emissions from paints, paint strippers, varnishes, wood finishes, caulking, adhesives, etc., can linger indoors for up to a week. Ventilate.

- Consult renovation experts on proper removal of lead paint or call the EPA at 800/532-3394 for detailed information. Older homes may have chipped or peeling lead paint—a dangerous source of lead for young children. A simple blood test can detect high levels of lead in children.

- Removing old carpet and padding can bring up large amounts of dust and whatever the dust is carrying. Ventilate the rooms well and use a good dust mask when removing a carpet.

- If you're thinking of buying new carpeting: pure nylon carpets are the strongest and one of the safer environmental carpet choices. Olefin or polypropylene is cheap and colorfast. However, it most likely has oil added to the fiber to survive the tufting process, and most American manufacturers do not spend the money to get the oil out. Make sure that Berber-type carpeting is not made from polypropylene or olefin. Wool carpets made before the 1960s are safe. Now, however, most quality wool is not domestic and is either sprayed with pesticides in other countries or is blended in this country with fibers that are not so environmentally friendly. Level loop carpets (tight weave) are better than plush or shag. You might also insist that the new carpet be opened up and aired out for a few days before installation.

BATHROOM

Spraying bathroom chemicals in an unventilated room results in mists that would never be allowed in a factory or laboratory given the strict health and safety laws regarding the use of hazardous chemicals. Many of these chemicals have not yet been tested for hormone disruption. Reducing exposure to these toxins in general is the best idea. Use your fans and open windows.

Air Fresheners

Approximately one-third of the homes in the TEAM studies had high levels of the chemical p-dichlorobenzene—a registered pesticide that is the active ingredient in moth repellents—even though only 10 percent of the people who lived in these homes said they used moth repellents. The researchers wondered if the villain might be toilet deodorizers and air fresheners, which were reported in use in 70 percent of the homes, so they tested all three types of air fresheners: liquid, spray, and solid. All contained p-dichlorobenzene. According to Wallace, this chemical has been demonstrated in tests by the U.S. National Toxicology Program to cause cancers in rats and mice. The pure white cakes commonly placed in urinals and public toilets to freshen the air are made up of 100 percent p-dichlorobenzene.

Showers and Baths

Believe it or not, relaxing in a hot shower or bath can be detrimental to your health. Many people today understand the importance of clean drinking water. Note the strong sales of bottled water. However, most of us are not aware of the fact that the greatest source of pollution from water does not come from what we drink but from what we inhale or absorb through our skin. Half of the chlorine in our tap water is released as *chloroform*, one of the simplest organochlorine siblings. When most people hear the word chloroform they think of the surgical anesthetic, used years ago, which was found to be toxic. Now chloroform is known as the shadow side of the process of water chlorination. It is a trihalomethane and these chemicals have not been tested yet for hormone disruption.

Chloroform travels throughout the house and pollutes the air of your home. It is released from water that is not heated (such as in the toilet or rinsing vegetables at the sink), but most is released into the air of our homes through the running and agitation of hot water, such as in showers, clothes washing, and dish washing. If the tap water in your house is chlorinated, every time you take a long shower or luxuriate in a bath, chloroform is released as a gas and you absorb it through your skin and inhale it through the steam, along with other volatile organic compounds.

A 1996 study showed that the inhaled breath of people who had taken a ten-minute shower or thirty-minute bath had a larger internal dose of volatile compounds (VOCs) than drinking half a gallon of tap water. Inhaling the steam in an enclosed shower stall gives the greatest dose of all. According to Dr. Wallace, the hotter the shower, the more the capillaries open up in the skin. The longer and hotter the shower, the more chloroform is absorbed through the skin. If the shower is cooler, say even 85°–90°F, the capillaries close off a little and this reduces the dermal exposure by a large percent, although there still is exposure through inhalation. Enclosed shower stalls obviously concentrate the chloroform more than open ones. Dr. Wallace does admit that this does not stop him from enjoying his hot showers, but he keeps the bathroom windows wide open.

Try these ways to minimize exposure in the bathroom.

- Avoid commercial air fresheners and toilet deodorants that contain p-dichlorobenzene (p-DCB). There are healthier alternatives. Or try the old-fashioned way: an open box of baking soda will absorb odors.

- Invest in a dual carbon/coconut shell filter at the main source of water into your house. In essence, this is a water filter for your whole house, not just for your kitchen sink or shower. These filters are expensive, costing between $1,000 and $2,000, but they remove a major source of home pollution from your showers, baths, dish washing, and clothes washing. If you cannot afford a house filter, buy a carbon-based water filter for your drinking and cooking water as well as one that attaches to or replaces your shower head. These cost a little over $100 and are well worth it. They even make travel models.

- If you don't have a water filter and your water is chlorinated, run the bathroom exhaust fan while showering. You need to do this anyway to control moisture and molds. Do relax in a bath but also open a window.

- After a long period (over twenty-four hours) of disuse, run your water taps for a few minutes to flush out contaminated water.

BEDROOM

In the TEAM studies, clothes that had been dry-cleaned were the most profound source of exposure to perchloroethylene, called perc. (It is also known as tetrachloroethylene.) Perc is used by machinists and mechanics as a metal degreaser for lubricated machine parts and, in dry cleaning, is used to dissolve oily stains caused by human sweat or other sources. It cleans your best dress or suit as effectively as it cleans airplane parts. Perc is known to be a thyroid-hormone disruptor. It is known to attack the central nervous system and is a suspected cause of a number of reproductive disorders as well as a carcinogen in rodent studies. Infertility in both men and women and menstrual disorders have been linked to perc exposure.

According to the EPA, the dry-cleaning industry ($6 billion a year in revenues) has more than 34,000 commercial dry-cleaning shops located in neighborhoods and malls, making it one of the largest groups of chemical users to have regular contact with the public. If you work at a dry-cleaning establishment and have constant headaches, consider the connection. An analysis in 1996 estimated that one out of every 6,700 people who wear dry-cleaned clothes at least once a week could be expected to get cancer from breathing fumes from the perc left in the fabric.

To minimize exposure in your bedroom, try the following:

- When you pick up clothes from the cleaners, remove the plastic and air out the clothes in the garage or on the back porch. It will take about a week to reduce these residues by a substantial amount. However, airing out dry-cleaned clothes even for a day or so before bringing them into the house will reduce exposure by about 20 percent.
- Don't patronize dry cleaners that use chlorinated solvents (perc). More than 100 establishments in the United States offer "professional multiprocess wet cleaning," an alternative to dry cleaning. The EPA has been working with the dry-cleaning industry to reduce exposure to perchloroethylene and to evaluate alternative technologies. Most dry cleaners, however, are locked into their use of perc because of their reliance on expensive equipment.
- Reduce your dependence on dry cleaning. Many clothes that are labeled "dry clean only" can actually be washed on delicate cycle in cold water.

- Usually perc is not found in water at levels high enough to worry about (although we don't know what even microscopic amounts of perc do in combination with chlorination by-products), except where wells have been contaminated. Some areas of the country have been known to have perc in the water supply. Since perc is carbon based, a carbon filter placed at the source of water for your home will remove this chemical and organic pesticides from tap water.

- Check labels for common consumer products that also contain perc, such as carburetor cleaners, engine solvents, and other automotive products that are often found in many American garages. Perc can make up 10 to 60 percent of the product by weight. Teenagers working on cars at homes with attached garages typically expose themselves and the whole family to elevated concentrations of perc.

- Buy T-shirts and other clothing made of 100 percent organic cotton or try unbleached, undyed, untreated cotton goods.

Mindy Pennybacker, in "The Hidden Life of T-Shirts," says that more than one billion T-shirts were produced in the United States during 1998, but "trace most T-shirts' life cycles—whether all cotton, synthetic, or a blend—and you'll find heavy hidden costs." To grow five pounds of cotton takes a pound of chemicals, and bioengineered cotton, such as Monsanto's "Roundup Ready" cotton (grown on an estimated 3 million acres in 1998), can use even higher quantities of toxic chemicals. The "miracle" synthetics such as polyester and nylon are made from fossil fuels and their manufacture dumps solvents, oils, acids, and caustics into our water. Chemical dyes use toxic heavy metals, and silk-screened logos are made from plastisol inks—a form of polyvinyl chloride (PVC), which is a major source of hormone-disrupting dioxins.

Kitchen

The kitchen—where we prepare our healthy meals—is frequently full of toxins. To minimize your exposure in the kitchen, try the following:

- Avoid super-strength cleaners. Use nontoxic cleaning products like baking soda, borax, and vinegar. Wear rubber gloves if you do use toxic products.

- Do not store chemical cleaners, ant-killing sprays, or other toxic chemicals under the sink where the heat from hot water pipes (or even heaters) may volatilize these compounds into the air you breathe. Removing these products from under the sink also ensures that your children cannot get at them.

- Filter your water or buy spring water. If you live in a place where radon gas or radioactive particles naturally occur in the water (if you're not sure about this, have your house tested), reverse osmosis is the only type of filtration that will clear out these particles. You then should take supplemental minerals, as filtered water removes the minerals that protect your heart and other parts of your body.

- Use the exhaust fan over gas stoves.

- Lead leaches from some types of ceramic dinnerware into foods and beverages. Avoid or limit to special occasions the use of antique or collectible housewares for food and beverages. Labels on ornamental ceramic products that say "For decorative purposes only" or "Not for food use" probably contain lead. Don't store acidic foods, such as fruit juices, in ceramic or lead crystal containers. Don't use lead crystal wine decanters and alcohol bottles. Also avoid home remedies or cosmetics that contain lead (Azarcon, Greta, Pay-loo-ah, Alkohl, Kohl, and hair-coloring products).

- Avoid cooking, microwaving, or storing food in plastic containers. High temperatures may cause packaging components such as paper, adhesives, and polymers to migrate into food. Remember, tiny amounts of chemicals in parts per trillion or parts per billion are being studied for their effects on biologic tissues. Use heat-resistant glass or lead-free ceramic containers. Some scientists feel that although pregnant women should avoid any possible exposure to the chemicals in plastic, this problem is not valid for adult males, and the data on how much plastic gets into the food is too controversial at this time to make a judgment. The latest Rubbermaid and Tupperware containers appear to be free of plasticizers, but we don't yet know enough about how plastic interacts with food when heated.

- Avoid polystyrene foam containers for fatty foods, alcohol, or hot foods or beverages.

- Avoid plastic cling wrap or minimize its direct contact with food. Reduce consumption of fatty foods packaged in plastic and heat-sealed containers. Since most endocrine disruptors are fat soluble, they tend to reside in meat and dairy products, such as cheese, ham, and beef. The packaging material may add more endocrine disruptors to what is already in the food itself. Buy plastic wraps made from polyethylene (has no plasticizers) such as Glad Crystal Clear Polyethylene. It's still smart not to have the wrap in direct contact with food.

- To prevent cockroach infestation, clean and fill any cracks and gaps in floors and walls. Use a least-toxic pest control company for serious pest problems.

LAUNDRY ROOM

When you take a shower, bathe, or wash clothes, the chemicals in your water will evaporate, especially at higher water temperatures, transforming waterborne contaminants into airborne vocs like chloroform or bromoform. Thus, cooking, humidifiers, dishwashers, clothes-washing machines, and bathing in the tub can release these volatile carbon compounds into

---

RECIPES FOR SAFE CLEANING

Oven cleaner: Make a paste of baking soda and water, apply to oven surfaces, and let stand a little while. Mechanical action is the key. Use a copper scouring pad for most surfaces. A razor blade is effective to get under large food deposits.

Window cleaner: Mix ½ cup vinegar, a few drops of liquid soap, and 1 quart of warm water in a spray bottle and use on glass surfaces. Rub with a lint-free cloth and polish with wadded up newspaper. For really dirty outdoor windows, wash with soapy water, rinse well, and squeegie dry.

For other recipes, contact the Washington Toxics Coalition, 4649 Sunnyside Ave. N, Ste. 540E, Seattle WA 98103, 206/632-1545.

our breathing space, where they get inhaled and absorbed. This is a major problem for women doing housework, infants, or people who clean homes for a living.

Here are a few ideas for minimizing exposure in the laundry room:

- Select soaps and detergents, especially liquid products, that do not contain nonyl phenol ethoxylates (NPES—derivatives of APES). Call the company for information on product ingredients.

- As an alternative to using detergent at all, consider chemical-free products with no phosphates, dyes, or fragrances. Try noncontaminating products, such as *EarthSmart* Laundry CD (from OneSource Worldwide Network, Inc.) or The Laundry Solution (from TradeNetMarketing, Inc., 1497 Main St., Ste. 301, Dunedin, FL 34698. Phone 813/738-1222; fax 813/738-0802). I have been using them and they clean as well as detergent.

- Use nonchlorine bleach. There are alternatives to chlorine. Using chlorine to bleach your clothes creates hormone-disrupting organochlorine compounds which are released into our waterways. I use Seventh Generation products for many of my cleaning needs. Contact the company at 800/456-1191.

- During and for several hours after using the washing machine, close the door to the laundry room and leave the window open.

OFFICE

Many people these days have offices in their home and can control the machinery and paper goods they purchase. If you work in an office outside the home, try suggesting the following ideas to whoever is in charge of purchases.

To minimize exposure in the office consider these tips.

- Buy unbleached paper products or those that don't use chlorine. To eliminate paper-related pollutants such as dioxins and furans, try treeless paper from hemp, kenaf, and other agriculturally based pulp sources (which are usually grown without pesticides and are chlorine- and acid-free).

- Check with the manufacturer to see if your computer monitor meets or exceeds regulations about emissions of radiation. Look for Energy Star compliant hardware.

READING PRODUCT LABELS ISN'T EASY, EVEN FOR GENIUSES

Nontoxic, green, environmentally safe, all natural, and *organic* (on products, not food) all sound simple and good, but it isn't necessarily so. Actually these terms can be murky and don't legally mean what most consumers think. Often they refer only to single ingredients. Why is it so confusing?

First, these terms refer to levels of acute (short-term) toxicity and not to low-dose exposure over time (which is how endocrine disruption works). Second, three different government agencies regulate labeling for various products, and each of the three agencies uses different labeling systems.

The Environmental Protection Agency (EPA) regulates pesticides for the lawn and garden, indoor insecticides, disinfectants such as chlorine, wood preservatives, and so on. The EPA requires a list of active ingredients but not the inactive ingredients. Thus, you don't know everything that is in a product. *Signal words* connote possible hazards of toxicity, corrosive action, harmful vapors, and/or flammable products. In increasing level of danger, words to watch for on EPA-regulated products are *caution, warning,* and *danger.*

The Food and Drug Administration (FDA) regulates over-the-counter medicines and personal-care products for the body, such as soaps and shampoos. The FDA does not use signal words. They do require a list of all a product's ingredients to be listed on the label. Therefore, this is one system that allows a consumer to identify hormone-disrupting compounds by reading the label.

The Consumer Product Safety Commission regulates products such as cleaning items. They use signal words but with slightly different meanings. The lack of signal words on a product connotes the lowest level of hazard but still suggests a hazard. The words *caution* and *warning* signify the next level of hazard, while *danger* warns of the highest level of hazard.

So what to do? As much as you can, try the following suggestions:

- Avoid products with the words *caution, warning,* or *danger* on the label.

- Avoid detergents that contain APES.

- Personal-care products must list ingredients. Avoid those with octoxynol and/or nonoxynol on the label.

- Avoid paints that do not state the amount of VOCs they contain. Two hundred and fifty grams per liter of paint is legally permitted but look for labels that state sixty or seventy grams per liter.

- You get more for your money with concentrated products, but concentrated disinfectants and pesticides could have more potential problems.

- Choose products with pumps rather than aerosol sprays and choose recyclable plastic rather than vinyl.

- Avoid phosphates.

- Avoid perfumes and dyes.

- Look for products that say *biodegradable* and/or *recyclable* (even though these terms leave room for some confusion).

- When you shop, stop and think. Be aware of a product's impact, both on the environment and on your body. Awareness is what will help the health of our children and our planet.

Many companies are responding to the environmental message and have bleach-free products that come in biodegradable or recyclable containers. The following are examples of products that have been tested and were found not to contain APES: Arm & Hammer, Country Save, Tide, and Wisk laundry detergents; Shout stain remover; PineSol; Murphy's Oil Soap; Soft Scrub (without bleach); and Bon Ami (without bleach). Dr. Bronner's Castille soap has been a long-time favorite of many health advocates.

For booklets on safe products write to Washington Toxics Coalition, 4649 Sunnyside Ave. N., Ste. 540 East, Seattle, WA 98103. Phone 206-632-1545; fax 206-632-8661; or E-mail info@watoxics.org.

- If you have a printer that uses carbon-based ink, vocs (volatile organic compounds) are being given off. When your computer warms up, it may volatilize persistent phthalates into the air. It is well worth putting money into an office air filter that will remove airborne contaminants.

- Office furniture can emit formaldehyde and vocs for years after purchase. Think about buying furniture made from certified sustainably harvested wood or recycled material finished with toxic-free paint and binding agents. Check out the Green Seal home page at www.greenseal.org for manufacturers of nontoxic furniture. Or buy used furniture that has had years to air out.

CIGARETTE SMOKE

Hard as it may be to believe, almost half of the total nationwide indoor personal exposure to benzene comes from cigarettes. There are 500,000 deaths per year from tobacco, making the numbers of deaths from breast and prostate cancer seem small. Many carcinogenic chemicals are in tobacco (such as styrene, toluene, xylenes, ethylbenzene, formaldehyde, and 1,3-butadiene), especially the benzopyrenes. Secondhand smoke accounts for more benzene exposure than the outdoor pollution caused by the entire industrial capacity of the United States.

How can something so small and personal contribute more to our exposure than companies venting this chemical into the air? Cigarettes are an incredibly efficient delivery system into the lungs. According to Dr. Wallace, "Every cigarette delivers benzene in mainstream smoke with near 100 percent efficiency to the smoker."

There is six to ten times more benzene in the bodies of smokers than in nonsmokers. Benzene is a bone marrow toxin. As the bone marrow is contaminated, it gives rise to faulty white blood cells (leukocytes), the hallmark of leukemia. Benzene is also suspected in multiple myeloma and non-Hodgkin's lymphoma. When a woman is pregnant, the fetus of a smoker gets much more benzene than the fetus of a mother who does not smoke. Two studies demonstrated that children of smokers died of leukemia two to four times more often than children whose parents did not smoke.

GARAGE

Garages tend to accumulate some of the nastier toxins. To lower your exposure, try the following.

- Car pool or minimize the use of your car. Npes (nonyl phenol ethoxylates) are used in oil and gas drilling, extraction, and production. Fuel combustion releases cadmium and mercury, two heavy metal hormone disruptors, into the environment.

- Keep your garage door open for an hour after you pull in your car or park outside and let the car cool down before pulling it into the garage. Don't idle the car in the garage.

When you pull your car into the garage and the car is still hot from running, the benzene that is in the gasoline is volatilized. Benzene was the first chemical ever identified as a human carcinogen in the 1700s in

---

INTEGRATED PEST MANAGEMENT (IPM)

American farmers used thirty-three times more pesticides in 1990 than they did in 1945, yet crop losses from pests during that time increased from 31 to 37 percent. In October of 1997, two American scientists—Ray F. Smith and Perry L. Adkisson—received the World Food Prize for developing an environmentally friendly alternative to chemical pesticides for crop protection, known as Integrated Pest Management. The U.S. Department of Agriculture has established a goal of having integrated programs in use on three-quarters of all American farms by the year 2000. And more and more towns and communities are using IPM instead of pesticides for parks and roadside greenery.

You can protect the health of your entire garden system through such practices as maintaining good soil, mulching, and growing flowers that draw natural predators—an integrated approach for having bugs stay in balance without the use of chemicals. For bug problems, the least toxic methods are tried first, like simply vacuuming bugs off plants or sophisticated pheromone traps.

People with multiple chemical sensitivity disorder (MCS) usually have an extreme sensitivity to pesticides. Neighbors who used pesticides like Malathion or Seven have been brought to court or before community organizations by MCS sufferers. The solution is often to bring in an IPM consultant. More and more nurseries are training their employees and educating their customers about integrated pest management.

---

chimney soot. It is a natural constituent of petroleum, which is refined to make gasoline. Gasoline is about 3 percent benzene. The benzene evaporates into the air and goes directly into the house through the seams around the door that connects the garage to the home.

One of the people who worked in Dr. Lance Wallace's EPA lab did an experiment at home. He parked his car on the street and let it cool down for an hour before bringing it into the garage. Just doing this greatly reduced the level of benzene in his home. Storing gasoline in the garage, even in metal cans, for use in lawn mowers, chain saws, or kerosene stoves is another source of benzene vapors. If possible, buy gasoline when you need to rather than storing it at home.

In the United States, nearly 85 percent of atmospheric benzene comes from cars; the remaining 15 percent is produced by industry, such as

---

WHY DON'T WE KNOW THIS ABOUT OUR HOMES?

Dr. Lance Wallace, an environmental scientist with a Ph.D. in physics, has worked at the EPA since 1977 and originated the TEAM studies. He has thought long and hard about why the importance of home pollution has not gotten out to the public, certainly not to the point that people are effectively acting on it. His conclusion is, in essence, that there is a whole structure out there designed to figure out and implicate outdoor pollution and to downplay indoor pollution: (1) People do not like to hear that they themselves are a major source of the problem. (2) Organizations that are trying to protect the environment have a vested interest in suing enemies with deep pockets (the chemical and petroleum industries) and play on the fears of people to retain their support. Wallace says that the environmental organizations don't jump on the issue of indoor pollution as they would lose the support of many of their members. (3) The laws are written so the EPA can't regulate indoor air and there are no funds to study it.

---

petroleum refineries and petrochemical plants. However, these two sources together account for less than half of your personal exposure to benzene. Active and passive cigarette smoke, outdoor exposure from lawn mowers and chain saws, indoor exposure from attached garages, driving, and refueling at the gas station account for the rest.

LAWN AND GARDEN AND OUTDOOR ACTIVITIES

We all want beautiful lawns and pretty flowers and shrubs to grace our homes, but there are better ways to accomplish this than by using pesticides. The EPA pegged U.S. pesticide sales at $11.3 billion in 1995, with estimates that U.S. consumers spent $1.2 billion for 71 million pounds of pesticides for use in their homes and lawns and gardens.

Try the following suggestions.

- Avoid pesticides. NPEs may be present but not indicated on the label. Don't recycle pesticide bottles. The plastic from recycled pesticide containers can leach small but detectable amounts of toxic compounds. Use natural lawn and garden maintenance methods (see sidebar on Integrated Pest Management).

- Use entryway mats to reduce the level of residues on carpet surfaces by 25 percent and carpet dust residues by 33 percent. Residues of lawn herbicides may be tracked into the house and deposited on indoor carpet surfaces or in household dust. A study examined the transport of two widely-used herbicides and found that 3 percent of the residues entered the carpet dust. Once indoors, the residues could remain for up to one year because natural degradation agents (sunlight, wind, rain, or soil microbes) were absent. Even homes in which the herbicide wasn't applied had detectable levels, probably due to drift while spraying other plots.

- Don't use old railway ties or telephone posts for garden projects. Wood products, including those that are pressure treated, are often treated with chemical pesticides (creosote, inorganic arsenicals, or pentachlorophenol) to preserve the wood. These chemicals can leach into the soil. Use woods that are naturally resistant to weathering and termites, such as redwood, cyprus, and cedar. There are also natural wood preservatives that are less toxic.

- Avoid areas freshly sprayed with pesticides. Inquire about spraying in parks, recreation grounds, and golf courses.

- If you golf, keep your hands, tees, and golf balls away from your mouth. Most golf courses are sprayed intensively, using four times more pesticide per acre than farms.

Pets

We all love our dogs and cats, but they do bring toxins into the home from outdoors. Fleas, in particular, are a problem. Try the following practices.

- Avoid flea shampoos and flea collars for pets. Look out for the ingredient carbaryl in flea/tick powders/dusts and in other household pesticides. To rid your pet of fleas, use a fine-toothed comb with petroleum or plant-based jelly, followed by an antibacterial, nontoxic herbal shampoo (if you have a very cooperative pet).

- Applying common flea pesticide treatments to carpets in the home creates levels twice above the legal limit, even when windows are open, and six times above the legal limit when windows are closed. The bottles all state that it is safe to return home several hours after the application. This is not true. If you do treat your rugs, go away for an overnight holiday and do not return for twenty-four hours from the time of application.

- Vacuum your pet's bedding and surrounding areas frequently.
- There are new spot application types of flea control that may have a better risk/benefit ratio.

ARTS AND HOBBIES

If you work with paints, pesticides, solvents, or toxins, shower and change shoes and clothes after use. Launder work clothes separately.

How Can You Help?

I would say that endocrine disruptors are one of the biggest threats to public health in the United States, probably worldwide. It's going to take a massive outcry by the American people to change the way we're doing things—from pesticide application to burning waste—in order to protect the next generation. A massive outcry is the only way we're going to be able to change the poisoning that's going on today.

—Lois Gibbs, Executive Director, Center for Health, Environment, and Justice

Even though I've tried to simplify the science that's involved, there is a lot of the information in this book that can be emotionally distressing. Frequently, the response to this type of information is to throw up our hands in despair, grab another beer (or whatever), turn up the volume on the latest sitcom, and say, "I can't take any more bad news!" It all seems so incomprehensible and overwhelming. Why bother?

We bother because we can't give up. What type of world are we passing on to our children? Our grandchildren? What can we do to relieve suffering, both our own and that of others? How can we live without hope?

Slavery, an institution that seemed entrenched as a backbone of the American economy, was abolished. When we learned about the terrible effects of lead, we made unleaded gasoline. Change does happen. Gandhi said: "Empires have come and gone. At the time they looked invincible, but all have fallen." Our dependence on harmful chemicals, new for the last fifty years, can change.

In 1982 Times Beach, Missouri, became a national symbol of a toxic-waste disaster when all the town's residents were evacuated and the entire town was bought by the government because of dioxin contamination. The cleanup was completed on schedule in 1997, bringing the second-largest Superfund project in the nation to a safe, successful conclusion. Now Times Beach is a state park.

We don't all need to be actively engaged in trying to solve the specific problem of hormone disruptors. Just small shifts in our actions, just a little effort in a more conscious direction, will cumulatively help. And those who are in a position to do more—leaders in global business, government, and science—open your eyes a little wider and see what you can do.

Part of the responsibility for our health rests squarely on our own shoulders—the way we lead our lives and the individual choices we make. We need to inspire and guide our families, and help our children understand the consequences of our actions by asking the right questions: *What are we putting in our mouths? Why do we not buy certain products? What's in our drinking water? What happens to our hazardous waste when we dispose of it?* But an equal share of responsibility lies with government and industry. How can we change what they think and what they do in relation to our health and that of our children?

As the last chapter showed, just because a product is widely used (or calls itself "natural") does not mean it is safe. If scientific studies suggest potential health hazards, even before they are proven to the point where the drug or product must be removed from the market, don't we have a right to know? Where do we draw the line between the consumer's right to know and government/industry reluctance to "needlessly" scare people? The FDA doesn't pull everything off the grocery shelves or out of pharmacies that can harm us. It takes many millions of dollars to test a chemical, so only the largest companies can afford to perform testing. It is up to industry—those who will profit by the production and sale of the chemicals or drugs—to run the tests and give the results to the FDA. We know that large companies, as well as the government, can make vested mistakes.

It was only at the end of the 1990s that tobacco companies were starting to be held liable for the deaths and disease smoking has caused. But years before the direct connection was established, there was compelling evidence to suggest that cigarettes were harmful, just like studies for several decades showed that DES didn't work and was harmful.

In the last few decades, a powerful grassroots movement for health reform has been traveling the globe, a collective voice demanding to be heard. Arlo Guthrie once quipped that Bob Dylan often "caught" more hit lyrics floating through the airways than he did, because Dylan always carried a pencil in his pocket. For more than a decade, researchers have been publishing articles about the devastating effects of certain substances in our environment, but these articles appeared in scientific journals and the information did not reach the public. These facts are now being "caught" in books like this one, in worldwide conferences, and through the courageous statements of scientists and activists. The message is that we can do more than simply cross our fingers and hope we won't get cancer or that future generations will be able to reproduce. But we do need to make changes. Now.

Consumer Be Aware

In the early 1990s the EPA commissioned several research laboratories to purchase 1,100 products and common household items from the shelves of stores. A laboratory analyzed the contents and found that the pollutants on the Superfund list or the list of Clean Air Act "air toxins" are the same ones found in the contents of these 1,100 consumer products. The concentration of some toxic substances in these products was often quite high, sometimes 10 to 60 percent by weight. Some products were labeled; some were not.

Obviously, the public is generally unaware of the composition of these ordinary household products—solvents, cleansers, cleaners, leather conditioners, glues, automotive products, etc. Since no U.S. agency checks the contents of consumer products, we might well wonder what compounds are found in beauty salon products, women's care products, and cosmetics. What are they actually made of? Does anyone know?

Corporations often say that it is consumer demand that makes them continue to produce and use toxic substances. As consumers, we have the power to nudge industry to reduce or stop the use of endocrine-disrupting chemicals and other pollutants.

One way we can influence what is produced in this country is by wisely choosing what we eat and what kinds of manufactured goods we buy, as we have seen in the last few chapters. Women purchase 80 percent of the products sold in the United States. When people demanded that packaging be recyclable, industry listened. More than we realize, *consumership is power*. We can come together on a grassroots level and inform others of the dangers in certain foods and goods so that they in turn can make choices based on this knowledge.

The Seventh Generation, a company dedicated to safe green products that I have used in my home for years, reminds us on their recycled paper napkin packages:

> *We can make a difference. If every household in the U.S. replaced just one 250 count package of virgin fiber napkins with 100 percent recycled ones, we could save: 819,000 trees; 3.2 million cubic feet of landfill space, equal to over 3,757 full garbage trucks; 336 million gallons of water, a year's supply for 9,605 families of four; and avoid 144,281 pounds of pollution.*

Here are some practical steps you can take to exercise your consumer rights.

- Call to find out what ingredients are used in products. Request full life-cycle information for that product, including how it was manufactured and how to dispose of it. Especially target the manufacturers of products that contain chemicals already known to be endocrine disruptors: plastics, paint, food, pesticides, batteries, paper, and soaps. Most companies have toll-free phone numbers for consumer feedback.

- Ask that your request or complaint be recorded and forwarded to the marketing manager.

- If you are told the information you seek is confidential, write a letter to your congressman requesting that laws be written and passed requiring the manufacturer to list any toxic pollutant (especially those on the Superfund list) by name on the label.

- Let the companies know you will switch brands if their product contains hormone disruptors.

- Get the company's commitment to send you a written response.

Industry can do a lot to help. It can systematically screen and retest the substances it produces and discharges as waste. It can provide consumers with product and hazard information. It can implement clean production and pollution prevention options. As a minimal priority, industry can adopt toxic-use reduction measures. It can fund research to develop safer products.

Before you "buy into" whatever it is that is being sold to you—a drug, a treatment center, the results of a study—be aware of the source of funding. For example, Zeneca, the company that makes Nolvadex (tamoxifen citrate), bought Salick, a company that runs breast-care centers. Merck, a pharmaceutical company that makes osteoporotic drugs, has been talking about opening osteoporosis clinics. The people who make Premarin may do menopause clinics! Research that says a chemical or drug is perfectly safe (when you've just read other studies that disagree) may have been funded by a chemical or drug company, no matter whose name is on the study.

A customer can sometimes make a business listen. The main reason businesses exist is to make money. Show a business that you won't patronize their product unless they do what you want and they will change. Economic pressure is a real key to cleaning up the environment and reducing our exposure to endocrine disruptors. "But it's not enough just not to buy them," Lois Gibbs, the executive director of the Center for Health, Environment, and Justice says. "Consumers should call the 800 number on the containers and say: I really like your shampoo [or whatever], and I really wanted to buy your shampoo, but it's in the wrong bottle. If you change your bottle, I will be a consumer of yours." Gibbs says that when corporations hear messages like that, especially about a container, they will change.

READING LABELS

Hazardous products line our kitchen, bath, utility, and garage shelves. Misuse or improper disposal of these products can pose a threat to health. The EPA defines a substance as hazardous if it is flammable, corrosive, toxic, or radioactive, or if it can react or explode when mixed with other substances.

How do you know if a product is hazardous? Check the label for the following terms.

- *Caution* or *Warning* indicates substances that are moderately or slightly toxic.

- *Danger* indicates substances that are extremely flammable, corrosive, or highly toxic.

- *Poison* indicates substances with extreme toxicity.

- The use of the term *nontoxic* is for advertising only. It has no regulatory definition by the federal government.

- Plastic with chlorine can be identified simply by looking at the bottom inside the recycle arrows. If the number *3* or a *V* is there, you know that its incineration could create dioxins. (If properly burned, it will not.)

- To buy paper that doesn't have chlorine in it, look on the side of the package to see if it says "bleached." It usually says what it's bleached with. Look for *chlorine-free paper* (made from all raw products, like tree or agricultural waste) or *processed chlorine-free paper*, which means that it has some recycled paper in it that may

---

CONSCIOUS CONSUMERS

Gary Cohen works with Health Care Without Harm, an international coalition that focuses attention on the elimination of environmental and public-health threats from health-care practices. Gary advises us to be "conscious consumers," not to bring toxic chemicals and foods into our homes. "Eat organically, buy environmentally safe household goods, live what you want the world to become, model to your children and community adults that care and feel that their consumership choices make a difference, act as though your actions count, and watch your world change."

I asked if he thought consumer lifestyle changes were sufficient. "No," he said, "but they are necessary. There is also community-based activism. Find out if a hospital in your town has medical incinerators dumping waste, if there are toxic chemical plants dumping waste, if your children's schools are surrounded by fields being sprayed so the children are exposed to pesticides. There is also a need for action on the international level—economic sanctions to enforce treaties and blocks."

People frequently ask Gary if his work with toxics over the last dozen years is depressing. "No," he says, "not at all. I am meeting people with resistance. People are resisting their own extinction. This is inspiring, empowering, and hopeful."

have some chlorine content. That's OK; it's the bleaching process with chlorine that creates the dioxin.

Labels only give information about acute or immediate effects. No information is given about chronic or long-term hazards of chemical products, so *no label gives information about endocrine-disrupting effects.*

WHO'S HOLDING THE BAG?

Baxter International, a large manufacturer of medical supplies, agreed to stop using IV bags and tubes made from PVC plastics and to find an alternative material. What brought this about? A group of shareholders petitioned the company after learning about the potential endocrine disruptor DEHP leaching from PVC and causing health problems. In a similar vein, a researcher at the Mayo Clinic found double the risk of non-Hodgkin's lymphoma in patients who received blood transfusions using PVC bags. The U.S. health-care industry uses more than 500 million IV bags each year.

Waste Management

What do we do with leftover chemicals after we use them? We usually throw them in the garbage can or toss them down the drain into the sewer system and let the city deal with them. However, the city doesn't deal with them. The chemicals go straight back into the environment via the sewage system into the water or into the ground water and right back to us. The disposal of these same chemicals by a laboratory or industry into regular sanitary waste or the sewer could easily result in a felony conviction for the person or company dumping the chemicals and fines in the millions of dollars.

Here are some ways to make sure chemicals are disposed of properly.

- The following items should be taken to a hazardous waste collection site (or call your community waste-collection agency for disposal procedures): automotive paint, batteries, brake fluid, dry-cleaning fluid, engine degreaser, epoxies and adhesives, flea powder, gasoline, herbicides, insecticides, mothballs, motor oil, oil-based paints, paint stripper, photographic chemicals, polishes containing nitrobenzene, and wood preservatives.

- Recycle used oil and antifreeze by taking them to service stations and other recycling centers. Never put used oil or other chemicals down storm drains or in drainage ditches or arroyos. One quart of oil can contaminate up to 2 million gallons of drinking water! Antifreeze is lethal in very small doses to pets, who lap up the sweet taste, go into convulsions, and die horrible deaths.

THE RIGHT TO KNOW

How do you know what chemicals are present in your workplace and in your children's schools? What's drifting in your windows and coming through your front door from your surrounding community?

You have the right to know which hazardous chemicals may be present in your home, workplace, and community from nearby factories or transport through your neighborhood. Tens of millions of American workers are routinely exposed in the workplace to toxic chemicals about which they have little or no information. People of color are almost 50 percent more likely than whites to live in communities with hazardous waste facilities.

The Right-to-Know Network (RTK Net) provides free access to databases, text files, and conferences on the environment, housing, and sustainable development. It was started in 1989 in support of the Emergency Planning and Community Right to Know Act (EPCRA), which mandated public access to the Toxic Release Inventory (TRI). It is operated by two nonprofit organizations—OMB Watch and The Unison Institute—and is funded by various government agencies and foundations.

RTK Net was established to empower citizen involvement in community and government decision making. Via RTK Net on-line, you can identify specific factories and their environmental effects. You can assess people and communities affected. RTK Net can be accessed via the Web, BBS, or Telnet. Community groups are often given an 800 number for free access. The RTK Net staff provides technical support and also conducts training around the country to teach people how to access and understand the data. http://www.rtk.net

There are other means of acquiring information.

Congress established the Toxic Release Inventory (TRI) in 1986 as part of the Emergency Planning and Community Right-to-Know Act. By law, manufacturers have to report annually any release or transfer of specific toxic chemicals. Since 1991, facilities must also report chemical recycling or burning for energy, on-site treatment, and source reduction efforts. According to the EPA, this disclosure has prompted a 42.7 percent decline in toxic releases. The TRI (toxic release inventory) data is available on microfiche, CD-ROM, diskette, and nine-track magnetic tape. The EPA has a gopher server (gopher.epa.gov), an FTP server (ftp.epa.gov), and a website (http://www.epa.gov) that includes all the EPA information available from RTK Net.

The Agency for Toxic Substances and Disease Registry (an agency of the U.S. Department of Health and Human Services) is directed by congressional mandate to perform specific functions concerning the effect on public health of hazardous substances in the environment. They maintain a website that includes an Internet HazDat Database for specific site and contaminant data. A Sensitive Map allows you to click on your state and find all the pertinent information about sites for that state. http://atsdr.cdc.gov:8080/haz-usa1.html

FEDERAL LEGISLATION

The U.S. government is very involved in examining the issue of endocrine disruption in regard to scientific research, government public-health policy, and industry regulation. In August 1996 Congress passed the Food Quality Protection Act (FQPA) and amendments to the Safe Drinking Water Act (SDWA), both of which contained provisions for screening and testing chemicals and pesticides for possible endocrine-disrupting effects. These two laws are responsible for a whole shift in the way government deals with environmental chemicals.

The FQPA, which was passed *unanimously* in Congress (much to the shock of the chemical industry, which contributes heavily to certain friendly congressmen), is the law that is turning around the ways in which we perceive and test chemicals. One of the people dedicated to environmental awareness is Lynn Goldman, who was head of the Office of Pesticides until the end of 1998. She was very concerned about developing the best science possible to meet the requirements of the new law and implementing practical protocols for assessing exposure. Up until now, the exposure we receive has been estimated based on the size of the field and the amount of pesticide used. The manufacturers had to do only a minimal amount of testing. If there wasn't an adverse effect when exposure occurred in adulthood, they didn't need to do more sensitive in utero and infancy tests based on parental exposure. With the passage of the FQPA, the amount of exposure must actually be measured.

Congress is also demanding that children, because of their vulnerability during development, have ten times more protection against possible endocrine-disrupting chemicals than adults. Plus, this law is taking real-life mixtures into account. It used to be that each pesticide was tested in isolation. But we eat food that has been sprayed with mixtures of pesticides, so this law says that pesticides must be tested as mixtures. This is why the EPA, which has to do the data, set up the EDSTAC committee to come up with recommendations for a screening and testing program, followed by EDSTP (the Endocrine Disruptor Screening and Testing Program) to carry it out.

In other words, this bill finally reverses the mind-set that chemicals are innocent until proven guilty. The Food Quality Protection Act is a holistic piece of legislation that is looking at the entire picture.

How did the Food Quality Protection Act come into being? In 1993–1994 the National Academy of Sciences started to publish papers about the risk to the young, showing that children were more vulnerable to chemical exposure than adults. Then breast cancer lobbyists brought this information to the attention of Congress, reaching the critical mass necessary to enact this excellent piece of legislation. I also feel it is fitting that as a DES daughter and a breast cancer survivor, I am writing about this for the public.

TRAC: A Sad Sidenote

The EPA's Tolerance Reassessment Advisory Committee (TRAC) was formed to help carry out the Food Quality Protection Act. In May of 1999, several public interest groups resigned from the committee because they felt that the pressures and demands of agribusiness interests regarding pesticide usage were hampering their work. Now most of the committee members come from chemical companies.

EDSTAC

As a result of its mandate from Congress, the EPA formed EDSTAC (Endocrine Disruptor Screening and Testing Advisory Committee) and charged it with designing a screening and testing program for endocrine-disrupting chemicals.

EDSTAC came from a more holistic viewpoint than had ever before been attempted in order to build scientific consensus: forty people who represented different groups and perspectives—research scientists; members of federal and state agencies; various sectors of industry; water providers; worker protection and labor organizations; national environmental groups; environmental justice groups; and public health groups— all sat down at the same table. This was revolutionary.

EDSTAC was well aware of how complex the issue of endocrine disruption really is. Its report (1998) recommended screening and testing substances in high and low doses that enhance, mimic, or inhibit estrogenic-, androgenic-, and thyroid hormone–related processes. They considered tests to detect "multiple hormone interactions, address endpoints in multiple species, and predict long-term or delayed effects." In order to jump-start the process, EDSTAC urged the EPA to begin work immediately on six mixtures:

1. contaminants in human breast milk
2. phytoestrogens in soy-based infant formulas
3. mixtures of chemicals most commonly found at hazardous waste sites
4. pesticide/fertilizer mixtures
5. disinfection by-products (such as chlorine)
6. gasoline

EDSTAC's thoroughness and straightforward approach to a highly complex and difficult task was impressive. It appears that the issue of endocrine disruption is stimulating an approach to chemicals and their testing and regulation that is more thorough than has existed up to this time. Unfortunately, by April 1999 reality had started to set in. The EPA peer review of the proposed program recommended that work on mixtures be moved to the back burner because of the complexity involved in testing, and low-dose testing remained "contentious," with industry being resistant to the idea. The EPA is grossly underbudgeted to implement the endocrine-disruptor screening program. Keep up to date on new developments through the EPA website (http://www.epa.gov/opptintr/opptendo/index.htm). Note: EDSTAC is only testing estrogen, androgen, and thyroid mimics, but there are *lots* of other hormones.

The Safe Drinking Water Act

The Safe Drinking Water Act (SDWA, 1974) sets safe levels for toxic substances in drinking water. For general information, contact the EPA Safe Drinking Water Hotline at 800/426-4791 (9:00–5:30 EST, Mon.–Fri.). For specific information on the Contaminant Candidate List and the contaminant identification process, contact the U.S. EPA, Office of Ground Water and Drinking Water, Mailcode 4607, Washington, DC 20460; phone 202/260-3029; fax 202/260-3762; or E-mail washington.evelyn@epamail.epa.gov.

FIFRA and FFDCA

There are two other pieces of legislation that are also looking at endocrine disruptors.

- The Federal Insecticide, Fungicide and Rodenticide Act (FIFRA, 1947, as amended) regulates the use of pesticides. FIFRA is a cost-benefit statute, meaning unreasonable adverse effects must also take into account socioeconomic factors as well as scientific judgments. To register a pesticide, industry conducts studies on its safety and submits them to the EPA, where they are evaluated by scientists and then used in risk assessments. Until new data based on FQPA is done, the risk assessments are based on single active ingredients. Presently there are approximately 600 registered pesticide active ingredients, and 1,800 inert ingredients. Under the new FQPA law, both active and inert ingredients must be tested.

- The Federal Food, Drug and Cosmetic Act (FFDCA, 1938, amended in 1958) regulates toxic additives to food and cosmetics and prohibits use of carcinogens. Pesticide tolerance levels for food are established under this act.

The EPA is not the only government agency working on the problem of hormone disruption. The EPA has been working in conjunction with the White House Office of Science and Technology Policy (OSTP) to stimulate cooperation and collaboration across the various federal agencies that have endocrine-disruptor concerns. For a list of these agencies, see Appendix D.

COMING TOGETHER

Dr. Dan Vallero is leading a team of scientists in NERL (the National Exposure Research Laboratory), the EPA laboratory that studies environmental exposures. Vallero and others at the EPA are part of a larger federal effort led by the White House Committee on Environment and Natural Resources.

Vallero says the federal government is "getting its act together" on endocrine disruptors. Historically, the EPA has been focused on researching each individual medium—air, water, soil, biota—but it has not done much in terms of looking at them together. With endocrine disruptors, there is no way to begin estimating exposure without looking at complete human and ecological systems. In his own research, Vallero is looking at how vinclozolin (a fungicide with known hormone-disrupting potential) moves from soil into groundwater and the atmosphere so he can figure out where it's likely to end up in the environment.

Dr. Vallero is impressed with the way ecologists and human health practioners and researchers, biological scientists (who normally see the world so differently), immunologists and endocrinologists, toxicologists, and engineers are bonding now over the issue of endocrine disruptors. "We're working on the same compounds," he said in our interview. "This has been an excuse for us to sort of work together. And that's relatively recent. So that may be the big bonus of all this endocrine disruptor stuff. No one has shut any doors in my face. I guess everyone benefits from this research. We can narrow down the list of potential disruptors while we begin to improve our understanding of how they behave in the environment."

CITIZEN ACTION

The people we elect to office must know that we consider the problem of hormone disruption to be a priority. We can inform our politicians of our concerns, and we can vote for those who support policy changes that put pressure on industry to stop using harmful chemicals and come up with safe substitutes. We can also encourage government to make industries that manufacture these chemicals pay taxes that contribute to cleaning up the environment. We can share some of this tax money with farmers to help them change the way they raise crops and enrich the soil.

Canaries on the Rim (Verso, 2000) by Chip Ward provides an example of how to bring about change on environmental issues by pursuing small winnable goals that lead to larger changes.

Here are some more ideas.

- Write to your elected representatives to remind them that it is the responsibility of the government to ensure that wildlife, the environment, and your health are protected from exposure to hormone-disrupting chemicals.

- Demand full disclosure when pesticides are used in public places, including parks, schoolyards, and roadsides. Find out who undertakes and regulates pesticide spraying in your town and write them.

- Call 202/224-3121 to urge your congressmen to support legislation for clean water.

- Demand legislation that would require industry to label hormonally active ingredients in products.

- Remember, we vote.

THE GLOBAL PICTURE

The light at the end of the tunnel is the glow of worldwide attention to the problem of endocrine disruption. Some U.S. government projects are underway in conjunction with European countries. Scientists have been reaching across the oceans to work hand-in-hand with their counterparts in many places around the world, especially now with scientific information able to travel so quickly through cyberspace.

It looks like endocrine disruption is finally gaining the international attention it deserves. The World Health Organization (WHO) released a statement in March 1998 about chemicals that disrupt hormonal activities. It said (in part):

There is a rapidly growing body of scientific evidence indicating that a number of substances interfere with the normal functions of the body governed by the endocrine system and have, thus, the potential of causing adverse effects to health. One of the most impressive consequences of such hormonal interference could be the decrease in sperm count and quality recently reported in a number of countries.

Indications for an increase in the incidence of some hormonally sensitive carcinomas, including female breast cancers, as well as testicular and prostate cancers, could also be linked to the effects of these chemicals, called "Endocrine disruptors."

From now on, these chemicals will be under permanent scrutiny *by a Steering Group of scientific experts, which met for the first time in Washington, D.C., USA, on 16–18 March 1998. . . . The scientific experts who compose the Steering Group will provide guidance for and participate in the development of a global inventory of research on endocrine-disrupting chemicals, as well as in the production of an international assessment of the "state of the science" on these substances. . . .*

THE PARTNERSHIP OF SCIENCE AND RELIGION

There are also other avenues of participating in the solution to the problem of endocrine disruption. The activities of more than 2,000 congregations of different faiths have been documented by the National Religious Partnership for the Environment in their booklet, *Models of Engagement: Profiles of Environmentally Active Congregations* in the areas of:

- advocacy—activities designed to influence public policy
- education—workshops, curriculum development, conferences, and innovative outdoor experiences for adults and children
- stewardship—making better use of buildings, grounds, and central community locations for education and to foster a positive impact on environmental sustainability

For example:

- In Baltimore, Maryland, the harvest from an organic farm run on eighty inner-city lots by members of St. John's Lutheran Church goes to the church soup kitchen.
- Each fall, the young people from Holy Trinity Church in St. Paul, Minnestoa, go to a tree farm and cover the trees with recycled corn sacks to protect them from insects and pesticides.
- Temple Adath Israel B'rith Shalom in Louisville, Kentucky, now uses recycled paper for its weekly bulletin, recycled toweling and office paper, reusable cups instead of Styrofoam, and biodegradable soaps.

- The Mothers of East L.A., including members of Resurrection Roman Catholic Church, successfully opposed a hazardous waste incinerator two miles downwind of East L.A. They also took on Chem Clear, a subsidiary of Union Pacific Corporation, and stopped the building of a factory near a local high school.
- In Columbia, Maryland, the extensive environmental program at St. John the Evangelist includes educating members about non-toxic household cleaners.

SHADES OF GRAY

Mirabai Bush is the director of the Center on Contemplative Mind in Society (sponsored by the Nathan Cummings Foundation and the Fetzer Institute). While exploring the use of contemplative practices for a wide range of society, Mirabai has been developing a program of mindfulness practices for one of the world's largest chemical companies.

As former chairperson of SEVA, an international, nonprofit, public-health organization, Mirabai spent many years working with the Mayan people in Guatemala to reclaim land that had been severely damaged by too many chemicals, and she acknowledged some strong negative feelings about chemical companies. To some extent, Mirabai had at first "demonized in my mind the corporate executives." After spending time with them, however, she said, "It's not as black-and-white as I originally thought. It's not that they think what they are doing is a bad thing and they keep doing it to make money. It's much more complex. They really think, based on the statistics of the population explosion, that chemical and biotech agriculture is necessary to feed the world of the future. They believe that genetically engineered food will save us and feed us all. These are good people, and I've come to respect them deeply, even while often disagreeing with them."

The executives were, Mirabai said, extraordinarily responsive to basic forms of insight meditation. "These are very smart people, with tremendous focus." What is important, she says, is the need for a new form of dialogue. "As we learn through contemplative practices to listen better and more clearly to our own bodies and minds, then extend this to being able to listen more clearly to others, this process could help communication among groups who need it, including chemical industry executives, world environmentalists, and government policy makers."

- Members of St. John's Episcopal Church in Elizabeth, New Jersey, situated in "cancer alley," engage in proactive, coalition-building activities to ban the planned construction and current operation of incinerators.

- The New Waverly Baptist Church in Dallas, Texas, is a stronghold of community action, advocating with the EPA to address the toxic effects of a local smelting plant (which eventually closed) and to bring in adequate health facilities and relocate residents.

The National Religious Partnership for the Environment is a federation of major American faith communities: the U.S. Catholic Conference, the Coalition on the Environment and Jewish Life, the National Council of Churches of Christ, and the Evangelical Environmental Network. Their goal is to integrate commitment to global sustainability and environmental justice permanently into all aspects of religious life. Paul Gorman, director of the organization, says, "There is no particular agenda here other than to be of service—in the name of life—because that is the joy of environmental work." You can reach the National Religious Partnership for the Environment at 1047 Amsterdam Ave., New York, NY 10025; phone 212/316-7441; fax 212/316-7547; website: http://www.nrpe .org. Contact them at 800/200-8858 for more information or to inform them of new stories.

Top Ten Actions to Reduce Your Exposure to Hormone-Disrupting Chemicals

(Adapted from the World Wildlife Foundation website: http://www.wwfcanada.org/reduce-risk/top10.html)

1. Eat lower on the food chain. Eat organic foods.

2. Do not microwave in plastic.

3. Do not use pesticides (inside, outside, or on pets and kids).

4. Quit smoking.

5. Treat dead batteries as hazardous waste.

6. Wash hands, floors, and windowsills frequently.

7. Avoid super-strength specialty cleaners.

8. Avoid mercury dental fillings.

9. Read labels and call 800 phone numbers for information on product formulations.

10. Write or call local, state, and federal politicians. Ask them to take action to reduce hormone-disrupting chemicals in our environment.

Never doubt that a small group of thoughtful, committed citizens can change the world; indeed it is the only thing that has.

—Margaret Mead

The Chemicals in Everyday Products

The following information is concerned only with those man-made chemicals that are known or strongly suspected to have hormone-disrupting effects. Keep in mind that there may be numerous chemicals out of the tens of thousands currently in production that affect the human hormone system but have yet to be identified, and accurate testing methods for identifying hormone disruptors are just now being developed.

PLASTICS

Plastics are made from combinations of different chemicals that contribute different properties. Some chemicals are used to make plastic soft, some to prevent it from yellowing. A number of the chemicals used in plastic are known to be hormone disruptors, and still other hormone disruptors (dioxins and furans) can be created when plastic is burned for disposal. A trillion pounds of plastics are manufactured every four years.

Phthalates are a class of compounds of some fifty related chemicals, which are used to make plastics more flexible and durable. They are the most abundant man-made environmental pollutants and have been found to be weakly estrogenic. Some plastics contain up to 40 percent phthalates by weight, which can leach or volatilize out as time passes.

Specific phthalates considered to be hormone disruptors follow.

- Di-ethylhexyl phthalate (DEHP) accounts for 90 percent of phthalate production. This additive is used in PVC plastic found in rainwear, footwear, upholstery material, shower curtains, floor tiles, children's toys, blood bags, and even beer bottle caps. It is also an ingredient in some paints, inks, and pesticides. DEHP is used in heat-seal coatings on metal foils (such as those found on yogurts) and in aluminum foil.

- Butyl benzyl phthalate (BBP) is used as a dispersant and carrier for insecticides, repellents, and perfumes and in the manufacture of flooring tiles, cellulose plastics, polyvinyl acetates, polyurethanes, and polysulfides. It is also used in vinyl products such as synthetic leathers, acrylic caulking, adhesive for medical devices, and cosmetics. BBP is approved for use as a component of paper and paperboard in contact with liquid, fatty, and dry foods.

- Di-n-butyl phthalate (DBP) is widely used in PVC and nitrocellulose polyvinyl acetate. It may contaminate food through its use as a plasticizer in coatings on cellophane and from its use in inks. It is found in carpet backing, paints, glue, insect repellents, hairspray, nail polish, and rocket fuel. (Doesn't it make you feel good to know that the same stuff you paint on your toenails has helped man get to the moon?)

- Diethyl phthalate (DEP) is a plasticizer in the clear film that is used in carton windows to display food. DEP may be used in blister packaging and may also be found in numerous articles such as toiletries, (especially nail polish), insect repellents, and adhesives, as well as in toothbrushes, car components, and toys.

Humans take in phthalates via various routes, especially through foods that have absorbed these chemicals from their packaging or from the manufacturing processes. Soft cheeses, chocolate bars, chips, cakes packaged in paper and cardboard, gravy granules, vegetable burger mix, vegetable fat, and sausages have been found to contain phthalates. Fifty-nine samples from fifteen various brands of baby milk, tested by the ministry in Britain, all revealed phthalates. A follow-up study in 1998 showed that the levels of phthalates were considerably lower than those in the 1996 study. Phthalates have been found in fruit juices and distilled water, leached from the plastic packaging. Levels of phthalates may by higher in the middle of foods than in the areas closest to the wrappings, suggesting that contamination occurs during processing. Phthalates are no longer used in the manufacture of cling film or most other food contact plastics in the United

Kingdom. Some food packagers in the United States have reportedly stopped using phthalates. However, aluminum foils, plastics, and ink used on food packages and cartons may all contain phthalates, which may get into our food.

Bisphenol A (BPA), a component of plastic, is one of the top fifty chemicals in production. In 1996 nearly 1.6 billion pounds of this bisphenol, which has a very similar molecular structure to DES, were produced. Dow Chemical has admitted to making over a billion dollars a year on this chemical. BPA is commonly used in the lacquer that coats metal products—in the lining of food cans (the plastic lining is colorless and can't be seen), bottle tops, and water supply pipes; in flame retardants; and in polycarbonate plastics that are used in many food and drink packaging applications.

Polymers of bisphenol A are used in some dental treatments as sealants for our children's teeth and in dental composites (the alternative to the mercury in amalgam fillings). Six different laboratories have demonstrated that bisphenol A is an estrogen, and there are at least two published in vivo studies showing that it is almost as potent as our natural hormones although not as potent as DES.

Polycarbonate plastics are clear, strong, and rigid. They are used as packaging for soft drinks, for water jugs and juice bottles, and for baby bottles and as plastic products used in hospitals and laboratories. Although generally believed to be safe, some experiments indicate this may not be the case. Dr. David Feldman from Stanford University discovered that the polycarbonate flasks used in an experiment were leaching bisphenol A when water was heated in the flasks. More disturbing, Professor Nicolas Olea tested eight brands of polycarbonate baby bottles by filling them with distilled water, sterilizing, and testing the water. Seven out of the eight bottles had leached 10 to 20 micrograms of BPA into the water. Perhaps going back to glass bottles will be an answer until industry comes up with nonhormonally active plastics (which do exist). Also baby formula may contain BPA if it comes packed in a tin can with a plastic lining.

DETERGENTS

A *surfactant*—short for *surf*ace *act*ive *agent*—is a chemical that functions in cleaning products to dissolve and remove oils and grease and to make water penetrate more readily. Soap is a surfactant, as are the synthetic detergents in most laundry and dishwashing products. Only products traditionally made from fat and lye are called soap, while all other surfactants are called *detergents*.

There are more than 100 different alkylphenols. Alkylphenol ethoxylates (APES)—along with their derivatives, the commonly used nonyl phenol ethoxylates (NPES)—are used as the "detergents" in many industrial processes and in everyday household products. Some 660 million pounds of APES are produced each year and ultimately released into the environment. Nonyl phenols bind easily to fats. However, it wasn't until Ana Soto's accidental discovery in 1991 that nonyl phenol was leaching from plastic and causing human breast cancer cells to grow that anyone was concerned about the health effects of alkylphenols.

APES are found in industrial detergents, such as those used for wool washing and metal finishing; various laboratory detergents (such as Triton X-100); domestic detergents, such as liquid laundry detergent and all-purpose cleaners; and personal care products, like some soaps, shampoos, and shaving foams. Some nonylphenol-containing products include the spermicides used with contraceptive diaphragms and in many condoms. Other uses of APES include: additives in latex paints and cosmetics, antioxidants and stabilizers in some plastics, and part of the formulation in some pesticides. They are used in the production of pulp and paper, oil, synthetic and natural textiles, and leather.

APES and NPES generally end up at sewage-treatment plants where they are only partially degraded (mainly becoming other alkylphenolic compounds) and then are dumped into rivers and the sea. Extensive research in Switzerland has shown that the breakdown compounds persist in rivers and sediment, and even in groundwater. Octyl phenol has been reported to have estrogenic activity in both in vitro and in vivo studies. Nonyl phenol and octyl phenol have been shown to affect the endocrine systems of exposed birds, fish, and mammals. It appears that it is the breakdown products rather than the surfactants themselves that disrupt hormones. There are better alternatives, such as alcohol ethoxylates.

By the year 2000, nonylphenols used in industrial cleaning were banned by fourteen European countries under the 1992 Paris Commission resolution. In the United States, analysis of drinking water has shown concentrations of alkylphenolic compounds at almost 1 microgram/liter. Surprisingly, the United States still allows these detergents to be used in domestic consumer products.

Persistent Organic Pollutants (POPs)

Persistent organic pollutants include dioxins, PCBs, pentachlorophenol (a heavy-duty fungicide used on textiles and as a wood preservative), as well as many pesticides (DDT, chlordane, and others) and a variety of other chemicals. They are among the most persistent chemicals ever produced. POPs are stored in fat and thus accumulate to higher concentrations with each step up the food chain. At the top of the food chain, polar bears, beluga whales, seals, and humans have measurable amounts of POPs in their fat.

What these substances have in common is that they are all chlorinated or brominated. Chlorine and bromine make these molecules resistant to being broken down, which is why chlorinated or brominated compounds are so persistent. Only about 1 percent of chlorine production is used for disinfecting water. Although this use of chlorine as a disinfectant has saved untold numbers of lives from waterborne diseases, there are questions about its safety. About 10 percent of chlorine is used for bleaching paper. Almost 85 percent of the pharmaceuticals manufactured in the world need chlorine at some stage of production. The majority of chlorine is combined with various carbon compounds (usually derived from petroleum) to make synthetic organochlorines. There are very few naturally occurring organochlorines. Today there are more than 15,000 chlorinated compounds in commerce.

Industry is scrambling to come up with chlorine alternatives. The paper and chemical industries are looking to substitute chlorine dioxide for chlorine. Chlorine dioxide is apparently a more effective disinfectant than chlorine and does not produce high levels of trihalomethanes, such as chloroform. The EPA tested chlorine dioxide in a pilot drinking-water-treatment plant and less toxic by-products were produced compared to chlorine. However, a number of other substances were produced about which nothing is known concerning toxicity to humans. There are other treatments being looked at for water disinfection.

Polychlorinated Biphenyls (PCBs)

PCBs, which are one type of POPs, are a whole family of related oily compounds that do not burn easily, which makes them excellent electrical insulators. They became important when the electrical industry mushroomed in the 1940s. However, their inability to burn makes them very stable and persistent compounds. As they became more widely used in products (lubricants, plasticizers, adhesives, carbonless copy paper, and as by-products formed in the manufacture of certain paints, plastics, and paper coatings), they became a permanent part of our environmental landscape. They were used for general weatherproofing and fire-resistant coatings to wood and plastic. They were even used in cosmetics.

PCBS (produced in the United States under the trade name Aroclor until they were banned and in Japan as Kanechlor) contain varying amounts of 209 possible congeners (related compounds), fifty of which have already been associated with health problems. Eleven different PCBS have an affinity to bind to the Ah receptor. A series of PCBS have been shown to bind to estrogen receptor sites and to mimic thyroid, estrogen, and other hormones, to decrease blood levels of the thyroid hormone, and to have toxic effects on the thyroid. It has been reported that almost one hundred percent of the salmon found in the PCB-contaminated Great Lakes have abnormally large goiters (enlargement of the thyroid gland).

According to Swedish researchers, high exposures to PCBS can cause serious damage to the lungs. One form of a PCB binds perfectly with the lung's uteroglobin protein. The only natural compound known to bind to uteroglobin is the hormone progesterone, and PCBS "bind with a thousand-fold higher affinity" than does progesterone. Hmmm. Makes one wonder if PCBS compete with progesterone elsewhere in the body and thereby play a role in unopposed estrogen.

The destruction wrought by PCBS was so obvious by 1976 that the U.S. Congress outlawed the manufacture, sale, and distribution of PCBS except in "totally enclosed" systems. They were, however, produced in Russia until 1990 and probably through 1998. Although the production of PCBS is now banned, they were once so widely used that PCBS have been found in almost every area of the global ecosystem—from the sediment at the bottom of the Hudson River to snow and seawater in the Antarctic. Since they are fat soluble and tend to bioaccumulate in organisms, PCBS are found in the blubber of dolphins, in the milk of Arctic seals, and in human breast milk. Fish, dairy, and poultry are the most consistent sources of PCBS in the food chain.

PCBS are released into the environment from poorly maintained toxic waste sites; illegal or improper dumping of PCB wastes, such as transformer fluids; leaks or emissions from electrical transformers containing PCBS;

and disposal of PCB-containing consumer products (such as old fluorescent lighting fixtures and electrical devices or old appliances with PCB capacitors) into municipal landfills rather than into landfills designed for hazardous wastes.

Dioxins and Furans

Dioxins and dioxin-like compounds—seventy-five halogenated (chlorinated or brominated) dibenzo-p-dioxins (PCDDs) and 135 dibenzofurans (PCDFs)—are a large family of chemicals that are not intentionally produced but are released into the environment as a by-product of chemical processes involving chlorine, such as bleaching pulp and paper, the production of some pesticides, the manufacture of PVC (vinyl) plastics, metal smelting, and waste incineration (which accounts for a large percentage of the dioxin in the air in urban regions). Smaller amounts of these compounds may be made during gasoline combustion, dry cleaning, and metal degreasing and refinishing. Other man-made sources of dioxin include motor vehicles (chlorinated chemicals are the antiknock additive in gasoline) and residential wood burning. A federal study released in the year 2000 indicates that a handful of rural households burning their garbage outside in barrels can spew as much dioxin as a large municipal incinerator.

More than 95 percent of all dioxins originate from human industrial activity; less than 1 percent stems from natural sources such as forest fires and volcanoes. Most dioxin is emitted through the air and then deposited on grass and trees and consumed by cows and other animals, or it is deposited in lakes and streams and ingested by fish. All these compounds are insoluble in water, love fatty substances, and are resilient against degradation, so they accumulate in the food chain. Ninety-five percent of our personal exposure is through meat, fish, and dairy products. Dioxin exposure is now so ubiquitous that ice in the center of Antarctica is contaminated.

Animal and human data show that these dioxin-like compounds affect developing tissues, and some of them may act like hormone disruptors at or near background exposure levels, meaning the amount we are exposed to through everyday living. Dioxins do not mimic estrogens or androgens, but they do amplify or reduce hormonal effects. They are also suspected of meddling with the thyroid hormone regulatory system in infants. Dioxin's interference with thyroid function may also disrupt liver enzyme activity. In October 1997, dioxin was upgraded to a known human car-

cinogen. Studies have shown that dioxin is one of the most potent carcinogens ever tested.

The massive three-volume EPA part I report in 1994 (*Estimating Exposure to Dioxin-like Compounds*) indicated that exposure to dioxin through
air, water, and foods was already at levels that could possibly cause adverse
health effects, including stunted fetal development, altered immune system, damage to the reproductive system, and cancer. Some of these
effects were happening from levels close to those found in our day-to-day
existence. (Of course, these results were disputed by some scientists who
said the EPA had inferred too much from animal studies.) The EPA identified medical and municipal waste incinerators as two of the top three
sources of air emissions of dioxin. Some hopsitals have stopped feeding
PVC to their incinerators or have moved to PVC-free materials, and 80 to
90 percent of hospital incinerators will be shut down over the next ten
years. There are new, effective technologies that are less polluting alternatives to incineration, such as microwaving or autoclaving, which steam-
sterilizes the waste. These high-tech solutions destroy the biologically
active components of hospital waste, and the remainder can be buried in
landfills, which don't create dioxins. Municipal incinerators are no longer
being built, and grassroots efforts are being made to shut down the ones
that exist already.

When dioxin enters cells, it binds to the Ah receptor and then turns
genes on or off "inappropriately." Dioxin has a high affinity for this receptor and is extremely persistent in the body. There are lots of Ah receptors in the liver, which suggests that dioxin affects the way the liver does
its job of handling chemicals. The EPA report mentioned that sensitive
individuals could experience subtle changes in liver enzyme activity, which
may affect how we handle other toxins, and reduced glucose tolerance,
which may be a contributing factor for diabetes. It appears that dioxin
affects the enzymes that break down estrogen, thus activation of the Ah
receptor can act as an antiestrogen or affect estrogen levels in other ways.
For example, dioxin can affect prolactin levels which indirectly affect
estrogens.

Of the seventy-five dioxins in the compound family, tetrachlorodibenzo-p-dioxin (TCDD) is the most potent and best studied. It is often
referred to as one of the most toxic man-made compounds known. Operation Ranch Hand was a military program spraying herbicides on the

jungles of Vietnam from 1962 to 1972. The herbicides were contaminated with dioxin. The Air Force has an ongoing study of the Vietnam vets who participated in the program. The Veteran's Administration currently recognizes seven diseases—skin diseases and cancers, such as soft-tissue sarcoma, Hodgkin's disease, multiple myeloma, respiratory cancers (lung, bronchus, larynx, trachea) and non-Hodgkin's lymphoma—related to exposure to Agent Orange and other herbicides. The birth defect spina bifida has been shown to be increased in children born to Vietnam vets. The dioxin-exposed group also showed abnormal functioning of the endocrine system. Vietnam vets who believe they or their children have health problems that may be related to their exposure to Agent Orange should call 1-800-827-1000.

International dioxin experts unanimously conclude that every one of TCDD's effects begins with the compound's binding to the Ah receptor in classic hormone activation style. Unlike natural hormones, which degrade in a few hours, TCDD molecules need seven years to reduce their concentration in humans by half.

The Japanese have forged ahead with government activity to set stricter air, water, and soil standards for dioxin and cut up to 90 percent of the country's dioxin output by 2002. They are mainly targeting garbage incinerators, which account for most of Japan's dioxin output. In the United States, the San Francisco Board of Supervisors was the first U.S. government body to adopt a resolution to eliminate dioxin wherever possible (March 22, 1999).

Pvc (polyvinyl chloride) contaminates us and our planet through its production, use, and disposal. Commonly called vinyl, pvc has been used widely in packaging, automobile parts and upholstery, home furnishings, children's toys, building materials, hospital supplies, and hundreds of other products. It was used for a period of time for water pipes, but ruptured easily.

Despite the fact that it is a highly versatile and relatively inexpensive material, pure pvc is almost useless by itself. To become the products we know and love, pvc has to be combined with a number of additives, including plasticizers (phthalates), stabilizers (containing heavy metals such as lead), fungicides, and other toxic substances. Additives can wash out of pvc and pass into other materials or be lost to air.

Pesticides

Synthetic pesticides include insecticides (for killing insects), herbicides (for killing plants), fungicides (for killing fungal diseases), and nematocides (for killing slugs and snails). Some interfere with nervous and digestive system enzymes, some with growth and reproductive hormones, and some are contact poisons. Only a few are specific to a particular pest. Rather, they work against any organism since all species share the same basic enzyme, hormone, and other body systems.

Approximately 70 percent of the pesticides used are applied to crops that humans and livestock eat. The rest are used in forestry and industrial applications, lawn and garden maintenance, on pets, for indoor pests, and on golf courses. On an acre-to-acre basis, pesticide use can be higher in urban areas than on farms.

One group of insecticides are organochlorines. While the DDT family is the best known, it is only one of a large number of related compounds used for a variety of pest control needs. Most are chemically stable, degrade slowly in humans, and persist for years in the general environment. Many have been banned from use in North America and Europe because of their adverse effects on wildlife reproduction and the concern over long-term effects on human fertility, reproduction, and development. However, in other parts of the world, especially in developing countries, their benefits in controlling the insects responsible for crop loss and human disease are thought to outweigh the risks.

DDT, although banned, is not yet gone from the United States by a long shot. The Palos Verdes Shelf, seventeen square miles of ocean floor south of Los Angeles, was declared a Superfund cleanup site in 1996; it is the world's largest deposit of DDT (the now-defunct chemical manufacturer Montrose Corp. dumped 110 tons of DDT there for over 25 years until 1971). As Michael Montgomery, the EPA's chief of Superfund cleanup in California said, "The levels of DDT are simply not acceptable for a recreational area that is so highly used and valued."

A number of organochlorines are still used in the United States, including lindane, malathion, endosulfan, methoxychlor, and dicofol. Those that have been banned, such as toxaphene, dieldrin, and DDT, are still persistent in the environment. Among the organochlorine pesticides tested on human breast cancer cells by Ana M. Soto and her associates at the Tufts University School of Medicine, toxaphene, dieldrin, and endosulfan had estrogenic properties comparable to those of DDT and chlordecone.

Fatty food is the main route of human exposure for these chlorinated insecticides. Concentrations in the fat have been found to be 300 to 500 times greater than in the blood.

Commercial and/or domestic pesticides that have known or suspected reproductive and endocrine disruptive effects include:

alachlor (herbicide)

aldicarb

amitrole (herbicide)

atrazine (herbicide used for corn crops)

benomyl (this, and its principal breakdown product, carbendazim, is a fungicide used on apples and bananas, among other food crops, and on flowers, trees, and grasses)

carbaryl

chlordane (termite killer)

cypermethrin (used on a variety of food crops)

DBCP (sterilized male workers at Occidental Petroleum; Dow knew it caused testicular atrophy in rats but didn't think it relevant to tell Occidental Petroleum.)

DDT

DDT metabolites

dicofol (used on cotton, citrus)

dieldrin (banned by EPA in 1974 with the exception of usage for termite control)

endosulfan (used on a variety of agricultural crops)

esfenvalerate

ethyl parathion

fenvalerate

h-epoxide

heptachlor (termite killer)

hexachlorobenzene (although banned in many countries in the 1970s, it continues to be released into the environment as a by-product and contaminant in many other chlorinated chemicals) kelthane

kepone

lindane (used to treat seeds and soil, and for beetle control in wood sources)

malathion (heavily sprayed around residential areas of the United States to kill mosquitoes; can help prevent life-threatening diseases until the bugs become resistant; flea/tick dip; used in food gardens)

mancozeb (fungicide)

maneb (fungicide)

methomyl

methoxychlor (widely used insecticide that replaced DDT; decreases progesterone and promotes endometriosis in rats)

metiram (fungicide)

metribuzin (herbicide)

mirex

nitrofen

oxychlordane

permethrin

synthetic pyrethroids

toxaphene

trans-nonachlor

tributyltin oxide (tributyltin compounds were used as antifouling paints on ships, small boats, and marine culture pen nets; now banned in many countries)

trifluralin (herbicide)

2,4,5-T and 2,4-D (crabgrass and dandelion killer, and herbicide widely used by U.S. forces in Vietnam)

vinclozolin (fungicide used for crops such as grapes, some fruits and vegetables, and ornamental plants)

zineb (fungicide)

ziram

PAHs

Most *polycyclic aromatic hydrocarbons* (PAHS) are toxic chemicals commonly produced from the incomplete combustion of petroleum products, wood, or tobacco. Many are carcinogenic. The name comes from the chemical structure—multiple rings of the aromatic solvent benzene. The term "aromatic" has nothing to do with smell, but with the chemical properties that give benzene its stability. Burnt toast, charred steak, French fries, smoke, wood ashes, used motor oil, and asphalt all contain PAHS, as do forest and brush fires and volcanoes.

Evidence suggests that PAHS directly interfere with the liver as well as the thyroid gland and its metabolizing enzymes. Alterations in thyroid hormone levels and neuro-behavioral performance were observed in human infants exposed in utero and through breastfeeding to relatively high levels of PAHS. Persistent PAHS can profoundly affect normal brain development in experimental animals, wildlife species, and human infants.

HEAVY METALS

Cadmium has been shown in laboratory tests to have a strong influence on the number of hormone receptors and receptor activity. Fifty percent of the world production of cadmium is used to make nickel/cadmium (NiCad) batteries. The rest shows up in coatings, pigments, and stabilizers in plastics and synthetic products and alloys. Cadmium is released from smelters and phosphate fertilizer production. Fossil fuels contain mercury and cadmium, which are released during combustion. Cigarette smoke also contains cadmium.

Lead is used in glazes, lead crystal, brass plumbing fixtures, solder, food cans, and lead batteries and as a stabilizer for PVC plastics. Lead persists in the environment from industrial activity, garbage incineration, and from the many years of use of leaded gasoline (which is still used in some parts of the world). Our greatest exposure comes from house dust, outside dirt, and drinking water. Old paint may be lead-based. It has been clearly shown that the higher the level of lead exposure in children, the greater the decrease in IQ.

Mercury is used in the production of chlorine, button-type batteries, fluorescent lights, pesticides, thermometers, polyurethane, most dental fillings, light switches, solvents, preservatives, paints, cosmetics, pharmaceuticals, seed dressings, and fossil fuels. Mercury is very toxic to humans, even in very small doses, affecting the central nervous system, kidneys, and liver. At hospitals, products that contain mercury (such as thermometers and batteries) end up with medical waste, which is put into red bags and burned in medical waste incinerators. Mercury has been clearly shown to get into the blood from dental amalgam fillings and from mother's milk into the suckling infant.

Aluminum (which is a light metal) is being investigated for its effects on development and behavior. Exposure comes from food (leaching from aluminum cooking pots and foil), water, pharmaceutical compounds, and in the environment as a result of acid rain leaching it from the soil. Aluminum laminate is a wash used on aluminum foil, which contains phthalates. Aluminum accumulates and persists in body tissue, so mother's exposure affects the fetus. Don't cook acidic foods like tomatoes or rhubarb in aluminum pots.

Natural Hormone Replacement and Hormone Potentiators

If you haven't heard about natural hormones, it's for one very good reason: they cannot be patented. That means there's no incentive for the pharmaceutical industry to spend millions of dollars to develop and test these hormones, then get approval by the FDA, then spend more money to promote them to doctors and patients. Many doctors simply don't know about the use of natural hormones. Medical literature includes hundreds of articles about patentable HRT for every one article about natural hormone therapy. In reality, the FDA stamp of approval tells us nothing about how good commercial drugs are compared with natural alternatives. It makes one stop and wonder about many of the other 87,000 chemicals manufactured since World War II, including those that are known endocrine disruptors. Although new technologies require new chemicals, there may be natural compounds that would work as well as some of the synthetics; however, there is no profit incentive to market them.

Hormone replacement therapy (HRT) refers to the use of synthetic hormones, while natural hormone replacement includes three natural estrogens in their optimal ratio along with progesterone, testosterone, DHEA, and other substances such as iodine, if needed. The real issue is hormone balance maintenance rather than estrogen replacement.

NATURAL HORMONES

Estrogens

Not all estrogens are created equal. If the human body overbalances estradiol and estrone with a large percentage of estriol, there must be a good reason, even if science hasn't yet discovered it. It makes sense, then, that physicians who prescribe natural estrogen prefer to use estriol alone or in a combination formula called triple estrogen (containing 80 percent estriol and 10 percent each of 17-beta-estradiol and estrone).

The hormones that are used in *natural* hormone replacement—"natural" estrone, estradiol, and estriol—today don't come from humans, as they did with the ancient Chinese. Nowadays, these hormones come from the wild yam (*Dioscorea composita*). If natural hormones come from a plant, why can't we just eat the wild yam and increase our estrogen or progesterone levels that way? Because human physiology doesn't include the enzymes that would convert the hormone precursors in the vegetable to hormones in our bodies.

So why are these hormones made from a wild yam considered more "natural" than the "synthetic" estrogen which is made from another "natural" source—horse urine? When analyzed biochemically, the hormone molecules produced from the wild yam are identical in every way to the hormones manufactured in the human body. Therefore, a "natural" hormone is not based on its origin but on its chemical structure. Synthetic estrogen is, in fact, different from any hormone ever found in nature, but altering the molecular structure is what allows a chemical to be patented.

When you buy natural products for relief of menopausal symptoms, you are increasing estrogenic activity in your body because most natural approaches to menopause use herbs that are estrogenic. Women have been led to believe that the wild yam added to some of these products produces progesterone in their bodies. This is not true. Although some women report an improvement from supplements containing wild yam, human beings can't convert the precursors in yam into actual hormones in their bodies. These products are increasing the estrogenic load on a woman's body without increasing the protective effect of progesterone at the same time. Are these women at higher risk for uterine cancer? It is probably best either to take herbs for just a short time to relieve symptoms, to include natural progesterone, or to add natural hormone potentiators.

Note: If you are interested in trying natural hormone replacement, find and work with a physician who understands and appreciates natural hormones. Triple estrogens or estriol alone are available in either cream or pill form only through prescription from medical doctors (MDS), osteopathic doctors (DOS), and, in some states, naturopathic doctors (NDS) and certified nurse practitioners (CNPS). With creams, the hormones pass through the circulation at least once before the breakdown process starts in the liver. When we swallow pills, the liver is always the first stop and some of the hormone gets broken down before it even gets used.

Dr. Jonathan Wright says, "This does not mean that Tri-Est is perfectly safe. To reduce a risk from even identical-to-natural estrogens, a woman should never take them without natural progesterone, DHEA, and possibly testosterone and thyroid hormones. If we're to supplement hormones at all, then all declining hormones should be supplemented, as they all work together."

Testosterone is the major androgenic hormone, and it is vital for both men and women. In both sexes, testosterone levels peak during youth and decline with age. Normal levels for women are 30–50 pg/ml. Research on the sexual effects of testosterone has shown that women who receive this hormone after menopause experience increased frequency of sexual intercourse, increased sexual desire, increased number of sexual fantasies, and an increased level of sexual arousal.

Many of the female hormones are derived from male hormones. Our bodies make estradiol from testosterone and estrone from androstenedione, another androgenic hormone. During perimenopause, testosterone appears to pick up part of the slack in estrogen production. When women who have had their ovaries removed are given testosterone, their levels of estrone and estradiol can rise significantly. According to research that has been going on for decades in Europe, there is some evidence that natural testosterone can reduce the risk of serious heart disease and improve osteoporosis.

Another hormone produced both by the ovaries and the adrenal glands is **dehydroepiandrosterone** (DHEA). DHEA is metabolized in the body into estrogen and testosterone. This means DHEA elevates the levels of many of the hormones that become deficient during menopause.

Studies done during the past decade have shown that DHEA improves the function of the immune system, helps prevent cancer and possibly heart disease, improves energy levels, benefits individuals with autoimmune diseases such as lupus, and reverses some of the manifestations of aging, such as loss of muscle mass and memory. There is also some evidence that DHEA supplementation is of value in the prevention and treatment of osteoporosis. Higher DHEA levels are associated with denser bones and several studies suggest it helps maintain bone mass. It appears that DHEA is able to enhance bone formation while it puts the brakes on bone resorption.

Women going through menopause usually have lower levels of DHEA than premenopausal women, and women with most types of breast cancer have been found to have abnormally low levels of DHEA. (It is not known if low levels of DHEA predispose a woman to breast cancer or if the lower levels are a direct result of having the disease.) Since the evidence to date suggests that DHEA does not cause cancer and may actually help to prevent it, and it is relatively free of side effects at physiologic dosages (acne and increased hair growth may occur on rare occasions), Dr. Jonathan Wright usually recommends DHEA supplements before considering testosterone therapy.

When progesterone and DHEA are administered together, a small proportion of each of these hormones gets converted to estrogen. Dr. Alan Gaby has found that, in some cases, hot flashes and other estrogen-related symptoms improve when a combination of progesterone and DHEA are taken. Since these hormones appear to be much safer than estrogen, he prefers to use them whenever possible. Sometimes Dr. Gaby recommends DHEA supplements before considering any other hormone therapy. However, since DHEA is converted to estrogen, any woman with estrogen-dependent illness (such as estrogen-receptor-positive breast cancer) should not take DHEA without a doctor's supervision. If it is used, it should be taken in fairly low dosages (3–5 mg).

The PEPI heart study data also showed that estrogen plus natural progesterone was far superior to estrogen plus synthetic progestins in producing an increase in "good" HDL cholesterol.

ALTERNATIVES TO ESTROGEN

Women who have had breast, uterine, or ovarian cancer (and other such estrogen-receptor-positive cancers) need to be especially cautious in their use of estrogens, patentable or natural. Most doctors strongly advise against using replacement therapies for at least three to five years following diagnosis. Women with these kinds of cancers are excellent candidates for herbs and natural hormone potentiators, although they should confer with their physicians before starting any program. Healthy women may want to try these alternatives to see if they relieve menopausal symptoms before going on a program of synthetic or natural hormone therapy.

Herbs

In some cases, menopausal symptoms may be relieved by the herbs dong quai and black cohosh. Black cohosh stimulates the ovaries and production of certain hormones that are useful in the perimenopausal (not the post-menopausal) woman. Thus, products containing high amounts of these herbs should just be used during perimenopause (whereas hormone potentiators may be used during both the peri- and postmenopausal years). Another herb, vitex, stimulates progesterone. Susan S. Weed's book *Menopausal Years: The Wise Woman Way* (Ash Tree Publishing, 1992) gives complete herbal remedies for all menopausal conditions. However, plant products such as cohosh, dong quai, vitex, and American ginseng may stimulate estrogen-dependent breast and uterine cancers. For women at risk, use other herbs or hormone potentiators (that use Korean ginseng). Homeopathic medications have been helpful for some women, too.

Hormone Potentiators

Hormone potentiators are nutritional products that act to gently slow down your body's normal breakdown process of hormones, causing a gentle elevation of your own natural hormones. A moderate potentiation of a number of hormones helps decrease menopausal symptoms while increasing a sense of well-being and vitality. Hormone potentiators are taken as pills or capsules, not creams, with PABA as the main ingredient.

Para-aminobenzoic acid (PABA) is a compound that is considered part of the vitamin B family, although it is not an essential vitamin (meaning we do not have to get it in our daily diet to survive). Inside the body, hormones are constantly being produced and broken down. Studies have shown that PABA helps safely slow down the speed of breakdown. This should gently maintain higher levels of estrogen in the body and, theoretically, could affect other hormones, such as progesterone, testosterone, and DHEA.

Different experiments have shown that this vitamin acts as a potentiator of female reproductive hormones. Young girls given PABA just before entering puberty displayed accelerated appearance of their secondary sex characteristics. Sixteen women with at least five years duration of infertility were given 400 mg/day of PABA for three to seven months, which resulted in pregnancy for 75 percent of the women.

Researchers and doctors began using PABA to decrease the amount of estrogen used to get therapeutic effects in menopausal women. In most of the studies, higher dosages of PABA also increased well-being, increased libido, lubricated the vaginal canal, and showed better hair growth on the head (many menopausal women start to suffer with thinning hair). HRT does not get these results. Other than testosterone, *PABA is the only agent associated with increased libido*, and not many women are anxious to take male hormones. Neither natural nor synthetic hormone therapy increases libido, even though both may decrease vaginal dryness, which lessens pain during sex. Studies showed elevated levels of PABA safely increased levels of natural hormones, such as adrenal and thyroid.

Note: Since PABA works at the liver to accomplish its actions, anyone with liver disease or elevated liver enzymes should not take PABA without the supervision of a doctor.

A number of studies (open trials, not using control groups) suggest **vitamin E** helps relieve menopausal symptoms. Since there were no control groups, there is the possibility that women experienced what is called the placebo effect—feeling better because they were taking something. There was only one placebo-controlled trial ever done; in that study, 50–100 mg/day of vitamin E was no more effective than a placebo. However, many women have reported feeling better simply by adding vitamin E to their daily diets.

Vitamin A helps maintain lubrication in the lining of the vaginal vault. One study suggested that vitamin A at very high dosages of 60,000 IU daily for two weeks stimulated the effects of estrogen and/or enhanced levels of internal production of 17-beta estradiol. However, women should not take more than the recommended daily dose of vitamin A without medical supervision, as too much vitamin A can be toxic.

Flavonoids and vitamin C work in tandem to help stabilize blood vessel walls. When blood vessel walls expand due to a drop in estrogen, hot flashes result. During peri- and postmenopause, when the estrogen levels are haphazard, it is hypothesized that vitamin C and flavonoids can take up the slack and help strengthen the walls of the blood vessels and decrease hot flashes.

Some flavonoids are estrogenic and bind to the estrogen receptors. Flavonoids are so effective they have been used to stop spotting in women. Doctors Sarfati and J. de Brux reported endometrial capillary resistance increased dramatically, and endometrial biopsy appeared the most normal in women given the highest dose of flavonoids with HRT.

Dr. Charles Smith published a double-blind study in which ninety-four women with menopausal hot flashes received different treatments during separate one-month periods. Flavonoids and vitamin C were superior to all the other preparations in relieving hot flashes, including low-dose estrogen preparations. The flavonoid/vitamin C combination works partially because the hesperidin (derived from citrus fruits) is structurally similar to estradiol and is a phytoestrogen.

Dr. Robert Atkins has reported that large doses of **folic acid** (10 mg/day) relieve menopausal symptoms in some cases. Studies also suggest that folic acid protects the cervical lining against precancerous changes.

When taken in dosages higher than can be obtained by diet alone, **pantothenic acid** (PA) has been shown to support activities of adrenal function.

Ginseng contains a phytoestrogen that binds to estrogen and progesterone receptor sites and has hormonelike effects on reproductive tissue. In the *American Journal of Obstetrics and Gynecology*, there was a report of a menopausal woman using a face cream from China that contained ginseng. She had normalization of FSH levels and proliferative endometrium noticeable on biopsy due to the cream. American ginseng has been shown to stimulate estrogen-dependent cells to grow (which may be due in part to spraying with pesticides). I used Korean ginseng in the hormone potentiator product I designed and had it tested on breast cancer cells; it did not stimulate them to grow.

LIFESTYLE AND FOOD CHANGES

Eighty percent of women improve the symptoms of menopause through diet. Try the following recommendations before opting for pharmaceutical or other solutions to menopausal symptoms.

1. *Eliminate or greatly reduce caffeine, refined sugar, salt, alcohol, and animal food sources.* Anecdotally, eliminating caffeine has provided relief from sore, swollen breasts (one sign of estrogen-

dominance) for many women. Coffee is the world's most herbi-cide- and pesticide-sprayed crop. According to a Norwegian study of 12,000 men and women, the more coffee they drank, the more homocysteine in their blood. This is an amino acid believed to promote hardening of the arteries, which increases the risk for heart attack and stroke. Moderate coffee drinking is OK; more than five cups of caffeinated beverages a day starts making a risky difference. However, if you have enough folate (a B vitamin) in your blood, it should greatly inhibit, if not stop, the production of homocysteine. Count how much tea, coffee, chocolate, colas, and other caffeinated soft drinks you consume. They add up.

2. *Exercise more.* Studies show that women who exercise about three-and-a-half hours a week have fewer hot flashes. Studies suggest that the more fit a woman is, the less horrific her menopausal symptoms are. However, in actuality, this is not always the case.

3. *De-stress.* A stressful lifestyle not only puts women more at risk of heart disease, cancer, high blood pressure, muscular aches, and headaches, but it also can increase the negative symptoms of menopause. Take time out each day to sit for five minutes of silence or to listen to your favorite music. Do something to make your life more user-friendly.

4. *Consume more vegetable-based protein food sources* such as beans, grains, seeds, and nuts. Soy products contain large amounts of phytoestrogens—plant substances with estrogen-like action. It is noteworthy that in Japan, where soy consumption is high, only 7 percent of menopausal women experience hot flashes, compared to 55 percent of women living in the United States. Of course, we have other dietary differences, too.

Increasing one's intake of soy products may eliminate the need for estrogen in some cases. Clinical reports from doctors suggest that drink-ing soy milk and taking soy powder help relieve symptoms better in the later stages than earlier in menopause. Women who are postmenopausal and have estrogen-dependent tumors should know that there is a contro-versy about soy. If you have allergic tendencies, you may want to consume soy products only several times a week rather than on a daily basis.

Natural Answers for Specific Peri- and Postmenopausal Problems

Heavy Menstrual Flow

- vitamin A and vitamin A–rich food
- natural form of Heme iron supplement and vitamin C

Have a doctor measure your ferritin levels to get an accurate reading of your iron levels. Iron supplements can cause constipation. Consume brussels sprouts, dark leafy greens, and broccoli with vitamin C–rich foods and/or vitamin C supplementation.

Fatigue

- PABA
- nutrients that support the adrenals such as vitamin C and pantothenic acid.

Breast Tenderness

- vitamin E
- kelp (a good source of iodine but iodine itself may be more effective)
- iodine (use with doctor's supervision)
- essential oils such as flaxseed, evening primrose, and fish oils
- B_6—this vitamin competes with the hormone prolactin at prolactin receptor sites (the hormone prolactin is associated with stress and breast pain)
- cut out or cut down caffeinated products (coffee, tea, colas, chocolate, and some medications)
- magnesium
- testosterone has been shown to decrease breast pain in some women

Libido

PABA and PABA-containing hormone potentiators have been found to enhance desire and enjoyment of sex.

Depression and Anxiety

- herbs such as skullcap, valerian, passion flower, St. John's wort
- nutrients such as magnesium, vitamin B_6, and certain amino acids (tryptophan and tyrosine)

Hot Flashes

- foods containing bioflavonoids (citrus fruits and buckwheat groats)
- soy products (tofu, soy milk, soy tempeh, soy cheese, miso soup)
- According to Dr. Wright, some women are helped by taking one tablespoon of organic, high lignan flaxseed oil a day. Whenever increasing oil intake, make sure to take vitamin E to protect against oxidation of the oil. An interesting note about vitamin E. One of the scientists at a conference told me he has been taking vitamin E ever since he noticed that companies that gave vitamin E to cattle right before they were slaughtered ended up with meat that stayed red for a much longer period of time and therefore brought top prices. This proved to him the antioxidant effect of vitamin E.
- Avoid hot caffeinated beverages, monosodium glutamate (MSG), and table salt. Substitute granulated kelp, potassium tablets, and herbs for salt. Request MSG-free foods in restaurants or, if you consume foods with MSG, increase vitamin B_6 supplementation for several days. Also avoid food additives and colorings, sugar, and alcohol.
- Watch out for excessive consumption of dairy products. Cow's milk products are high in salt, fat, and naturally occurring milk sugar. They are often the source of food allergies/sensitivities and are potentially high in EDCs, especially cheese. Dark leafy greens, raw seeds and nuts, and soy products are better sources of calcium.
- Try goat's milk products. Why? Because postmenopausal women are at risk for heart disease. Cow's milk has more cholesterol than goat's milk. Goat's milk is naturally pasteurized, while the commercial pasteurization of cow's milk creates factors that enhance the laying down of cholesterol inside arteries.

- Decrease saturated and processed fats.

- Eat a bigger breakfast and a smaller lunch and dinner.

- Try helpful herbs in capsules or teas, such as black cohosh, ginseng, dong quai, licorice, unicorn root, and fennel.

- Try natural hormone potentiators, such as products that contain PABA, bioflavonoids, and supportive nutrients.

- Consider natural progesterone and DHEA.

WEIGHT GAIN AND MENOPAUSE

We live in a society, so they say, where you can never be too rich or too thin. Even if this is true, the average woman still tends to gain five to ten pounds during menopause. A study at MIT followed a group of menopausal women who did not change their diet or exercise habits. Within two years they gained an average of between five and eight pounds. This weight gain was independent of whether they took HRT or not.

What to do? Maintain regular exercise, get your thyroid checked, and eat less. Eating less is the strongest factor associated with a decreased risk of cancer and increased longevity. Many doctors have found that some women become borderline hypothyroid (underactive) during peri- and postmenopause. Get checked by a doctor with a complete blood screen, a thorough physical, and an underarm temperature test (Dr. Broda Barnes's test). Consume more sea vegetables such as hiziki and nori seaweeds. Use granulated dulse and kelp (various forms of sea vegetables) as salt substitutes and eat more deep-sea fish such as haddock and tuna.

DES DAUGHTERS

DES daughters, who are now entering the age where breast and ovarian cancers tend to manifest, may be at heightened risk for these diseases. There are adequate clues to warrant careful observation. The bottom line is: tell your doctor you are a DES daughter before he or she prescribes HRT. Studies suggest 67 percent of pregnant women were not told they were given DES. Order hospital birth records if you have suspicions. Call DES Action (800-DES-9288) for more information.

Lists and Charts

A List of DES and Other Pharmaceutical Estrogens

Some people don't realize they are DES children because their mothers were given a drug that wasn't called DES. Following are some names under which DES and other nonsteroidal estrogens have been sold in the United States:

Nonsteroidal Estrogens

Benzestrol
Chlorotrianisene
Comestrol
Cyren A.
Cyren B.
Delvinal
DES
DesPlex
Dibestil
Dienestrol
Dienoestrol
Diestryl

Diethylstilbenediol
Diethylstilbestrol dipalmitate
Diethylstilbestrol diphosphate
Diethylstilbestrol dipropionate
Digestil
Domestrol
Estilben
Estrobene
Estrobene DP
Estrosyn
Fonatol
Gynben

Gyneben
Hexestrol
Hexoestrol
Hi-Bestrol
Menocrin
Meprane
Mestilbol
Microest
Mikarol
Mikarol forti
Milestrol
Monomestrol
Neo-Oestranol I
Neo-Oestranol II
Nulabort
Oestrogenine
Oestromenin
Oestromon
Orestol
Pabestrol D.
Palestrol

Restrol
Stil-Rol
Stilbal
Stilbestrol
Stilbestronate
Stilbetin
Stilbinol
Stilboestroform
Stilboestrol
Stilboestrol DP
Stilestrate
Stilpalmitate
Stilphostrol
Stilronate
Stilrone
Stiles
Synestrin
Synestrol
Synthoestrin
Vallestril
Willestrol

Nonsteroidal Estrogen-Androgen Combinations

Amperone
Di-Erone
Estan
Metystil

Teserene
Tylandril
Tylosterone

Nonsteroidal Estrogen-Progesterone Combination

Progravidium

Vaginal Cream Suppositories with Nonsteroidal Estrogens

Avc cream with dienestrol
Dienestrol cream

THE ASSOCIATION BETWEEN BREAST CANCER AND PESTICIDES IN HUMAN STUDIES

POSITIVE ASSOCIATION	NEGATIVE ASSOCIATION
Aronson (2000) found a clear association between levels of PCBS in breast fatty tissue and the development of breast cancer in 217 cases versus 213 controls.	Mendonca (1999) found no significance between organochlorines and breast cancer in 177 cases versus 350 controls.
Hoyer (1998) measured blood levels in 1976 and analyzed 240 women who during the seventeen-year follow-up developed breast cancer. Found dieldrin positively associated with increased risk for breast cancer.	Zheng (1999) conducted two studies on the same 304 breast cancer cases that did not support association between fat tissue levels of DDE, DDT, and HCB with breast cancer risk.
Kettles (1997) showed a statistically significant increase in breast cancer risk with medium and high levels of triazine exposure (herbicide used on corn, etc.) in 120 counties in Kentucky, representing 1.9 million women.	Helzlsouer (1999) conducted a large study following a group of women who had donated blood in the 1970s and 1980s and found no association between blood levels of DDE or PCBS with the development of 346 cases of breast cancer up to twenty years later.
Dewailly (1994) found moderately elevated levels of lindane in twenty women with breast cancer. Women with ER+ breast cancer had substantially higher levels of DDE.	Moysich (1998) studied 154 postmenopausal women with newly diagnosed breast cancer. There was no evidence of a link between blood levels of PCBS and three EDCS and breast cancer. A small number of the women who had children but had never breast-fed did have association between levels of PCBS and breast cancer.

POSITIVE ASSOCIATION	NEGATIVE ASSOCIATION
Melius (1994) discovered that women who lived within 1 kilometer of a chemical plant were 60 percent more likely to develop breast cancer after menopause than women who did not live near such a plant.	Hunter (1997) studied blood levels of 240 women who were diagnosed with breast cancer within two years after blood samples were taken. This showed that higher levels of DDE and PCBS did not increase the risk of getting breast cancer. The data also suggested a nonsignificant trend toward these chemicals protecting against getting cancer.
Wolff (1993) found elevated levels of DDE in blood in fifty-eight women with breast cancer.	Lopez-Carrillo (1997) compared blood levels of DDE in 141 women with breast cancer to 141 women without. This study did not support a causal relationship between this chemical and breast cancer.
Falck pilot study (1992) found higher PCBS (50–60 percent higher) in fat tissue in twenty-five breast cancer patients.	Van't Veer (1997) found no association between DDE and breast cancer among 606 women from five European countries on the basis of DDE samples removed from their fat. The authors mention that the lower levels of DDE may be caused by the disease itself (if true, may make conclusions of this kind of study very murky).
Weston (1990) suspected that a 30 percent drop in breast cancer incidence in Israel was related to a ban on three pesticides.	Adami (1995) found that women exposed to PCBS and DDT at work did not have higher association with breast cancer.

POSITIVE ASSOCIATION	NEGATIVE ASSOCIATION
H. Mussalo-Rauhamaa (1990) found an elevated level (50 percent higher) of a lindanelike compound (beta-HCH) in fourty-four breast cancer patients.	Cantor (1995) conducted a study of 33,509 women who had died of breast cancer and did not find an association of breast cancer and PCBS and found perhaps even a protective effect with insecticides. They did find a positive association with endocrine-disrupting metals, several solvents, and styrene.
Najem (1985) discovered in two studies that death from breast cancer increased the closer the women lived to toxic dump sites.	Ahlborg (1995) found no association between exposure to DDT at work and an increased risk of breast cancer.
Chiazze (1977) found women who breathed vinyl chloride vapors at work had increased death rates from breast cancer.	Krieger (1994) studied blood levels of 150 women with breast cancer (fifty African Americans, fifty whites, and fifty Asian Americans) and found no significant association of DDE and PCBS with breast cancer. This was the first study to compare blood levels from before the time of breast cancer diagnosis (thirty years) and the time the women contracted the disease. However, when the groups were looked at separately, whites and African-American women with breast cancer had higher levels of DDE than women without breast cancer. There was a trend toward higher levels of chemicals and breast cancer in whites and African-American women that was not statistically significant.

POSITIVE ASSOCIATION	NEGATIVE ASSOCIATION
Wasserman (1976) found organochlorine compounds (PCBS and insecticides) higher concentration in fat and tumor tissue in nine women with breast cancer.	Key (1994) conducted a meta-analysis of less than 1,000 women. It failed to demonstrate a strong relation between DDT and PCBS and breast cancer risk.

Resources

ON-LINE INFORMATION ABOUT ENDOCRINE DISRUPTORS

Environmental Concepts Made Easy

http://www.tmc.tulane.edu/ecme/eehome/default.html

Produced by the Center for Bioenvironmental Research (CBR) of Tulane and Xavier Universities in New Orleans, directed by John McLachlan. Full of easily digested information on environmental estrogens. Intended for use by students, journalists, and researchers, it includes a huge bibliography.

Our Stolen Future

http://www.osf-facts.org

This website about the book *Our Stolen Future* includes summaries and references for new research that has come out since the book was published.

World Wildlife Fund

http://www.wwfcanada.org/hormone-disruptors/index.html

Dr. Theo Colborn's home base. Easy-to-follow information on endocrine disruption and preventative measures. WWF also has a series of videos featuring leading scientists in the field of endocrine disruption. Available for undergraduate and graduate level studies.

The Liberty Tree Alliance

http://www.libertytree.org/trenches/endo/endo.html

A national association of writers, scientists, and activists concerned with the preservation of the natural world. Writer Carolyn J. Strange reviews the subject of endocrine disruption; suggests Web resources; lists activist groups involved in the issue; and provides quotes, opinions, and comments from various sources.

DES RESOURCES

DES Action USA

1615 Broadway #510
Oakland, CA 94612
510/465-4011 or 800/DES-9288
desact@well.com
http://www.desaction.org

DES Cancer Network

514 10th St. NW, Ste. 400
Washington, DC 20004
800/DES-NET4 or 202/628-6330
Fax 202/628-6217
desnetwrk@aol.com

DES Sons Network

104 Sleepy Hollow Pl.
Cherry Hill, NJ 08003
609/795-1658

Registry for Research on Hormonal Transplacental Carcinogenesis

The University of Chicago
5841 S. Maryland Ave. (MC 2050)

Chicago, IL 60637

312/702-6671

Fax 312/702-0840

This registry was created to register cases of clear-cell adenocarcinoma of vagina or cervix in women born since 1948 or adenocarcinoma of Fallopian tube or endometrium.

Helfand's Outreach Campaign

Pamela Calvert

Judith Helfand Productions

2112 Broadway #402A

New York, NY 10023

212/875-0456

Fax 212/501-0889

A Healthy Baby Girl

Women Make Movies

462 Broadway #500

New York, NY 10013

212/925-0606

Fax 212/925-2052

babyg@www.com.

Dry Cleaning

For brochures, fact sheets, case studies, televideo conferences, educational videos, and pollution-prevention manuals about wet and dry cleaning, contact:

EPA's Pollution Prevention Information Clearinghouse (PPIC)

U.S. Environmental Protection Agency

410 M St., SW (3404)

Washington, DC 20460

202/260-1023

Fax 202/260-0178

Food and Water

To keep informed about organic food legislation, check out the Wild Oats website (www.wildoats.com) or call 800/494-WILD, 800/357-2211 (Citizens for Health), or 800/253-0681 (Pure Food Campaign).

To get information on bottled-water standards—or to find out what's in the water you buy—contact the Food and Drug Administration, Federal Office Building #9, Room 5807, 200 C St. SW, Washington, DC 20004, 888/INFO-FDA.

For information on your tap water, call the EPA's Safe Drinking Water Hotline, 800/426-4791.

Home Environment

This forty-hour course is offered free in the Seattle area.

Training Manual for the Master Home Environmentalist Program (ed. Philip Dickey). Published by the American Lung Association of Washington (1997). To order the manual ($150 or free if you take the course) call the American Lung Association at 206/441-5100. Includes the Home Environmental Assessment List (HEAL) for evaluating the pollution in your home and a booklet that lists household products by name and evaluates their toxicity.

Environmental Health Clearinghouse

2605 Meridian Pkwy., Ste. 115
Durham, NC 27713
Fax 919/361-9408
eheath@niehs.nih.gov
http://infoventures.com/e-hlth

The Environmental Health Clearinghouse has put together many packets of information—fact sheets, journal articles, and research findings—that focus on safe indoor and outdoor habitats. The authors are toxicologists, freelance writers, epidemiologists, and consumer advocates. They indicate the possible adverse health effects of commonly used household chemicals and home building products, and/or suggest less toxic or nontoxic alternatives.

Pesticides and Pest Control

Common Sense Pest Control: Least Toxic Solutions for Your Home, Garden, Pets and Community. William Olkowski, et al. Tauton Press, Newtown, 1991. Considered by experts to be one of the best bug books.

For questions about the health effects of pesticides, product information, cleanup procedures, etc., call the National Pesticide Telecommunication Network at 800/858-7378 (24 hours a day).

Farm Chemicals Handbook '97. Information about all pesticides registered in the United States, including trade and common names, active ingredients, registered uses, toxicity, and basic manufacturers. Detailed descriptions of laws and regulations pertaining to pesticides, including the Clean Air Act, the Food Quality Protection Act, the Endangered Species Act, and many others.

Meister Publishing Co.
37733 Euclid Ave.
Willoughby, OH 44094
800/572-7740 or 216/942-2000
Fax 216-942-0662

Growing Doubt: A Primer on Pesticides Identified as Endocrine Disruptors and/or Reproductive Toxicants, Charles Benbrook, 1996. Overview of pesticide impacts on the endocrine system; reviews scientific literature on 20 pesticide active ingredients identified as endocrine disruptors and/or reproductive toxins; describes pesticide-use trends, routes of exposure, and health effects for each chemical examined; and calls on the U.S. government to implement research programs to identify other endocrine-disrupting pesticides.

National Campaign for Pesticide Policy Reform
7370 Cactus Thorn Ln.
Tucson, AZ 85747
520/647-7036
Fax 520/647-7547
ncppr@igc.org

Northwest Coalition for Alternatives to Pesticides
P.O. Box 1393
Eugene, OR 97440
541/344-5044

Pesticide Action Network North America (PANNA)
116 New Montgomery, #810
San Francisco, CA 94105
415/541-9140
Fax 415/541-9253
panna-info@igc.apc.org
http://www.panna.org/panna

PRODUCT INFORMATION

A Consumer's Dictionary of Household, Yard, and Office Chemicals, Ruth Winter, Crown Publishers, 1992. Winter also wrote *A Consumer's Dictionary of Cosmetic Ingredients* and *A Consumer's Dictionary of Food Additives*.

Your Health and the Indoor Environment: A Complete Guide to Better Health Through Control of the Indoor Atmosphere, Randall Earl Dunford, NuDawn Publishing, 1991.

Are You Poisoning Your Pets? A Guidebook on How Our Lifestyles Affect the Health of Our Pets, Nina Anderson and Howard Peiper, Safe Goods, 1995; or call 800/903-3837.

The Safe Shopper's Bible: A Consumer's Guide to Non-toxic Household Products, Cosmetics, and Food, David Steinman and Samuel S. Epstein, Mac-Millan, 1995.

Office Green Buying Guide, Kathleen Gray, Green Seal, 1996. Published by the nonprofit group that evaluates green products, this guide is available by becoming a member of Green Seal. Call 202/331-7337.

Co-op America's National GreenPages, Co-op America, 1996. A directory of more than 1,400 socially and environmentally responsible businesses offering products and services. Call 800/58-GREEN.

Prescriptions for a Healthy House: A Practical Guide for Architects, Builders, and Homeowners, Paula Baker, John Banta, and Erica Elliot.

Catalogs That Carry Nontoxic Products

Seventh Generation 800/456-1177
RealGoods www.realgoods.com

Consumer Product Safety Commission

Office of the Secretary
5401 Westbard Ave.
Bethesda, MD 20207
800/638-2772

This office can supply a list of local laboratories that will test for a wide category of pollutants.

GOVERNMENT AGENCIES (OTHER THAN THE EPA) CONCERNED WITH HORMONE DISRUPTORS

Department of the Interior (DOI) has wildlife management, steward-ship, and research responsibilities. In particular, two subagencies of DOI—the Fish and Wildlife Service and the new Biological Resources Division of U.S. Geological Survey—are interested in endocrine disruptors (www.doi.gov/doitext.html).

Department of Health and Human Services (HHS) has many sub-agencies that are knowledgeable in relevant areas of science or policy (www.hhs.gov/about).

Agency for Toxic Substances and Disease Registry (ATSDR) is a gov-ernment agency of the U.S. Department of Health and Human Services. Its website has much valuable information about toxins and toxicology, including the ATSDR/EPA list of "Top 20 Hazardous Substances" and the newsletter "Hazardous Substances & Public Health." The agency is man-dated to perform specific functions concerning the effect on public health of hazardous substances in the environment (atsdr.cdc.gov.html).

Food and Drug Administration (FDA) has numerous people with expertise in endocrine disruption in general and the issue of phytoestrogens in particular. The FDA/NCTR (National Center for Toxicological Research) is studying the effects of antiestrogens and estrogens on reproductive development and is working to establish an in vitro model for uterine growth and determine estrogen responsiveness to this system (www. fda.gov/nctr/index.html).

Centers for Disease Control (CDC) has many departments interested in endocrine disrupter issues (www.cdc.gov), as does the **National Center for Environmental Health** (NCEH) (www.cdc.gov/nceh), which conducts epidemiological studies all over the United States.

National Institute for Environmental Health Sciences (NIEHS) conducts and sponsors research in epidemiology, cellular and molecular pharmacology, and environmental toxicology. NIEHS has long been developing and validating new methods for toxicological research and testing programs. (www.niehs.nih.gov) NIEHS maintains a hot line: 800/ NIEHS94 (643-4794) for answers or help in tracking down the best available data on environmental health issues (envirohealth@infoventures.com; infoventures.com/e-hlth).

NIEHS introduced CHEHSIR, a publicly accessible database, to ensure that federal research agencies, researchers at universities, community groups, and the public have access to information on all research conducted or funded by the federal government that is related to adverse health effects for children resulting from exposure to environmental agents and safety risks.

National Institute for Occupational Safety and Health (NIOSH) does research designed to help set recommended worker exposure standards (www.cdc.gov/niosh/homepage.html). They work closely with the Department of Labor's **Occupational Safety and Health Administration** (OSHA), the policy side of the standards setting (www.osha.gov). They are the only federal agency that conducts research on reproductive effects of worker exposure to chemicals and pesticides.

Agency for Toxic Substances and Disease Registry (ATSDR) conducts health assessments of communities impacted by hazardous waste sites (www.atsdr1.atsdr.cdc.gov:8080/atsdrhome.html or 800/447-1544). In 1996 ATDSR started a Child Health Initiative that established a Child

Health Workgroup composed of nationally recognized experts in child health and environmental medicine (atsdr1.atsdr.cdc.gov:8080/child/chw 497.htm). Contact the ATDSR Information Center at 1600 Clifton Rd. NE, MS E57, Atlanta, GA 30333, 404/639-6357.

National Toxicology Program (NTP) is an inter-agency research program with representatives from NIEHS, NIOSH, FDA, EPA, OSHA, and the Consumer Product Safety Commission (CPSC). It develops screening and testing procedures for certain chemicals and pesticides and can provide information about potentially toxic chemicals to health regulatory and research agencies, scientific and medical communities, and the public (ntp -server.niehs.nih.gov).

Department of Agriculture (USDA) has a couple of offices involved in endocrine disruptor–related issues. The EPA is also working collaboratively with the Department of Agriculture and private sector groups to reduce pesticide use and risks. Nationwide, their goal is to expand the use of integrated pest management (IPM) to cover 75 percent of U.S. crop acreage by the year 2000 (www.usda.gov).

Food Safety and Inspection Service (FSIS) is responsible for the inspection of meat and poultry in the United States (www.usda.gov/ agency/fsis/homepage.htm). Through the National Residue Program, USDA identifies chemicals and pesticides likely to be in meat and poultry and then determines ways to eradicate them. Recently, substances chosen have been from lists of potential endocrine disrupters. The **Office of Public Health and Science** monitors chemical and pesticide residues in meat, poultry, and eggs and designs specific testing procedures for meat and poultry (www.usda.gov/fsis.ophs/ophshome.htm).

Endocrine Disruption Research Workgroup of the Committee on Environment and Natural Resources (CENR) is compiling an inventory of research related to endocrine disruption (www.epa.gov/endocrine/ project.html).

Special Report on Environmental Endocrine Disruption: An Effects Assessment and Analysis, 1997, Environmental Protection Agency (EPA), reviews scientific literature on endocrine disruptors and covers a range of health effects. Specify order number EPA/630/R96/012. Us EPA, ORD Publications, Mailstop G-72, 26 W. Martin Luther King Dr., Cincinnati, OH 45268; 513/569-7562; fax 513/569-7566. Report is online at www.epa.gov/ord/whatsnew.htm.

Organizations Working for Chemical Regulation

Consumers Union of the United States
101 Truman Ave.
Yonkers, NY 10703
914/378-2000

Environmental Defense Fund
1875 Connecticut Ave. NW
Washington, DC 20009
202/387-3500
Fax 202/234-6049
rks@edf.org

Environmental Working Group
1718 Connecticut Ave. NW, Ste. 600
Washington, DC 20009
202/667-6982

National Coalition Against the Misuse of Pesticides
701 E St. SE, Ste. 200
Washington, DC 20003
202/542-5450

Greenpeace
1436 U St. NW
Washington, DC 20009
202/462-1177
Fax: 202/462-4507
rick.hind@green2.greenpeace.org

Mothers and Others for a Livable Planet

40 West 20th St.
New York, NY 10011
212/242-0010

National Audubon Society

666 Pennsylvania Ave. SE, Ste. 200
Washington, DC 20003
202/547-9009

Natural Resources Defense Council

1350 New York Ave. NW, Ste. 300
Washington, DC 20005
202/783-7800

INTEREST GROUPS

Center for the Study of Environmental Endocrine Effects

11 Dupont Circle
Washington, DC 20036
202/797-6368
Fax 202/939-6969
http://www.endocrine.org

This is an industry-sponsored site that provides the latest information on scientific research and governmental policy developments.

Children's Environmental Health Network

5900 Hollis St., Ste. E
Emergyville, CA 94608
510/450-3818 x137
Fax 510/450-3773
http://www.cehn.org

Institute for Evaluating Health Risks

(specializing in pesticides and dioxin toxicity)
1629 K St. NW, Ste. 402
Washington, DC 20005

202/289-8721
Fax 202/955-3814
http://www.igc.apc.org/ncppr

Physicians for Social Responsibility
11 Garden St.
Cambridge, MA 02138
617/497-7440
Fax 617/876-4277

W. Alton Jones Foundation
232 E. High St.
Charlottesville, VA 22902
804/295-2134
Fax 202/861-8378

The following two groups are watchdogs of the EPA:
Environmental Defense Group

257 Park Ave. South
New York, NY 10010
800/684-3322
www.edf.org

Natural Resources Defense Council
40 W. 20th St.
New York, NY 10011
212/727-2700
http://www.nrdc.org
nrdcinfo@nrdc.org

RESEARCH AND MEDICAL SOCIETIES

American Chemical Society
1155 16th St. NW
Washington, DC 20036
202/872-6041
Fax 202/872-4370

American College of Occupational and Environmental Medicine

55 W. Seegers Rd.
Arlington Heights, IL 60005
847/228-6850 x152
Fax 847/228-1856
http://www.apha.org

National Association of Physicians for the Environment

6410 Rockledge Dr., Ste. 412
Bethesda, MD 20817
301/571-9791
Fax 301/530-8910
nape@ix.netcom.com

Society of Environmental Toxicology and Chemistry

1010 N. 12th Ave.
Pensacola, FL 32501-3307
904/469-1500
Fax 904/469-9778
setac@setac.org

Society of Toxicology

1767 Business Center Dr., Ste. 302
Reston, VA 20190
703/438-3115
Fax 703/438-3113
www.toxicology.org

BREAST CANCER

For scientific reading:

"Endocrine Disrupters and Breast Cancer: A Connection or Not?" Edited by D. L. Davis. *Environmental Health Perspectives* 105 (3), (1997).
A monograph based on papers presented at the Workshop on Hormones, Hormone Metabolism, Environment, and Breast Cancer, New Orleans, Center for Bioenvironmental Research, 1995.

For general reading:

Environmental Links to Breast Cancer Handbook and *Environmental Links to Women's Breast Cancer: The Global Agenda*, both available from Women's Environment & Development Organization (WEDO), 355 Lexington Ave., 3rd Floor, New York, NY 10017.

World Resources Institute (WRI)

Dr. Devra Davis has an excellent resource on breast cancer here.

1709 New York Ave. NW
Washington, DC 20006
202/662-3771
Fax 202/662-2511
www.wri.org

RESOURCES FOR NATURAL HORMONES

Nutrition and Healing, a monthly newsletter written by Dr. Jonathan Wright. Call 1-800/528-0559.

Compounding pharmacies in your area can be located by contacting:

International Academy of Compounding Pharmacists (IACP)

P.O. Box 1365
Sugar Land, TX 77487
800/927-4227
Fax 713-495-0602

Professional Compounding Centers of America, Inc. (PCCA)

800-331-2498
Fax 800-874-5760
www.compassnet.com/~pcca

Medical doctors or osteopaths who are members of the American College for Advancement in Medicine (ACAM) are knowledgeable in the use of natural hormones. For a referral to an ACAM doctor, contact:

ACAM

23121 Verdugo Dr., Ste. 204
Laguna Hills, CA 92653
800-532-3688
www.acam.org

Osteopathic physicians differ from MDs mainly in their emphasis on a "whole person" and a preventative approach to the practice of medicine. To find an osteopath, contact:

American Osteopathic Association

142 E. Ontario St.
Chicago, IL 60611-2864
312-380-5800
www.am-osteo-assn.org

Naturopathic medicine is based on the belief and observation that the human body possesses enormous power to heal itself when given the correct natural materials and energies. To locate a naturopathic physician, contact:

American Association of Naturopathic Physicians (AANP)

2366 Eastlake Ave., Ste. 322
Seattle, WA 98102
206/298-0125
www.infinite.org/naturopathic.physician

Notes

INTRODUCTION

"infertility . . ." M. Perloe and E. S. Sills, "Infertility" from www.ivf.com/ fertview.html.

"in Erice, Sicily, for a work session . . ." "Work Session on Environmental Endocrine-Disrupting Chemicals: Neural, Endocrine, and Behavioral Effects," Erice, Sicily, November 1995, in *Toxicology and Industrial Health* 14(1&2): 1998.

CHAPTER 1

"six-mile-long train . . ." "How Much Is a Part per Million?" Extoxnet, Pesticide Information Project of Cooperative Extension Offices.

"the hormone is said to be *bound* to the receptor . . ." G. L. Green, "Mechanistic Complexities in Endocrine Modulation: Estrogen Receptor Structure Modulators, Modulators and Targets," Human Diet and Endocrine Modulation Conference at Fairfax, VA. (Nov. 19–21, 1997).

"Most commercially available laboratory animals . . ." J. Spearow, "Genetic Variation in Susceptibility to Endocrine Disruption by Estrogen," a lecture at Environmental Hormones: Past, Present, Future, New Orleans, LA (Oct. 18–20, 1999)

"response to the same chemicals . . ." E. J. Clark, D. O. Norris, and R. E. Jones, "Interactions of Gonadal Steroids and Pesticides (DDT/DDE) on Gonaduct Growth of Larval Tiger Salamanders, Ambystoma Tigrinum," *General and Comparative Endocrinology* 109:94-105 (1998).

"effect in the animal . . ." Personal communications with F. vom Saal and Dr. John McLachlan.

CHAPTER 2

"The hypothesis is that . . ." From the PBS documentary *Fooling with Nature*, PBS Video (June 2, 1998).

"messages coming from outside . . ." A. O. Cheek et al., "Environmental Signaling: A Biological Context for Endocrine Disruption," *Environmental Health Perspectives* 106(1):5–10 (1998).

"detected by accident, not by intent . . ." P. Montague, "Warning on Male Reproductive Health," *Rachel's Environment and Health Weekly* No. 438 (Electronic edition, April 20, 1995).

"accelerated with the war against bugs . . ." D. Fagin, M. Lavelle, and the Center for Public Integrity, *Toxic Deception: How the Chemical Industry Manipulates Science, Bends the Law, and Endangers Your Health*, Birch Lane Press, 1996.

"1,000 tons a year . . ." R. Maynard, "Sperm Alert," *Living Earth* 188:89 (1995).

"exported in 1992 . . ." J. Raloff, "The Pesticide Shuffle," *Science News* 149: 174–75 (March 1996).

"burning PVC plastic . . ." *National Dioxin Survey: Tier 4: Combustion Sources*, U.S. EPA (1986).

"least recyclable of all plastics . . ." "Pvc: The Poison Plastic," Greenpeace, 1436 U Street NW, Washington, DC 20009.

"authors of study to stay independent of industry . . ." "The Ties That Bind," *U.S. News and World Report*, 12(March 6, 2000).

"defined as the 'science of poisons' . . ." D. C. Klaassen, M. O. Amdur, and J. Doull, eds., *Casarett and Doull's Toxicology* (3d ed.), MacMillan, 1986.

"opening scene of *Macbeth* . . ." B. Weiss, "Behavioral Toxicology: A New Agenda for Assessing the Risks of Environmental Pollution," in *Psychopharmacology: Basic Mechanisms and Applied Interventions*, J. Grabowski and G. R. VandenBos, eds., American Psychological Association (1992).

"what they do to the endocrine system . . ." S. Steingraber, *Living Downstream*, Addison-Wesley, 1997, p. 99.

"fit into various receptors . . ." J. D. McKinney, "Interactive Hormonal Activity of Chemical Mixtures," *Environmental Health Perspectives* 105(9):896–97 (1997).

"any dose of hormone disruptors, no matter how low . . ." D. M. Sheehan et al., "No Threshold Dose for Estradiol-Induced Sex Reversal of Turtle Embryos: How Little Is Too Much?" *Enivronmental Health Perspectives* 107(2):155–59 (1999).

"blown in from distant lands . . ." J. M. Blais et al., "Accumulation of Persistent Organochlorine Compounds in Mountains of Western Canada," *Nature* 395:585–88 (1998).

"coauthor of *Our Stolen Future* . . ." T. Colburn, D. Dumanoski, and J. P. Myers, *Our Stolen Future*, Dutton, NY (1996).

Chapter 3

"from our external environment . . ." D. M. Sheehan et al., "No Threshold Dose for Estradiol-Induced Sex Reversal of Turtle Embryos: How Little Is Too Much?" *Environmental Health Perspectives* 107(2):155–59 (1999).

"not just a female hormone . . ." R. A. Hess, D. Bunick, K. H. Lee, J. A. Taylor, K. S. Korach, and D. B. Lubahn, "A Role for Estrogens in the Male Reproductive System, *Nature* 390:509–12 (1997).

"both males and females . . ." R. Sharpe, "Do Males Rely on Female Hormones?" *Nature* 390:447–48 (1997).

"Dr. David Crews . . ." J. Travis along with Judy Bergeron and John McLachlan, "Modus Operandi of an Infamous Drug," *Science News* 155:124–26 (1999).

"eggs will hatch out females . . ." D. Crews et al., *Developmental Genetics* 15:29–312 (1994).

"Similar findings have been reported . . ." D. M. Fry and T. K. Toone, "DDT-Induced Feminization of Gull Embryos," *Science* 213:922–24 (1981).

"painted two kinds of PCBs on turtle eggs . . ." "Gender-Bending PCBs," *Science News* 145:239 (Nov. 8, 1994).

"Just the right amount of testosterone . . ." J. A. Raloff, "A New Breadth to Estrogen's Influence," *Science News* 151:116 (1997).

"As a side note . . ." R. W. Goy and B. S. McEwen, *Sexual Differentiation of the Brain*, MIT Press (1980).

"The gene Wnt-7 alpha . . ." A. Swain et al., "Mammalian Sex Determination: A Molecular Drama," *Genes and Development* 13:755–67 (1999).

"Environmental Estrogens . . ." J. A. McLachlan (Ed.), proceedings of the symposium *Estrogens in the Environment II: Influences on Development*, Raleigh, NC (April 1985).

"health disorders such as breast cancer . . ." C. Lamartiniere, in M. Eubanks, "Hormones and Health," *Environmental Health Perspectives* 105 (5):482–87 (1997).

"soy may not be beneficial . . ." Personal conversation with C. Hughes, who says that genistein, which is one of the major phytoestrogens in soy, is ¹⁄₂₀th the potency of natural estradiol at the alpha receptor and is ⅓ the potency at the beta receptor. This implies that phytoestrogens may have more effect than once thought (Jan. 1999).

"Dr. Siesta Mosselman . . ." S. Mosselman et al., "ER Beta: Identification and Characterization of a Novel Human Estrogen Receptor," *FEBS Letters* 19; 392(1): 49–53 (1996).

"membrane ER . . ." M. Razandi, A. Pedram, G. L. Greene, and E. R. Levin, "Cell Membrane and Nuclear Estrogen Receptors Derive from a Single Transcript: Studies of ERa and ERb Expressed in CHO Cells," *Molecular Endocrinology* 13(2):307–19 (1999).

"estrogen works in more than one way . . ." Z. Chen et al., "Estrogen Receptor Mediates the Nongenomic Activation of Endothelial Nitric Oxide Synthase by Estrogen," *Journal of Clinical Investigation* 103:401–06 (1999).

"For a substance to act like an estrogen . . ." T. I. Oprea, "A Receptor-Ligand View of Endocrine Disruption," *Fiziologia (Physiology)*, 7(2):413 (1997).

"our natural estrogen . . ." B. Hileman, "Environmental Estrogens Linked to Reproductive Abnormalities, Cancer," *Chemical and Engineering News* (Jan. 1994).

"Suddenly the first chemical . . ." A. M. Soto et al., "The Pesticides Endosulfan, Toxaphene, and Dieldrin Have Estrogenic Effects on Human Estrogen-Sensitive Cells," *Environmental Health Perspectives* 102 (4):380–83 (1994).

"affinity with the estrogen receptor . . ." K. S. Korach and J. A. McLachlan, "The Role of the Estrogen Receptor in Diethylstilbestrol Toxicity," *Archives of Toxicology Supplement* 8:33–42 (1985).

"DES has a metabolite nicknamed DQ . . ." K. Chae, J. Lindzey, J. A. McLachlan, and K. S. Korach, "Estrogen-Dependent Gene Regulation by an Oxidative Metabolite of Diethylstilbestrol, Diethylstilbestrol-4′, 4″-Quinone," *Steroids* 63:149–57 (1998).

"Even a weak estrogen . . ." J. M. Bergeron et al., "Developmental Synergism of Steroidal Estrogens in Sex Determination," *Environmental Health Perspectives* 107:93–97 (1990).

"more active (and possibly more destructive) metabolites . . ." D. Kupfer, "Effects of Pesticides and Related Compounds on Steroid Metabolism and Function," *Critical Review in Toxicology* 4:83–124 (1975).

"hormone disruptors inhibit progesterone . . ." K. G. Osteen et al., "Dioxin (TCDD) Can Block the Protective Effect of Progesterone in Nude Mouse Model of Experimental Endometriosis," American Society for Reproductive Medicine annual meeting (November 1996).

"weighted toward more estrogenic signaling . . ." W. G. Foster et al., "Hexachlorobenzene (HCB) Suppresses Circulating Progesterone Concentrations During the Luteal Phase in the Cynomolgus Monkey," *Journal of Applied Toxicology* 12:13–17 (1992).

"Dr. John McLachlan says . . ." From McLachlan interview, Jan. 1998.

"shut down production of melatonin . . ." J. Raloff, "EMF's Biological Influences: Electromagnetic Fields Exert Effects on and Through Hormones," *Science News* 153:29–31 (1998).

"in the Western world . . ." P. T. Ellison et al., "The Ecological Context of Human Ovarian Function," *Human Reproduction* 8:2248–58 (1993).

"GnRH is a hormone . . ." Dr. Knobil, "Neuro-Endocrine Control of Primate Reproduction," a lecture at the Human Diet and Endocrine Modulation conference in Fairfax, VA (Nov 19–21, 1997).

"Thus, women with more fat . . ." Danish researcher J. Clemmensen's observations are referred to as *Clemmensen's hook*. Davis and coworkers suggest that the renewed surge in breast cancer after menopause, especially in obese women, might be linked with xenoestrogens and with the production of endogenous estrogens that would be created in those with proportionally more body fat.

"fourteen drinks per week . . ." S. A. Smith-Warner et al., "Alcohol and Breast Cancer in Women: A Pooled Analysis of Cohort Studies," *Journal of the American Medical Association* 279:535–40 (Feb. 18, 1998). M. E. Reichman et al., "Effects of Alcohol Consumption on Plasma and Urinary Hormone Concentrations in Pre-menopausal Women," *Journal of the National Cancer Institute* 85(9):722–26 (1993).

"estrogen becomes toxic to the body . . ." J. R. Lee with V. Hopkins, *What Your Doctor May Not Tell You About Menopause*, Warner Books, 1996.

"my researcher sent me a study . . ." H. W. Simpson, C. S. McArdle, K. Griffiths, A. Turkes, and G. H. Beastall, "Progesterone Resistance in Women Who Have Had Breast Cancer," *British Journal of Obstetrics and Gynaecology* 105:345–51 (1998).

"estrogenic metabolite of DDT . . ." D. Kupfer, "Effects of Pesticides and Related Compounds on Steroid Metabolism and Function," *Critical Reviews in Toxicology* 4:83–124 (1975).

"Monkey studies showed . . ." W. G. Foster et al., "Hexachlorabenze (HCB) Suppresses Circulating Progesterone Concentrations During the Luteal Phase in the Cynomolgus Monkey," *Journal of Applied Toxicology* 12:13–17 (1992).

"Then, in the mid-1990s . . ." K. G. Osteen et al., "Dioxin (TCDD) Can Block the Protective Effect of Progesterone in Nude Mouse Models of Experimental Endometriosis," American Society for Reproductive Medicine Annual Meeting (November 1996).

"circulating unopposed estrogen . . ." I. Jatoi, "Neoadjuvant Progesterone Therapy for Primary Breast Cancer: Rational for a Clinical Trial," *Clinical Therapeutics* 19(1):56–61 (1997).

"menstrual timing of their surgery . . ." I. S. Fentiman, "Timing of Surgery Has Major Impact on Survival Rates for Premenopausal Breast Cancer Patients," *Cancer* 86:2053–2058 (1999).

"leading cause of early miscarriages . . ." Fax communication with Dr. John Lee, June 25, 1999.

"progesterone production was low . . ." B. C. Cambell et al., *Hormone Research* 37(45):132–36 (1992)

"I found a study . . ." A. L. Southern et al., "The Effect of 2,2-bis(2-Chlorophenyl-4-Chlorophenyl)-1,1,Dichloroethane (o.p′-DDD) on the Metabolism of Infused Cortisol-7-H," *Steroids* 1(11) (1996).

CHAPTER 4

"They were wrong . . ." R. Mittendorf and A. L. Herbst, "Managing the DES-Exposed Woman: An Update," *Contemporary Obstetrics/Gynecology* 61–80 (1994).

"in utero exposure to an endocrine disruptor . . ." R. Newbold, "Cellular and Molecular Effects of Developmental Exposure to Diethylstilbestrol: Implications for Other Environmental Estrogens," *Environmental Health Perspectives* 103(Suppl. 7):83–87 (1995); R. M. Giusti, K. Iwamoto, and E. E. Hatch, "Diethylstilbestrol Revisited: A Review of the Long-Term Health Effects," *Annals of Internal Medicine* 122(10):778–88 (1995); R. R. Newbold, J. A. McLachlan, "Transplacental Hormonal Carcinogenesis: Diethylstilbestrol as an Example," *Progress in Clinical and Biological Research* 394:131–47 (1996).

"Why didn't it surprise me . . ." A. Direcks and E. Hoen, "DES: The Crime Continues," in: *Adverse Effects, Women and the Pharmaceutical Industry* (ed. K. McDonnell), International Organization of Consumer Unions (1986).

"What was basically ignored . . ." A. A. Lacassagne, "Comparative Study of the Carcinogenic Action of Oestrogenic Hormones," *American Journal of Cancer* 28:735–40 (1938); A. A. Lacassagne, "Hormonal Pathogenesis of Adenocarcinoma of the Breast," *American Journal of Cancer* 27:212–28 (1936).

"In 1939 and 1940 . . ." A. A. Lacassagne, "Confirmation par des experience de traitement a l'oestrone, du rule preponderant de la lere dans la transmission hereditaire du carcinome de la mammalle," *Comp. Rendu Soc Biol* 132:222–25 (1939).

"One study showed that 64 percent . . ." F. Cahen, E. Dubreuil, and J. C. Pons, "Prenatal Exposure to Diethylstilbestrol and the Mother-Daughter Relationship," *European Journal of Obstetrics, Gynecology, and Reproductive Biology* 65(2):181–87 (1996).

"DES was manufactured by 267 companies . . ." B. C. Tilley and A. B. Barnes et al., "A Comparison of Pregnancy History Recall and Medical Records," *American Journal of Epidemiology* 121(2):269–81 (1985). Twenty-nine percent of DES mothers could not remember if they took DES, and an additional 8 percent said they did not take DES when it was recorded in their charts that they in fact had.

"two theoretical studies . . ." W. Smith and G. V. S. Smith. "The Influence of Diethylstilbestrol on the Progress and Outcome of Pregnancy as Based on a Comparison of Treated with Untreated Primagrovadis," *American Journal of Obstetrics and Gynecology* 58:994 (1994). A second influential study by Dr. Karnaky reported that DES, when injected into the wall of the cervix, stopped uterine contractions. Karnaky extrapolated this as proof that the drug might protect against threatened miscarriages.

"Though a few studies did report helpful effects . . ." D. Robinson and L. B. Shettles, "The Use of Diethylstilbestrol in Threatened Abortion," *American Journal of Obstetrics and Gynecology* 63:1330 (1952).

"Two huge reviews . . ." A. G. King, "Threatened and Repeated Abortion," *Obstetrics and Gynecology* 1:104 (1953); J. W. Golziehler and B. B. Benigno, "The Treatment of Threatened and Recurrent Abortion: A Critical Review," *American Journal of Obstetrics and Gynecology* 75:1202 (1958).

"DES actually seemed to increase the rate . . ." J. Travis, "Modus Operandi of an Infamous Drug: Mutant Mice Provide Clues to How DES Wreaked Havoc in the Womb," *Science News* 155:124–26 (1999).

"Dr. Arthur L. Herbst . . ." A. L. Herbst, H. Ulfelder, and D. C. Poskanzer, "Adenocarcinoma of the Vagina: An Association of Maternal Stilboestrol Therapy with Tumor Appearing in Young Women," *New England Journal of Medicine* 284:878–81 (1971). A. L. Herbst, D. Anderson, M. M. Hubby et al., "Risk Factors for the Development of Diethylstilboestrol-Associated Clear Cell Adenocarcinoma: A Case Control Study," *American Journal of Obstetrics and Gynecology* 154:814–22 (1971).

"It never prevented miscarriages . . ." W. J. Dieckmann et al., "Does the Administration of Diethylstilbestrol During Pregnancy Have Therapeutic Value?" *American Journal of Obstetrics and Gynecology* 66(5):1062–81 (1961).

"sterility, impotence, and breast growth . . ." O. Schell, *Modern Meat*, Vintage Books, Random House, 1985, pp. 283–84.

"Estrogen-like compounds . . ." J. Robbins, *A Diet for a New America*, Stillpoint, 1987, p. 313.

"not tested for DES in meat since 1991 . . ." E. Olsen, "Searches for Sources of Tainted Beef Sent to Switzerland," *New York Times* (Feb. 4, 2000).

"Most DES Sons . . ." J. Raloff, "DES Sons Face No Fertility Problems," *Science News* 147:324 (1995).

"Yet a Canadian research team proposed . . ." L. J. Brandes et al., "Stimulation of Malignant Growth in Rodents by Antidepressant Drugs at Clinically Relevant Doses," *Cancer Research* 52:3796–800 (1992); L. J. Brandes et al., "Enhanced Cancer Growth in Mice Administered Daily Human-Equivalent Doses of Some H_1-Antihistamines: Predictive in Vitro Correlates," *Journal of the National Cancer Institute* 86(10):770–74 (1994).

"growth of preexisting cancer . . ." S. Nemecek, "Backfire: Could Prozac and Elavil Promote Tumor Growth?" *Scientific American* 271(3):22 (1994).

"Thomas A. Gasiewicz . . ." T. A. Gasiewicz, "Exposure to Dioxin and Dioxin-like Compounds as a Potential Factor in Developmental Disabilities," *Mental Retardation and Developmental Disabilities Research Reviews* (1998).

CHAPTER 5

"If we design a compound . . ." From "Minute Doses Cause Huge Effects," www.wwfcanada.org/hormone-disruptors.

"irreversible abnormalities . . ." Statement from the work session on Environmental Endocrine-Disrupting Chemicals: Neural, Endocrine, and Behavioral Effects, Erice, Sicily, November 1995, in *Toxicology and Industrial Health* 14(1&2) (1998).

"DDE levels in the umbilical cord . . ." W. J. Rogan et al., "Polychlorinated Biphenyls (PCBs) and Dichlorodiphenyl Dichloroethene (DDE) in Human Milk: Effects of Maternal Factors and Previous Lactation," *American Journal of Public Health* 76(2):172–77 (1986).

"90 percent of the level . . ." Ueki M. Osaka Medical College, at April 13 scientific meeting, http://www.tmc.tulane.edu/ecme/EEHome /newsviews/whatsnew/junnews.html

"Once pollutants do cross the placenta . . ." H. Bern, "The Fragile Fetus," in *Chemically-Induced Alterations in Sexual and Functional Development: The Wildlife/Human Connection* (T. Colborn and C. Clement, Eds.), Princeton Scientific Publishing Co., 1992, pp. 9–15.

"mothers with limbless children . . ." "New Toxicological Patterns" from http://www.wwfcanada.org/hormone-disruptors/

"eleven out of 380 children," from http://www.itn.co.uk/Britain/brito81106. htm

"exposure is sufficient to be a cause for concern . . ." L. Needham, "Human Health Outcomes Related to Dioxin Exposure," lecture from Environmental Hormones: Past, Present, Future. New Orleans, LA (Oct. 18–20, 1999).

"sex hormone-binding globulin," D. Sheehan and M. Young, "Diethylstilbestrol and Estradiol Binding to Serum Albumin and Pregnancy Plasma of Rat and Human," *Endocrinology* 104:1442–46 (1979); F. S. vom Saal et al., "Estrogenic Pesticides: Binding Relative to Estradiol in MCF-7 Cells and Effects of Exposure During Fetal Life on Subsequent Territorial Behavior in Male Mice," *Toxicology Letters* 77:343–50 (1995); S. C. Nagel et al., "Relative Binding Affinity-Serum Modified Access (RBA-SMA) Assay Predicts the Relative In Vivo Bioactivity of the Xenoestrogens Bisphenol A and Octylphenol," *Environmental Health Perspectives*

105:70–76 (1997); F. S. vom Saal et al., "Prostate Enlargement in Mice Due to Fetal Exposure to Low Doses of Estradiol and Diethylstilbestrol and Opposite Effects at High Doses," *Proceedings of the National Academy of Sciences* 94:2056–61 (1997); S. C. Nagel, F. S. vom Saal, K. Sharpe-Timms, and W. V. Welshons, "Mechanisms of Fetal Vulnerability to Xenoestrogens," *Poster Session Abstracts* at Estrogens in the Environment IV: Linking Fundamental Knowledge, Risk Assessment, and Public Policy, 13 (July 21, 1997).

"sex hormone-binding proteins," vom Saal, Welshons, and Nagel were the first to set up assays that specifically looked at how much estrogenic activity of a xenoestrogen was reaching the cell.

"Xenoestrogens, therefore, circulate freely," T. Colborn, F. S. vom Saal, and A. M. Soto, "Developmental Effects of Endocrine-Disrupting Chemicals in Wildlife and Humans," *Environmental Health Perspectives* 101:378–84 (1993).

"100 times more potent than natural estradiol," W. S. Branham et al., "The Postnatal Ontogeny of Rat Uterine Glands and Age-Related Effects of 17B-Estradiol," *Endocrinolgy* 117(5):2229–237 (1985).

"apple-shaped people, as opposed to the pear-shaped ones," G. De Pergola et al., "Body Fat Accumulation Is Possibly Responsible for Lower Dehydroepiandrosterone Circulating Levels in Premenopausal Obese Women," *International Journal of Obesity* 20: 1105–110 (1996); D. Goodman-Gruen et al., "Sex Hormone-Binding Globulin and Glucose Tolerance in Postmenopausal Women," The Rancho Bernardo Study, *Diabetes Care* 20(4):645–47 (1997).

"The genome . . ." NIEHS News, *Environmental Health Perspectives* 105(6) (1997).

"Every single cell in the body . . ." C. Bernes, *Persistent Organic Pollutants: A Swedish View of an International Problem* (translated by M. Naylor), Swedish Environmental Protection Agency (1998).

"xenohormones can damage DNA," C. Dees et al., "Estrogenic and DNA-Damaging Activity of Red No. 3 in Human Breast Cancer Cells," *Environmental Health Perspectives* 105(3):625–32 (1997); L. Shuanfang et al., "Developmental Exposure to Diethylstilbestrol Elicits Demethylation of Estrogen-Responsive Lactoferrin Gene in Mouse Uterus," *Cancer Research* 57:4356–359 (1997).

"steroids also play an important role," C. Bernes, *Persistent Organic Pollutants: A Swedish View of an International Problem* (translated by M. Naylor). Swedish Environmental Protection Agency (1998).

"Pregnant rats fed one meal . . ." R. Peterson, R. Moore, T. Mably, D. Bjerke, and R. Goy, "Male Reproductive System Ontogeny: Effects of Perinatal Exposure to 2,3,7,8-Tetrachlorodibenzo-*p*-Dioxin," in *Chemically Induced Alterations in Sexual and Functional Development* (Eds. T. Colborn and C. R. Clement) Princeton Scientific Publishing, 1992.

"75 percent reduction in sperm counts . . ." "Thalidomide, Dioxin: Timing of *In-Utero* Exposure Is Key, Many Ways to Disrupt the Hormone System": http://www.wwfcanada.org/hormone-disruptors/

"exposure to estrogenic compounds in the womb . . ." R. Santti, "Urethral Dyssynergia: An Estrogen-Related Condition?" lecture from Environmental Hormones: Past, Present and Future, New Orleans, LA (Oct. 18–20, 1999).

"weak environmental estrogenic compounds . . ." R. A. Hajek et al., "During Development, 17-Alpha Estradiol Is a Potent Estrogen and Carcinogen," *Environmental Health Perspectives* 105(3):577–81 (1997).

"numerous general population surveys . . ." J. E. Davies et al. "The Role of Social Class in Human Pesticide Pollution," *American Journal of Epidemiology* 96:(5)334-41 (1972); J. E. Davies et al., "An Epidemiological Application of the Study of DDE Levels in Whole Blood," *American Journal of Public Health* 59:435–41 (1969); R. T. Rappolt et al., in *Pesticide Symposia*, ed. by W. B. Deichman, Halos & Associates, 1970, pp. 7–11; W. S. Hoffman et al., "Relation of Pesticide Concentrations in Fat to Pathological Changes in Tissues," *Archives of Environmental Health* 15:758–65 (1967).

"minimum of a dozen chemical contaminants . . ." *Our Stolen Future*, p. 106, Dutton, 1996.

"Mother's milk is 3 percent fat. . . ." W. Rogan et al., "Polychlorinated Biphenyls (PCBS) and Dichlorodiphenyl Dichloroethene (DDE) in Human Milk: Effects of Maternal Factors and Previous Lactation," *American Journal of Public Health* 76(2):172–77 (1986).

"breastfeeding substantially increases the child's exposure . . ." K. H. Niessen et al., "Chlorinated Hydrocarbons in Adipose Tissue of Infants and Toddlers: Inventory and Studies on Their Association with Intake of Mothers' Milk," *European Journal of Pediatrics* 142:238–43 (1984).

"cumulative body burden of chemicals . . ." S. Patandin et al., "Dietary Exposure to Polychlorinated Biphenyls and Dioxins from Infancy Until Adulthood: A Comparison Between Breast-Feeding, Toddler, and Long-Term Exposure," *Environmental Health Perspectives* 107(1):45–51 (1999).

"poisonous substances in food . . ." "Action Levels for Poisonous or Deleterious Substances in Human Food and Animal Feed," Industry Activities Section, Center for Food Safety and Nutrition, Food and Drug Administration, Washington, DC: FDA (1992, 1994).

"Breast milk is the food . . ." K. H. Niessen et al., "Chlorinated Hydrocarbons in Adipose Tissue of Infants and Toddlers: Inventory and Studies on Their Association with Intake of Mothers' Milk," *European Journal of Pediatrics* 142:238–43 (1984).

"chemicals such as PCBS . . ." "A Dutch Study Indicated That Rotterdam Preschoolers Who Were Breastfed Had 3.6 Times as Many PCBS in Their Blood Plasma as Children Who Had Been Fed Formula," *Science News* 152(22):344 (1997).

"DDT was banned . . ." P. Furst, C. Furst, and K. Wilmers, "Human Milk as a Bioindicator for Body Burden of PCDDS, PCDFS, Organochlorine Pesticides, and PCBS," *Environmental Health Perspectives* 102(1):187–93 (1994).

"higher levels of DDE . . ." W. J. Rogan et al., "Polychlorinated Biphenyls (PCBS) and Dichlorodiphenyl Dichloroethene (DDE) in Human Milk: Effects of Maternal Factors and Previous Lactation," *American Journal of Public Health* 76(2):172–77 (1986).

"Only 5 percent of the Caucasian mothers . . ." W. J. Rogan et al., "Polychlorinated Biphenyls (PCBS) and Dichlorodiphenyl Dichloroethene (DDE) in Human Milk: Effects of Maternal Factors and Previous Lactation," *American Journal of Public Health* 76(2):172–77 (1986).

"A remarkable overlap . . ." B. C. Gladen and W. J. Rogan, "DDE and Shortened Duration of Lactation in a Northern Mexican Town," *American Journal of Public Health* 85:504–09 (1995).

"Two German Studies," H. Drexler et al., "The Mercury Concentration in Breast Milk Resulting from Amalgam Fillings and Dietary Habits," *Environmental Research* 77(2):124–29 (1998); G. Drasch et al., "Mercury in Human Colostrum and Early Breast Milk: Its Dependence on Dental

Amalgam and Other Factors," *Journal of Trace Elements in Medicine and Biology* 12(1):23–27 (1998).

"A study by Nagayama and coworkers . . ." J. Nagayama et al., "Postnatal Exposure to Chlorinated Dioxins and Related Chemicals on Thyroid Status in Japanese Breast-Fed Infants," *Chemosphere* 37(9–12):1789–93 (1998).

"Korrick and coworkers . . ." S. A. Korrick et al., "High Breast Milk Levels of Polychlorinated Biphenyls (PCBS) Among Four Women Living Adjacent to a PCB-Contaminated Waste Site," *Environmental Health Perspectectives* 106(8):513–18 (1998).

"Ayotte and Dewailley . . ." P. Ayotte et al., "Health Risk Assessment for Inuit Newborns Exposed to Dioxin-like Compounds Through Breast-feeding," *Chemosphere* 32(3):531–42 (1996).

"PCBS in the blood of Swedish women . . ." L. Rylander et al., "The Impact of Age, Lactation and Dietary Habits on PCB in Plasma in Swedish Women," *The Science of the Total Environment* 207:55–61 (1997).

"soft, discolored molars . . ." S. Alaluusua et al., "Developing Teeth as Biomarker of Dioxin Exposure," *Lancet* 353:9148–206 (1999).

"phytoestrogens found in breast milk . . ." L. J. C. Bluck and S. A. Bingham, Letter to the Editor, *Clinical Chemistry* 43 (5):851–52 (1997).

"biological activity in the infant . . ." M. McCarthy, "Soy-Based Formulas Linked to Excess Estrogens," *New York Times* (July 6, 1997).

"hormone-dependent diseases . . ." K. Setchell, D. R. Linda, J. Cai, and J. E Heubi, "Exposure of Infants to Phytoestrogens from Soy-Based Infant Formula," *Lancet* 350:23–27 (1997).

"unmonitored human infant experiment . . ." D. M. Sheehan, Letter to the Editor, National Center for Toxicology Research, *Clinical Chemistry* 43 (5):850 (1997).

"most ideal food for infants . . ." W. J. Rogan, "Pollutants in Breast Milk," *Archives of Pediatric and Adolescent Medicine* 150:981–89 (1996).

"come from in utero exposure . . ." "Public Health Briefs," *American Journal of Pediatric Health* 74(4):379 (1984); S. P. Porterfield and L. B. Hendry, "Impact of PCBS on Thyroid Hormone Directed Brain Development, *Toxicology and Industrial Health* 14(1/2):103–20 (1998).

"benefits of breastfeeding . . ." W. J. Rogan, "Pollutants in Breast Milk," *Archives of Pediatric and Adolescent Medicine* 150:981–89 (1996).

"Dispose of . . ." "Baby Alert: New Findings About Plastics," *Consumer Reports*:28–29 (May 1999).

"Don't have dental sealants . . ." J. Raloff, "Dental Sealant Safety Reconsidered," *Science News* 152:324 (1997). "Dangerous Dental Sealants," *Environmental Health Perspectives* 104 (4):373–4 (1996).

"mercury from the mother's fillings . . ." H. Drexler and K. H. Schaller, "The Mercury Concentration in Breast Milk Resulting from Amalgam Fillings and Dietary Habits," *Environmental Research* 77(2):124–29 (1998); G. Drasch et al., "Mercury in Human Colostrum and Early Breast Milk: Its Dependence on Dental Amalgam and Other Factors," *Journal of Trace Elements in Medicine and Biology* 12(1):23–27 (1998).

"risk of malformed fetuses . . ." S. Khattak et al., "Pregnancy Outcome Following Gestational Exposure to Organic Solvents," *Journal of the American Medical Association* 281 (March):1106–09 (1999).

"tobacco go into the amniotic fluid . . ." C. Poirot, "Just One Puff," *The New Mexican*, Health/Science: C-1 (Feb. 6, 1998).

CHAPTER 6

"safe lifetime exposures . . ." A. Schecter et al., "Congener-Specific Levels of Dioxins and Dibenzofurans in U.S. Food and Estimated Daily Dioxin Toxic Equivalent Intake," *Environmental Health Perspectives* 102:962–66 (1994).

"fetus's brain and cognitive ability . . ." S. Schantz, D. Rice, and R. F. Seegal all have written and emphasized that postnatal exposure is sufficient to cause adverse impairments in cognitive function.

"first four years of life . . ." A. Fausto-Sterling, *Myths of Gender: Biological Theories About Women and Men*, Basic Books, (1992) p. 73.

"decreased learning capabilities . . ." "NIEHS News," *Environmental Health Perspectives* 102(8):628 (1994).

"prevents the penetration of toxins . . ." "Los Angeles Times Report: Pesticide Residue Harmful to Kids," *The New Mexican* A-5 (January 30, 1998).

"signals that normally control development . . ." T. Colborn, M. J. Smolen, and R. Rolland, "Environmental Neurotoxic Effects: The Search for New Protocols in Functional Teratology," *Toxicology and Industrial Health* 14 (1/2):9–23 (1998).

"total dietary intake of pesticides . . ." G. Aklend, et. al., "The Three Interacting Factors Associated with Children's Dietary Exposures: Environmental Concentrations, Food Contamination, and Children's Behaviors," Preprints of *Extended Abstracts* 39(2):119–21. Paper presented before the Division of Environmental Chemistry American Chemical Society, New Orleans, LA (Aug. 22–26, 1999).

"environmental chemicals than adults have . . ." R. Jackson, "Assessing Children's Health," Preprints of *Extended Abstracts* 39(2):134. Paper presented before the Division of Environmental Chemistry American Chemical Society, New Orleans, LA (Aug 22–26, 1999).

"Natural Resources Defense Council . . ." "Threats to Children," *Pesticide and Toxic Chemical News* (Nov. 26, 1997).

"presumption of greater toxicity. . ." P. J. Landrigan et al., *Pesticides in the Diets of Infants and Children*, National Academy Press, 1993, p. 9.

"number-one cause of hospitalization . . ." J. Chuda and N. Chuda, Checnet Children's Health Environmental Coalition Network. nancy@checnet.org

"auditory system in the fetus . . ." F. S. Goldey et al., "Developmental Exposure to Polychlorinated Biphenyls (Aroclor 1254) Reduces Circulating Thyroid Hormone Concentrations and Causes Hearing Deficits in Rats," *Toxicology and Applied Pharmacology* 135(1):77–88 (1995).

"Precocious puberty . . ." M. E. Herman-Giddens et al., "Secondary Sexual Characteristics and Menses in Young Girls Seen in Office Practice: A Study from the Pediatric Research in Office Settings Network," *Pediatrics* 99(4):505–12 (1997).

"earlier puberty in rodents . . ." Frederick vom Saal and Susan Nagel exposed pregnant mice to bisphenol A at the same levels that cause breast cancer cells to grow. Certain female mice went through puberty five days earlier. Keystone Symposium on Endocrine Disruptors (B5) in Tahoe City, CA (Jan. 31–Feb. 5, 1999).

"Dr. William Kelce . . ." Keystone Symposium on Endocrine Disruptors (B5) in Tahoe City, CA (Jan. 31–Feb. 5, 1999).

"70 percent of girls with early breast growth . . ." I. Colin et al., "Identification of Phthalate Esters in the Serum of Young Puerto Rican Girls with Premature Breast Development (Thelarche)," poster session from Environmental Hormones: Past, Present, and Future, New Orleans, LA, Oct. 18–20, 1999.

"home and garden pesticides . . ." J. R. Davis, R. C. Brownson, R. Garcia, B. H. Bentz, and A. Turner, "Family Pesticide Use and Childhood Brain Cancer," *Archives of Environmental Contamination and Toxicology* 24:87–92 (1993).

"Studies continue to prove . . ." J. M. Pogoda and S. Preston-Martin, "Household Pesticides and Risk of Pediatric Brain Tumors," *Environmental Health Perspectives* 105(11):1214–20 (1997).

"anti-lice pesticide shampoo . . ." D. L. Davis et al., "Policy Issues in Environmental Epidemiology: Making the Connection Between Exposure and Human Disease," Hazardous Waste Conference, 1993. http://atsdr1 .atsdr.cdc.gov:8080/cx1d.html

"Research on boys from the University of Edinburgh . . ." J. M. Williams, L. C. Dunlop, "Pubertal Timing and Self-Reported Delinquency Among Male Adolescents," *Journal of Adolescents* 22(1):157–71 (Feb. 1999).

"analyzed girls seen in doctors' offices . . ." J. Rieder, S. M. Coupy, "Update on Pubertal Development," *Current Opinions in Obstetrics and Gynecology* 11(5):457–62 (Oct. 1999).

"weigh 20 percent more than normal . . ." K. L. Howdeshell et al., "Exposure to Bisphenol A Advances in Puberty," *Nature* 401(67 55):763–4 (1999).

"Guillette and her team reported . . ." E. A. Guillette et al., "An Anthropological Approach to the Evaluation of Preschool Children Exposed to Pesticides in Mexico," *Environmental Health Perspectives* 106(6):347–53 (1998).

"Dr. Elizabeth Guilette said . . ." Telephone conversation with Dr. Guillette (Nov. 19, 1999).

"In 1995, the Environmental . . ." R. Wiles and K. Davies, "Pesticides in Baby Food," Environmental Working Group (1995).

"interesting marketing challenge . . ." "Gerber Goes Organic with Baby Food Line," *The New Mexican* (Oct 30, 1997).

"fish from the Great Lakes . . ." J. L. Jacobson and S. W. Jacobson, "Intellectual Impairment in Children Exposed to Polychlorinated Biphenyls In Utero," *New England Journal of Medicine* 335(11):783–89 (1996).

"(PCB-induced) handicaps . . ." J. Raloff, quoted in "Emerging Science on the Impacts of Endocrine Disruptors on Intelligence and Behavior": http://www.wwfcanada.org/hormone-disruptors/

"background PCB exposure . . ." W. J. Rogan, Pre-meeting comments for EPA workshop report on developmental neurotoxic effect associated with exposure to PCBS, EPA/630/004, A128–A130 (1993); S. Schantz, "Developmental Neurotoxicity of PCBs in Humans: What Do We Know and Where Do We Go From Here?" *Neurotoxicology and Teratology* 18(3):217–27 (1996).

"school report cards . . ." B. Gladen and W. Rogan, "Effects of Perinatal Polychlorinated Biphenyls and Dichlorodiphenyl Dichloroethene Transplacentally and Through Human Milk," *Journal of Pediatrics* 113:991-95 (1988); W. J. Rogan et al., "Polychlorinated Biphenyls (PCBS) and Dichlorodiphenyl Dichloroethene (DDE) in Human Milk: Effects of Maternal Factors and Previous Lactation," *American Journal of Public Health* 76(2) (1986).

"PCB exposure . . ." J. L. Jacobson, S. W. Jacobson, and H. E. B. Humphrey, "Effects of Exposure to PCBs and Related Compounds on Growth and Activity in Children," *Neurotoxicology and Teratology* 12:319–26 (1990).

"in utero exposure to PCBS . . ." S. Schantz, "Developmental Neurotoxicity of PCBs in Humans: What Do We Know and Where Do We Go from Here?" *Neurotoxicology and Teratology* 18(3):217–27 (1996).

"Bernard Weiss, a neurotoxicologist . . ." J. Raloff, "Because We Eat PCBs," *Science News Online* (Sept. 14, 1996).

"higher levels of DDT in their bodies compared to white women . . ." Irva Hertz-Picciotto, "In Utero Exposures to Organochlorines and Child Development in a Birth Cohort from the 1960s," talk from "Human Health Outcomes Related to Dioxin Exposure" lectures from Environmental Hormones: Past, Present, Future conference, New Orleans, LA (Oct., 18–20, 1999).

"rat offspring were 'hyperreactive' . . ." H. Daly, "Laboratory Rat Experiments Show Consumption of Lake Ontario Salmon Causes Behavioral Changes: Support for Wildlife and Human Research Results," *Journal of Great Lakes Research* 19(4):784–88 (1993).

"Even with low fish consumption . . ." E. Lonky, T. Reihman, J. Darvill, J. Mather, and H. Daly, "Neonatal Behavioral Assessment Scale Performance in Humans Influenced by Maternal Consumption of Environmentally Contaminated Lake Ontario Fish," *Journal of Great Lakes Research* 22(2)198–212 (1996).

"Researchers from the University of Wisconsin . . ." W. P. Poreter, et al., "Endocrine, Hormone, and Behavioral Effects of Aldicarb (Barbameate), Cotrazine (Tricazyne), and Nitrate (Fertilizer) Mixtures at Ground Water Concentrations" *Toxicology and Industrial Health* 15 (1–2):133–50 (1999).

"irreversible changes in adult brain function . . ." P. Eriksson, "Developmental Neurotoxicity of Environmental Agents in the Neonate," *Neurotoxicology* 18(3):719–26 (1997).

"impaired on cognitive tests . . ." D. C. Rice, "Behavioral Effects of Postnatal Exposure to a PCB Mixture in Juvenile Monkeys," *Toxicologist* 15:243 (1995).

"higher among delinquents than nondelinquents . . ." D. Mann, "Experts Demand More Study of Environmental Toxins' Effect on Children," *The New Mexican* C:1 (May 28, 1999).

"1980–81 the Jacobsons . . ." J. L. Jacobson and S. W. Jacobson, "Intellectual Impairment in Children Exposed to Polychlorinated Biphenyls In Utero," *New England Journal of Medicine* 335(11):783–89 (1996).

"Daly and Lonky . . ." E. Lonky et al., "Neonatal Behavioral Assessment Scale Performance in Humans Influenced by Maternal Consumption of Environment Contaminated Lake Ontario Fish," *Journal of Great Lakes Research* 22(2):198–212 (1996).

"1978–82, Rogan and Gladen . . ." W. J. Rogan, EPA workshop on PCB/EPA 630/or:A128–A130 (1993).

"1989, Dutch PCB/Dioxin Study . . ." S. Patandin et al., "Effects of Environmental Exposure to Polychlorinated Biphenyls and Dioxins on Cognitive Abilities in Dutch Children at 42 Months of Age," *Journal of Pediatrics* 134:33–41(1999).

"A review by Tilson . . ." H. A. Tilson et al., "Cross Species Study Reveals Perinatal Exposure in All Species Frequently Associated with Impairments in Cognitive and Psychomotor Activity," *Neurotoxicology and Teratology* 12:239–48 (1990).

"The offspring of exposed mothers . . ." Statement from the Director of Environmental and Occupational Health at the National Cheng Kung University Medical Center, Taiwan.

"Times Beach, Missouri . . ." D. S. Cantor et al., "In Utero and Postnatal Exposure to 2,3,7,8,-TCDD in Times Beach, Missouri: Impact on Neurophysiological Functioning," Dioxin 93: Thirteenth International Symposium on Chlorinated Dioxin and Related Compounds, Vienna, Austria, 1993.

"Dr. Hauser studied the children . . ." P. Hauser, J. M. McMillin, and V. S. Bhatara, "Resistance to Thyroid Hormone: Implications for Neurodevelopmental Research on the Effects of Thyroid Hormone Disruptors," *Toxicology and Industrial Health* 14(1/2):85–101 (1998).

"A German study . . ." N. Osius et al., "Thyroid Hormone Level in Children in the Area of a Toxic Waste Incinerator in South Essen," *Gesundheitswesen* 60(2):107–12 (1998).

"Sher and team . . ." E. S. Sher et al., "The Effects of Thyroid Hormone Level and Action in Developing Brain: Are These Targets for the Actions of PCBs and Dioxins?" *Toxicology and Industrial Health* 14(1/2):121–58(1998).

"Bonacci and coworkers . . ." R. Bonacci et al., "Relevance of Estrogen and Progesterone Receptors Enzyme Immunoassay in Malignant, Benign, and Surrounding Normal Thyroid Disease," *Journal of Endocrinology Investigation* 19:159–64 (1996).

"Porterfield . . ." S. P. Porterfield and L. B. Hendry, "Impact of PCBs on Thyroid Hormone Directed Brain Development," *Toxicology and Industrial Health* 14(1/2):103–20 (1998).

"researchers on lead . . ." D. C. Rice, "Neurotoxicity of Lead, Methylmercury, and PCBs in Relation to the Great Lakes," *Environmental Health Perspectives* 103(9):71–87 (1995).

"lead affects estrogenic signaling . . ." N. N. Tchernitchin et al., "Effect of Subacute Exposure to Lead on Responses to Estrogen in the Immature

Rat Uterus," Bulletin of Environmental Contamination and Toxicology 60:759–65 (1998).

"Yu-Cheng mothers . . ." Statement from the Director of Environmental and Occupational Health at the National Cheng Kung University Medical Center.

"consistent with the animal data . . ." T. A. Gasiewicz, "Exposure to Dioxin and Dioxin-like Compounds as a Potential Factor in Developmental Disabilities," *Mental Retardation and Developmental Research Reviews* 3:230–38 (1997).

"American Council on Science and Health (ACSH) . . ." C. E. Koop, "A Scientific Evaluation of Health Effects of Two Plasticizers Used in Medical Devices and Toys: A Report from the American Council on Science and Health," *MedGenMed* (June 22, 1999).

"We Should be Concerned . . ." Health Care Without Harm press release. "Clean Bill of Health, or Misdiagnosis?" (1999), www.noharm.org

"or blood components." Raloff J. response in Letters. *Science News* 155:387 (June 19, 1999).

"phthlalates out of toys . . ." National Environmental Trust, E-wire press release, June 22, 1999.

"Dutch children exposed to . . ." Koopman-Esseboom et al., "Effects of Polychlorinated Biphenyl/Dioxin Exposure and Feeding Type on Infants' Mental and Psychomotor Development," *Pediatrics* 97(5):700–06 (1996).

"In another Dutch study . . ." S. Patandin et al., "Effects of Environmental Exposure to Polychlorinated Biphenyls and Dioxins on Cognitive Abilities in Dutch Children at 42 Months of Age," *Journal of Pediatrics* 134:33–41 (1999).

"IQ deficits at age three-and-a-half . . ." J. S. Lakind, et al., "Dietary Exposure to PCBs and Dioxins, *Environmental Health Perspectives* 107(10):A495–97 (1999).

"childhood developmental disorders . . ." S. L. Swan, "Response to Commentaries," *Neurotoxicology and Teratology*, 18:3:271–76 (1996).

"metabolism of thyroid hormone . . ." A. G. Schuur et al., "Inhibition of Thyroid Hormone Sulfation by Hydroxylated Metabolites of Polychlorinated Biphenyls," *Chemical-Biological Interactions* 109(1–3):293–97 (1998);

Y. Kato et al., "Reduction of Thyroid Hormone Levels by Methylsulfonyl Metabolites of Polychlorinated Biphenyl. *Archives of Toxicologoy* 72(8):541–44 (1998).

"experimental animals, wildlife species, and . . ." A. Brouwer et al., "Interactions of Persistent Environmental Organohalogens with the Thyroid Hormone System: Mechanisms and Possible Consequences for Animal and Human Health," *Toxicology and Industrial Health* 14(1–2):59–84 (1998).

"other permanent neurological problems . . ." Learning Disabilities Association of America, "Brain Development: Toxins and Brain Teratogens," 4156 Library Rd., Pittsburgh, PA. 15234; ph: 412/344-1515.

"Dr. Hauser . . ." P. Hauser, J. M. McMillin, and V. S. Bhatara, "Resistance to Thyroid Hormone: Implications for Neurodevelopmental Research on the Effects of Thyroid Hormone Disruptors," *Toxicology and Industrial Health* 14(1/2):85–101 (1998).

"thyroid hormone in infants . . ." J. Magayama et al., "Postnatal Exposure to Chlorinated Dioxins and Related Chemicals on Thyroid Hormone Status in Japanese Breast-Fed Infants," *Chemosphere* 37(9–12):1789–93 (1998).

"damage to their offspring . . ." G. Csaba and A. Inczefi-Gonda, "Transgenerational Effect of a Single Neonatal Benzpyrene Treatment on the Glucocorticoid Receptor of the Rat Thymus," *Human and Experimental Toxicology* 17:88–92 (1998); G. K. Nelson et al., "Exposure to Diethylstilbestrol During a Critical Developmental Period of the Mouse Reproductive Tract Leads to Persistent Induction of Two Estrogen-Regulated Genes," *Cell Growth Differentiation* 5:595–606 (1994).

"nonexposed males . . ." B. E. Walker, "Tumors of Female Offspring of Mice Exposed Prenatally to Diethylstilbestrol," *Journal of the National Cancer Institute* 73:133–40 (1984).

"granddaughters of DES-exposed mother mice . . ." R. R. Newbold et al., "Increased Tumors but Uncompromised Fertility in the Female Descendants of Mice Exposed Developmentally to Diethylstilbestrol," *Carcinogenesis* 19(9):1655–63 (1998).

"males exposed to DES . . ." V. S. Turusov et al., "Occurrence of Tumors in Descendants of CBA Male Mice Prenatally Treated with Diethylstilbestrol," *International Journal of Cancer* 50:131–35 (1992).

"The Society for the Advancement of Women's Health Research . . ." *Women's Health and the Environment: Findings of National and Regional Roundtable Meetings* report (1993).

"lindane promoted tumor growth . . ." R. Bigsby. "Molecular and Pharmacokinetic Mechanisms of Xenestrogen Action." Talk presented at Keystone Symposium on Endocrine Disruptors (B5) in Tahoe City, CA (Jan. 31–Feb. 5, 1999).

"lead poisoning symptoms . . .": http://www.tmc.tulane.edu/ecme/leadhome/protect.html

CHAPTER 7

"undescended testicles . . ." A. L. Herbst, "The Effects in the Human of Diethylstilbestrol (DES) Use During Pregnancy," R. W. Miller et al. (eds.), *Unusual Occurrences as Clues to Cancer Etiology* Japanese Scientific Society Press, pp. 67–75 (1988).

"small penis size . . ." A. M. Niculescu, "Effects of In Utero Exposure to DES on Male Progeny," *Journal of Obstetrics and Gynecologic Neonatal Nursing* 14(6):468–70 (Nov.–Dec. 1985).

"abnormal semen . . ." R. J. Stillman, "In Utero Exposure to Diethylstilbestrol: Adverse Effects on the Reproductive Tract and Reproductive Performance in Male and Female Offspring," *American Journal of Obstetrics and Gynecology* 142(7):905–21 (1982).

"lower sperm counts . . ." R. M. Sharpe and N. E. Skakkebaek, "Are Oestrogens Involved in Falling Sperm Counts and Disorders of the Male Reproductive Tract?" *Lancet* 341(8857):1392–95 (May 29, 1993); MRC Reproductive Biology Unit, "Gestational and Lactational Exposure of Rats to Xenoestrogens Results in Reduced Testicular Size and Sperm Production," *Environmental Health Perspectives* 103(12):1136–43 (1995). The DES-exposed rats had lower sperm production and changes in testicular and prostate size, and exposure to two different kinds of plastics got the same results.

"possibly prostatic disease . . ." C. Y. Yonemura, G. R. Cunha, Y. Sugimura, and S. L. Mee, "Temporal and Spatial Factors in Diethylstilbestrol-Induced Squamous Metaplasia in the Developing Human Prostate: Persistent Changes After Removal of Diethylstilbestrol," *Acta Anatomica*

(Basel) 153(1):1–11 (1995); L. Pylkkanen et al., "Prostatic Dysplasia Associated with Increased Expression of C-myc in Neonatally Estrogenized Mice. *Journal of Urology* 149(6):1593–601 (1993).

"(on the epididymis) . . ." J. A. McLachlan, "Rodent Models for Perinatal Exposure to Diethylstilbestrol and Their Relation to Human Disease in the Male," in A. L. Herbst and H. A. Bern (eds.), *Developmental Effects of Diethylstilbestrol (DES) in Pregnancy*, Thieme-Stratton Inc. (1981).

"major depressive disorder (MDD) . . ." R. D. Pillard, L. R. Rosen, H. Meyer-Bahlburg et al., "Psychopathology and Social Functioning in Men Prenatally Exposed to Diethylstilbestrol (DES)," *Psychosomatic Medicine* 55(6):485–91 (1993).

"90 percent of the alligator population disappeared . . ." T. Colborn, D. Dumanoski, and J. Peterson Myers, *Our Stolen Future*, Dutton (1996).

"males had almost no testosterone . . ." J. Raloff, "The Gender Benders," *Science News* 145:24–27 (1994).

"estrogenic chemicals in the lake . . ." P. M. Vonier, D. A. Crain, J. A. McLachlan, L. J. Guillette, and S. F. Arnold, "Interaction of Environmental Chemicals with the Estrogen and Progesterone Receptors from the Oviduct of the American Alligator," *Environmental Health Perspectives* 104:1318–322 (1996).

"Guillette said . . ." From Guillette's lecture at Keystone Symposium on Endocrine Disruptors (B5) in Tahoe City, CA (Jan. 31–Feb. 5, 1999).

"England's sewage effluent . . ." J. P. Sumpter and S. Joblin, "Vitellogenesis as a Biomarker for Oestrogenic Contamination of the Aquatic Environment," *Environmental Health Perspectives* 103(7):173–78 (1995).

"Treated and untreated waste . . ." Results of federal research at 25 sites around the country, reported at the annual meeting of the Society of Environmental Toxicology and Chemistry (1996).

"injected DDT into male fish . . ." T. Hesman, "DDT Treatment Turns Male Fish into Mothers," *Science News*, 157:87 (Feb. 2000).

"level of TCDD exposure . . ." J. Raloff, "Perinatal Dioxin Feminizes Male Rats," *Science News* 141:359 (1992).

"the 1976 Seveso accident . . ." P. Mocarelli et al., "Change in Sex Ratio with Exposure to Dioxin," *Lancet* 348:409 (1996).

"parent birds bring food that has been sprayed . . . " D. Michael Fry, et al., "Disruption of Brain Development and Reproductive Behavior of Birds," in a lecture at the Environmental Hormones: Past, Present, and Future conference in New Orleans, LA (Oct. 18–20, 1999).

"After a period of time . . ." National Health and Nutritional Examination Survey (NHANES III), 1988–94.

"reproductive health of large populations . . ." B. B. Allan et al., "Declining Sex Ratios in Canada," *Canadian Medical Assocation Journal* 156(1):37–41 (1997).

"number of newborn males had declined significantly . . ." H. Moller, "Change in Male/Female Ratio Among Newborn Infants in Denmark," *Lancet* 348:828–29 (1996).

"unexplained defects in male reproduction . . ." D. Davis et al., *Journal of the American Medical Association* 279(13):1018–23 (1998).

"some sperm were hyperactive . . ." E. Carlsen, A. Giwercman, N. Keiding, and N. E. Skakkebaek, "Evidence for Decreasing Quality of Semen During Past 50 Years," *British Medical Journal* 305:609–14 (1992).

"biomarker of reproductive dysfunction . . ." J. Pajarinen, "Incidence of Disorders of Spermatogenesis in Middle-Aged Finnish Men, 1981-1991: Two Necropsy Series," *British Medical Journal* 314 (1997).

"doubled within eight years . . ." I. M. Thompson et al., "Increased Incidence of Testicular Cancer in Active Duty Members of the Department of Defense," *Urology* 53:806–07 (1999).

"300 percent more testicular cancer . . ." A. Giwercman, E. Carlsen, N. Keiding, and N. E. Skakkebaek, "Evidence for Increasing Incidence of Abnormalities of the Human Testis: A Review," *Environmental Health Perspectives* 101(2):65–71 (1993).

"victims are getting younger . . ." L.H. Klotz, "Why Is the Rate of Testicular Cancer Increasing?" *Canadian Medical Association Journal*, 160(2):213–14 (Jan. 26, 1999).

"Nordic and Baltic countries . . ." J. Toppari et al., "Male Reproductive Health and Environmental Xenoestrogens," *Environmental Health Perspectives* 104(4):741–803 (1996); H. K. Weir, L. D. Marrett, and V. Moravan, "Trends in the Incidence of Testicular Germ Cell Cancer in Ontario by Histologic Subgroup, 1964–1996," *Canadian Medical Associa-*

tion Journal, 160(2):201–05 (1999); R. Bergstrom et al., "Increase in Testicular Cancer Incidence in Six European Countries," *Journal of the National Cancer Institute* 88(11):727–33 (1996).

"Men with decreased sperm count . . ." H. Moller et al. "Risk of Testicular Cancer in Subfertile Men: Case-Control Study." *British Medical Journal* 318(7183):559–62 (1999).

"accumulated body burden of endocrine disruptors." Shanna Swan, "Assessing the Impact of Environmental Hormones on Human Reproduction: Is a New Paradigm Required for Epidemiology?," a lecture at Environmental Hormones: Past, Present, and Future, New Orleans, LA (Oct. 18–20, 1999).

"Undescended testicles . . ." J. Garcia-Rodriquez, "Exposure to Pesticides and Cryptorchidism: Geographical Evidence of a Possible Association," *Environmental Health Perspectives* 104(10):1090–95 1996.

"hypospadias increased . . ." I. S. Weidner et al., "Cryptorchidism and Hypospadias in Sons of Gardeners and Farmers," *Environmental Health Perspectives* 106(12):793–96 (1998).

"severe reproductive problems . . ." W. R. Kelce, "Developmental Effects and Molecular Mechanisms of Environmental Antiandrogens." Keystone Symposium on Endocrine Disruptors (B5) in Tahoe City, CA (Jan. 31–Feb. 5, 1999).

"sperm production are correlated . . ." A. Giwercman, E. Carlsen, N. Keiding, and N. E. Skakkebaek, "Evidence for Increasing Incidence of Abnormalities of the Human Testis: A Review," *Environmental Health Perspectives* 101(2):65–71 (1993).

"suppress other hormones . . ." From interview with W. Welshons (1999).

"long-term exposure to estrogen . . ." "Reproductive Tract Abnormalities," http://www.wwfcanada.org/hormone-disruptors/

"circulating free estradial . . ." F. vom Saal et al., "Prostate Enlargement in Mice Due to Fetal Exposure to Low Doses of Estradiol or Diethylstilbestrol and Opposite Effects at High Doses," *Proceedings of the National Academy of Science USA* 4:94(5)2056–61 (1997).

"research has recently been replicated." C. Gupta, "Reproductive Malformation of the Male Offspring Following Maternal Exposure to Estrogenic Chemicals." Proceedings of Society of Experimental Biology and Medicine in press (2000).

"prostate problems start in the womb . . ." W. Y. Chang et al., "Neonatal Estrogen Stimulates Proliferation of Periductal Fibroblasts and Alters the Extracellular Matrix Composition in the Rat Prostate," *Endocrinology* 140:405–15 (1999).

"Adult bald eagles . . ." "New Toxicological Problems," http://www.wwfcanada.org/hormone-disruptors/

"Should we be upset . . ." From the BBC documentary *Horizon: Assault on the Male*, written and produced by Deborah Cadbury.

"Parisian sperm bank . . ." J. Auger et al., "Decline in Semen Quality Among Fertile Men in Paris During the Past 20 Years," *New England Journal of Medicine* 332(5):281–85 (1995); J. Ginsburg, S. Okolo, G. Prelevia, and P. Hardiman, "Residence in the London Area and Sperm Density," *Lancet* 343(8891):230 (1994).

"U.S. sperm banks refuted . . ." H. Fisch and E. Goluboff, "Geographic Variations in Sperm Counts: A Potential Cause of Bias in Studies of Semen Quality," *Fertility and Sterility* 65(5):1044–46 (1996).

"decline was worldwide . . ." H. Fisch and E. Goluboff et al., "Semen Analyses in 1,283 Men from the United States over a 25-Year Period: No Decline in Quality," *Fertility and Sterility* 65(5):1009–14 (1996).

"fifty-six studies on sperm . . ." S. H. Swan, E. P. Elkin, and L. Fenster, "Have Sperm Densities Declined: A Reanalysis of Global Trend Data," *Environmental Health Perspectives* 105(11):1228–32 (1997).

"led to reduced fertility . . ." H. Fisch and E. Goluboff et al., "Semen Analyses in 1,283 Men from the United States over a 25-Year Period: No Decline in Quality," *Fertility and Sterility* 65(5):1009-14 (1996).

"You only need one . . ." "Sperm Counts Have Declined in the Last 60 Years, Study Says," *The New Mexican* A-1-2 (Nov. 24, 1997).

"drastically lowered sperm count . . ." D. Whorton et al., "Infertility in Male Pesticide Workers," *Lancet* ii:1259–61 (1977); M. D. Whorton et al., "Testicular Function in DBCP-Exposed Pesticide Workers," *Journal of Occupational Medicine* 21:161-66 (1979); M. Whorton, "The Effects of the Occupation on Male Reproductive Function," A. Spira and E.

Jouannet (eds.), *Human Fertility Factors*, INSERM, Paris 103:339–50 (1981).

"higher sperm counts . . ." H. Fisch et al., "Semen Analyses in 1,283 Men from the United States over a 25-Year Period: No Decline in Quality," *Fertility and Sterility* 65(5):1009–14 (1996).

"hostile environment . . ." D. Cadbury, *Feminization of Nature*, Hamish Hamilton, London, (1997).

"low doses of EDCs . . ." S. Swan, lecture at the Keystone Symposium on Endocrine Disruptors in Tahoe City, CA (Jan. 31–Feb. 5, 1999). Studies from P. Foster, R. Sharpe, and F. vom Saal show decreased sperm counts can be deliberately produced by exposure to EDCs at specific times. E. Gray's work showed a 58 percent decrease in sperm count when rats were given dioxin on day 15 and a 24 percent decrease when given dioxin on day 8.

"the insecticide kepone . . ." P. S. Guzelian, "Comparative Toxicology of Chlorodecone (Kepone) in Humans and Experimental Animals," *Annual Review of Pharmacology and Toxicology* 22:89–113 (1982).

"nonexposed control groups . . ." G. M. Egeland et al., "Total Serum Testosterone and Gonadotropins in Workers Exposed to Dioxin," *American Journal of Epidemiology* 139(3):272–81 (1994).

"A study by the Occupational . . ." M. M. Quinn et al., "Investigation of Reports of Sexual Dysfunction Among Male Chemical Workers Manufacturing Stilbene Derivatives," *American Journal of Industrial Medicine* 18(1):55–68 (1990).

CHAPTER 8

"Landi and Bertazzi . . ." M. T. Landi, "2.3.7.8.-Tetrachlorodibenzo-p-Dioxin Plasma Levels in Seveso 20 Years After the Accident," *Environmental Health Perspectives* 106(5):273–77 (1998).

"pharmaceutical drugs . . ." L. Neergaard, "Drugs May Be Prescribed by Sex," Associated Press (May 15, 1999).

"high-school female athlete . . ." R. J. Barnard et al., "The Estrogen-like Effect of Herbicides: A Patient Report," *Clinical Pediatrics* 633 (1998).

"Dr. John Lee . . ." J. R. Lee, *What Your Doctor May Not Tell You About Menopause*, Warner Books, 1996.

"part of large cohorts . . ." the largest cohorts are National Cooperative Diethylstilbestrol Adenosis (DESAD) Project, the original "Dieckmann" cohort, the DES Mother's Study, the Connecticut Mother's Study, the British Research Medical Council (BRMC) Study, the British Randomized Trial, and the Registry for Research on Hormonal Carcinogenisis.

"DES daughters . . ." National Cancer Institute, *DES Daughters* (booklet), 1995.

"oddly sized vagina, cervix . . ." H. Hricak et al., "Cervical Incompetency: Preliminary Evaluation with MR Imaging," *Radiology* 174(3):821–25 (1990). J. M. Emens, "Continuing Problems with Diethylstilboestrol," *British Journal of Obstetrics and Gynaecology* 101:748–50 (1994).

"reduced fertility . . ." M. J. Berger and M. M. Alper, "Intractable Primary Infertility in Women Exposed to Diethylstilbestrol In Utero," *The Journal of Reproductive Medicine* 31(4):231–35 (1986); Krumholz, et al., "Problems of a DES-Exposed Woman in her Child-Bearing Years," *Journal of Clinical Outcomes Management* (Obstetrics and Gynecology Edition) (Nov 1995).

"problems with pregnancy . . ." H. Barber, "An Update on DES in the Field of Reproduction.," *International Journal on Fertility* 31:130–34 (1986); A. L. Herbst, E. K. Senekjian, and K. W. Frey, "Abortion and Pregnancy Loss Among Diethylstilbestrol-Exposed Women," *Seminars in Reproductive Endocrinology* 7(2):124–29 (1989); A. L. Herbst, H. Ulfelder, and D. C. Poskanzer, "Adenocarcinoma of the Vagina," *New England Journal of Medicine* 284(16):878–81 (1971).

"vaginal or cervical cancer . . ." J. Boyd et al., "Molecular Genetic Analysis of Clear Cell Adenocarcinomas of the Vagina and Cervix Associated and Unassociated with Diethylstilbestrol Exposure In Utero," *Cancer* 77(3):507–13 (1996).

"menstrual irregularities . . ." D. Schechter et al., "Menstrual Cycle Functioning in Women with a History of Prenatal Diethylstilbestrol Exposure," *Journal of Obstetrics and Gynecology* 12:51–66 (1991).

"adenosis . . . of the vagina . . ." P. C. O'Brian et al., "Vaginal Epithelial Changes in Young Women Enrolled in the National Cooperative Diethylstilbestrol Adenosis (DESAD) Project," *Journal of Obstetrics and Gynecology* 53(3):300–07 (1979).

"adversely affects the immune system . . ." K. N. Moller et al., "Increased Occurrence of Autoimmune Disease Among Women Exposed In Utero to Diethylstilbestrol," *Fertility and Sterility* 49(6):1080–82 (1988); S. D. Holladay, B. L. Blaylock et al., "Selective Prothymocyte Targeting by Prenatal Diethylstilbestrol Exposure," *Cellular Immunology* 152(1): 131–42 (1993); S. C. Ways, J. F. Mortola et al., "Alterations in Immune Responsiveness in Women Exposed to Diethylstilbestrol In Utero," *Fertility and Sterility* 48(2):193–97 (1987); D. L. Wingard and J. Turiel, "Long-Term Effects of Exposure to Diethylstilbestrol," *Western Journal of Medicine* 149:551–54 (1988).

"some data do not support . . ." D. D. Baird, A. J. Wilcox, and A. L. Herbst, "Self-Reported Allergy, Infection, and Autoimmune Diseases Among Men and Women Exposed In Utero to Diethylstilbestrol," *Journal of Clinical Epidemiology* 49(2):263–66 (1996).

"greater risk for anorexia . . ." Gustavson et al., "Increased Risk of Profound Weight Loss Among Women Exposed to Des In Utero," *Behavioral and Neural Biology* 55 (1991).

"predisposed them toward depression . . ." H. F. L. Meyer-Bahlburg and A. A. Ehrhardt, "A Prenatal-Hormone Hypothesis for Depression in Adults with a History of Fetal Des Exposure," *Hormones and Depression*, Raven Press, 1987.

"identity confusion, and guilt . . ." E. J. Saunders, "Physical and Psychological Problems Associated with Exposure to Diethylstilbestrol (des)," *Hospital and Community Psychiatry* 39(1):73–77 (1988).

"exhibit more masculine behavior . . ." H. F. L. Meyer-Bahlburg et al., "Perinatal Factors in the Development of Gender-Related Play Behavior: Sex Hormones Versus Pregnancy Complications," *Psychiatry* 51:260–71 (1988). A study that contradicts this is J. D. Lish et al., "Prenatal Exposure to Diethylstilbestrol (des): Childhood Play Behavior and Adult Gender-Role Behavior in Women," *Archives of Sexual Behavior* 21(5):423–40 (1992); J. D. Lish et al., "Gender-Related Behavior Development in Females Exposed to Diethylstilbestrol (des) In Utero: An Attempted Replication," *Journal of the American Academy of Child and Adolescent Psychiarty* 30(1):29–37(1991).

"sex-partner relationships . . ." H. F. L. Meyer-Bahlburg et al., "Sexual Activity Level and Sexual Functioning in Women Prenatally Exposed to Diethylstilbestrol," *Psychosomatic Medicine* 47(6):497–511 (1985); D. A. Smith and B. E. Walker, "Evidence of Hypothalamic Involvement in the Mechanism of Transplacental Carcinogenesis by Diethylstilbestrol," *Cancer Letters* 67(1):55–59 (1992).

"orientation to parenting . . ." A. E. Ehrhardt, H. F. L. Meyer-Behlburg et al., "The Development of Gender-Related Behavior in Females Following Prenatal Exposure to Diethylstilbestrol (DES)," *Hormones and Behavior* 23:526–41 (1989).

"bisexuality and homosexuality . . ." A. E. Ehrhardt, H. F. L. Meyer-Bahlburg et al., "Sexual Orientation after Prenatal Exposure to Exogenous Estrogen," *Archives of Sexual Behavior* 14(1) (1985); H. F. L. Meyer-Bahlburg, A. Ehrhardt et al., "Prenatal Estrogens and the Development of Homosexual Orientation," *Developmental Psychology* 31(1):12–21 (1995). "Daughters of Moms Who Took DES Also Show Bisexuality," *Newsday* (Feb. 6, 1995).

"indirectly elevate estrogen . . ." J. Menczer, M. Dulitzky, G. Ben-Baruch, and M. Modan, "Primary Infertility in Women Exposed to Diethylstilbestrol In Utero," *British Journal of Obstetrics and Gynaecology* 93:503–07 (1986); J. Assies, "Hyperprolactinaemia in Diethylstilbestrol-Exposed Women," *Lancet* 337:983 (1991); J. R. Cunningham, G. P. Gidwani, M. S. Gupta et al., "Prolactin-Secreting Pituitary Adenoma: Occurrence Following Prenatal Exposure to Diethylstilbestrol," *Cleveland Clinic Quarterly* 49:249–54 (1982); D. L. Wingard and J. Turiel, "Long-Term Effects of Exposure to Diethylstilbestrol," *Western Journal of Medicine* 149:551–54 (1988).

"cancers later in life . . ." Boyd et al., "Molecular Genetic Analysis of DES," *Cancer* 77:507–13 (1996); S. Li et al., "Developmental Exposure to Diethylstilbestrol Elicits Demethylation of Estrogen-Responsive Lactogerrin Gene in Mouse Uterus," *Cancer Research* 57:4356–59 (1997).

"more prone to breast . . ." E. S. Boylan and R. E. Calhoon, "Transplacental Action of Diethylstilbestrol on Mammary Carcinogenesis in Female Rats Given One or Two Doses of 7, 12-dimethylbenz(a)anthracene," *Cancer Research* 43:4879–84 (1983). If DES was given in the second trimester of pregnancy, it produced tumors earlier. The authors suggest

DES may affect breast and other estrogen-sensitive tissue in DES daughters.

"ovarian cancers later . . ." M. A. Seoud, O. Tawfik, and V. Hunter, "Peritoneal Papillary Serous Carcinoma in a Woman with a History of Utero DES Exposure," *Gynecologic Oncology* 50(3):371–73 (1993); B. E. Walker and L. A. Kurth, "Multigenerational Carcinogenesis from Diethylstilbestrol Investigated by Blastocyst Transfers in Mice," *International Journal of Cancer* 61:249–52 (1995); B. E. Walker, "Tumors of Female Offspring of Mice Exposed Prenatally to Diethylstilbestrol," *Journal of National Cancer Institute* 73:133–40 (1984).

"development of gynecologic cancers . . ." M. A. Seoud, O. Tawfik, and V. Hunter, "Peritoneal Papillary Serous Carcinoma in a Woman with a History of Utero DES Exposure." *Gynecologic Oncology* 50(3): 371–3 (1993).

"German researchers . . ." I. Gerhard and B. Runnebaum, "The Limits of Hormone Substitution in Pollutant Exposure [in German]," *Zentralbl Gynakol* 114(12):593–602 (1992).

"Health Effects in Women . . ." K. Morgan, Center for Bioenvironmental Research at Tulane and Xavier Universities, 1997.

"under the age of twenty-five . . ." A. Chandra and E. H. Stephen, "Impaired Fecundity in the United States (1982–1995)," *Family Planning Perspectives* 30: 34–42 (1998).

"smoking makes the pollutants . . ." April 14 issue of Miljoaktuellt. http://www.omi.tulane.edu/ecme/eehdme/newsviews/whatsnew/junnews.html (June 2,1999).

"pregnant while on the birth-control pill . . ." K. A. Thayer, S. Benson, and F. S. vom Saal, "Prenatal Exposure to Clinically Relevant Levels of Ethinyl Estradiol Increases Prostate Weight in Adult Male Mice," *Poster Session Abstracts* at Estrogens in the Environment IV: Linking Fundamental Knowledge, Risk Assessment, and Public Policy, 32 (July 21, 1997).

"receptors in the fetus . . ." D. A. Crain et al., "Cellular Bioavailability of Natural Hormones and Environmental Contaminants as a Function of Serum and Cytosolic Binding Factors," *Toxicology and Industrial Health* 14(1/2):261–73 (1998).

"drinking estrogen metabolites . . ." J. Raloff, "Drugged Waters: Does It Matter That Pharmaceuticals Are Turning Up in Water Supplies?" *Science News* 153:187–89 (1998).

"exposed fetuses . . ." A. B. Barnes, "Maternal Progestins as a Possible Cause of Hypospadias," *New England Journal of Medicine*, 300(2):75–78 (1979); J. Schardein, *Chemically Induced Birth Defects*, 2nd. ed., Marcel Dekker, 1993.

"give a warning . . ." E. Bumiller, "Reality Shapes an Editor's Fashionable Life," *New York Times* Metro B-2 (March 31, 1998).

"About half of these women . . ." H. W. Jones et al., "Current Concepts: The Infertile Couple," *New England Journal of Medicine* 329: 1710–15 (1993).

"smaller than normal . . ." D. A. Barsotti, R. J. Marlar, and J. R. Allen, "Reproductive Dysfunction in Rhesus Monkeys Exposed to Low Levels of PolychlorinatedBiphenyls (Aroclor 1248)," *Cosmetologica Toxicology* 14: 99–103 (1976).

"The Women's Environmental and Development Organization . . ." WEDO Press Releases: "Risks, Rights and Reforms: A 5-Country Survey Assessing Government Actions Five Years After the International Conference on Population and Development." Presented at the UN during 32nd Commission on Population and Development (1999).

"Fertility was significantly decreased . . ." A. P. Beard, P. M. Bartlewski, and N. C. Rawlings, "Endocrine and Reproductive Function in Ewes Exposed to the Organochlorine Pesticides Lindane or Pentachlorophenol," *Journal of Toxicology and Environmental Health* 56(1):23–46 (1999).

"an article from *Cancer Research* . . ." J. A. Gustafsson, "Properties, Distribution, and Function of ER-beta." Speech at the Keystone Symposium on Endocrine Disruptors (B5) in Tahoe City, CA (Jan. 31–Feb. 5, 1997).

"researchers in Italy . . ." D. Taruscio et al., "Human Endogenous Retroviruses and Environmental Endocrine Disruptors: A Connection Worth Exploring: Letter to the Editor," *Teratology* 58:27–29 (1998).

"6 million women in this country . . ." J. M. Wheeler, "Epidemiology and Prevalence of Endometriosis," *Infertility and Reproductive Medical Clinics of North America* 3:545–49 (1992).

"It's 11 P.M.: Do You . . ." P. Montague, "How We Got Here—Part I: The History of Chlorinated Diphenyl (Pcbs)," *Rachel's Hazardous Waste News* 327:1 (1993).

"Dr. Mayani . . ." A. Mayani, S. Barel, S. Soback, and M. Almagor, "Dioxin Concentrations in Women with Endometriosis," *Human Reproduction* 12(2):373–75 (1997).

"Pcbs in the blood . . ." I. Gerhard, "Grenzen der Hormonsubstitution bei Schadstoffbelastung und Fertilitatsstorungen," *Zentralblatt fur Bynakologie*, 114:593–602 (1992).

"Endometriosis appears . . ." P. R. Koninck et al., "Dioxin Pollution and Endometriosis in Belgium," *Human Reproduction* 9(6):1001–02 (1994).

"Osteen and associates . . ." K. G. Osteen et al., "Does Disruption of Immune and Endocrine Systems by Environmental Toxins Contribute to Development of Endometriosis?" Seminars in Reprodroduction and Endocrinology 15(3):301–08 (1997).

"Sherry Rier . . ." S. E. Rier et al., "Immunoresponsiveness in Endometriosis: Implication of Estrogenic Toxicants," *Environmental Health Perspectives* 103 (1995); S. E. Rier et al., "Endometriosis in Rhesus Monkey (Macaca mulatta) Following Chronic Exposure to 2.3.7.8-Tetrachlorodibenzo-p-Dioxin," *Fundamental Applications in Toxicology* 21(4):433–41 (1993).

"Cummings and research team . . ." A. M. Cummings, J. L. Metcalf, and L. Birnbaum, "Promotion of Endometriosis by 2,3,7,8-Tetrachlorodibenzo-p-Dioxin in Rats and Mice: Time-Dose Dependence and Species Comparison," *Toxicology and Applied Pharmacology* 138:131–39 (1996).

"Exposure to dioxin . . ." M. S. Riccci et al., "Estrogen Receptor Reduces spyiAi Induction in Cultured Human Endometrial Cells," *Journal of Biological Chemistry* 272(6):3430–438 (1999).

"Lebel and team . . ." G. Lebel et al., "Organochlorine Exposure and the Risk of Endometriosis," *Fertility and Sterility* 69(2):221–28 (1998).

"Human and animal studies . . ." A. Mayani, S. Barel, S. Soback, and M. Almagor, "Dioxin Concentrations in Women with Endometriosis," *Human Reproduction* 12(2):373–75 (1997); S. E. Rier, D. C. Martin, R. E. Bowman, and J. L. Becker, "Immunoresponsiveness in Endometriosis:

Implications of Estrogenic Toxicants," *Environmental Health Perspectives* 103(7):151–56 (1995).

"the 1994 EPA Dioxin Reassessment . . . " External Review Draft and Dioxin Reassessment, 6 volumes released by the U.S. EPA office of Research and Development EPA/600/BP-92/001 (June, 1994).

"protective effects of progesterone . . ." K. G. Osteen et al., "Dioxin (TCDD) Can Block the Protective Effect of Progesterone in Nude Mouse Model of Experimental Endometriosis," American Society for Reproductive Medicine Annual Meeting (1996).

"considered autoimmune diseases . . ." M. L. Ballweg, "Immunotherapy for Endometriosis: The Science Behind a Promising New Treatment," *Endometrium and Endometriosis*, Blackwell Science, Inc. (1997).

"interaction between dioxin . . . " M. S. Ricci, et al., "Human Endometrial Cells as a Model System to Study Dioxin Disruption of Steroid Hormone Function," *In Vitro Cellular and Developmental Biology–Animal* 35:183–89 (1999).

"pre- and postmenopausal women . . ." V. S. Buttram et al., "Uterine Leiomyomata: Etiology, Symptomatology, and Management," *Fertility and Sterility* 36:433–35 (1981).

"animals that spontaneously make fibroids . . ." C. Walker et al., "Leiomyomas: Endocrine Interactions and Potential Sites of Disruption," talk and presentation at Keystone Symposium on Endocrine Disruptors (B5) at Tahoe City, CA (Jan. 31–Feb. 5, 1999).

"Summary of National Health . . . (table)" K. Morgan, Center for Bioenvironmental Research, Tulane and Xavier Universities, July 17, 1997.

"increased fibroid growth . . ." L. C. Hodges et al., "Organochlorine Pesticides Alter Endocrine Signaling in Uterine Leiomyoma-Derived Cells," presented at Keystone Symposium on Endocrine Disruptors (B5) at Tahoe City, CA (Jan. 31–Feb. 5, 1999).

"Kelly Morgan . . ." K. Morgan, "Fibroids Incidence, Race, and the Environment," Center for Bioenvironmental Research at Tulane and Xavier Universities (1997).

"observations made by the researchers . . ." S. P. Saxena et al., "DDT and Its Metabolites in Leiomyomatous and Normal Human Uterine Tissue," *Archives of Toxicology* 59:453–55 (1987).

"9.2 out of every 1,000 women . . ." F. Parazzini, "Reproductive Factors and Risk of Uterine Fibroids," *Epidemiology* 7(4):440–42 (1996).

"Risk factors for fibroids . . ." F. Parazzini et al., "Epidemiologic Characteristics of Women with Uterine Fibroids: A Case-Control Study," *Obstetrics and Gynecology* 72:853–57 (1988).

"unopposed estrogen . . ." R. K. Ross et al., "Risk Factors for Uterine Fibroids; Reduced Risk Associated with Oral Contraceptives," *British Medical Journal* 293(6543):359–62 (1986).

"younger age at menarche . . ." L. Marshall et al., Nurses Health Study II Research Group, "Reproductive History and Risk of Clinically Confirmed Uterine Leiomyomata in Premenopausal Women," *American Journal of Epidemiology* 143(11):S5 (1996).

"estrogenic compounds in the environment . . ." P. A. Gunjjar, M. Finucane, and B. Larsen, "The Effect of Estradiol on *Candida albicans* Growth," *Annals of Clinical and Laboratory Science* 27(2):151–56 (1997).

CHAPTER 9

"breast cancer risk . . ." A. H. Wu, C. Pike, and D. O. Stram, "Meta-analysis: Dietary Fat Intake, Serum Estrogen Levels, and the Risk of Breast Cancer," *Journal of the National Cancer Institute* 91:529–34 (1999).

"which estrogens to test . . ." G. A. Colditz, "Relationship Between Estrogen Levels, Use of Hormone Replacement Therapy, and Breast Cancer," *Journal of the National Cancer Institute* 90 (11):814–23 (1998).

"between environmental estrogens . . ." Presented at the 88th Annual Meeting of the American Association for Cancer Research, Highlights from the AACR Conference, *Oncology* 11(9):1383 (1997).

"46,000 U.S. women . . ." F. M. Visco, Letter from the National Breast Cancer Coalition, 1707 L St. NW, Ste. 1060, Washington, DC 20036.

"prenatal DES exposure . . ." T. C. Rothschild, E. S. Boylan et al., "Transplacental Effects of Diethylstilbestrol on Mammary Development Tumorigenesis in Female ACI Rats," *Cancer Research* 47:4508–516 (1987); B. E. Walker and L. A. Kurth, "Pituitary Tumors in Mice Exposed Prenatally to Diethylstilbestrol," *Cancer Research* 53(7):1546–49 (1993); H. Bern and F. Talamantes, "Neonatal Mouse Models and Their

Relation to Disease in the Human Female," in A. L. Herbst and H. A. Bern (eds.), *Developmental Effects of Diethylstilbestrol (DES) in Pregnancy*, Thieme-Stratton Inc., pp. 129–47 (1981); D. Vassilacopoulou and E. S. Boylan, "Mammary Gland Morphology and Responsiveness to Regulatory Molecules Following Prenatal Exposure to Diethylstilbestrol," *Teratogenesis, Carcinogenesis, and Mutagenesis* 13(2):59–74 (1993).

"chemical carcinogens . . ." H. A. Bern and F. J. Talamantes, "Neonatal Mouse Models and Their Relation to Disease in the Human Female," in: A. L. Herbst and H. A. Bern (eds.), *Developmental Effects of Diethylstilbestrol (DES) in Pregnancy*, Thieme-Stratton Inc., pp. 129–47 (1981).

"secondary exposures . . ." M. Rustia and P. Shubik, "Effects of Transplacental Exposure to Diethylstilbestrol on Carcinogenic Susceptibility During Postnatal Life in Hamster Progeny," *Cancer Research* 39(11):4636–44 (1979); W. C. Beckman, R. R. Newbold, C. T. Teng, and J. A. McLachlan, "Molecular Feminization of Mouse Seminal Vesicle by Prenatal Exposure to Diethylstilbestrol: Altered Expression of Messenger RNA," *Journal of Urology* 151(5):1370–78 (1994).

"Below seventy-six, however . . ." S. Love, "What We Really Know About Breast Cancer and HRT," interview by B. Horrigan, *Alternative Therapies* 3(5):82–90 (1997).

"increase in DCIS . . ." P. A. Wingo, L. A. G. Ries, H. M. Rosenberg, D. S. Miller, and B. K. Edwards, "Cancer Incidence and Mortality, 1973-1995: A Report Card for the U.S.," *Cancer* 82(6):1197–207 (March 15, 1998).

"inherited genetic defects . . ." J. P. Struewing et al., "The Risk of Cancer Associated with Specific Mutations of BRCA1 and BRCA2 Among Ashkenazi Jews," *New England Journal of Medicine* 336(20):1401–420 (1997).

"Dr. Generosa Grana . . ." NIH, NIEHS Conference: Estrogens in the Environment IV: Linking Fundamental Knowledge, Risk Assessment, and Public Policy (July 1997).

"role in initiating cancer . . ." T. Tsutsui and J. C. Barrett, "Neoplastic Transformation of Cultured Mammalian Cells by Estrogens and Estrogen-like Chemicals," *Environmental Health Perspectives* 105(3):619–24 (1997).

"environmental pollutants acting like . . ." J. D. Yager and J. G. Liehr, "Molecular Mechanisms of Estrogen Carcinogenesis," *Annual Review of Pharmacology and Toxicology* 36:203–32 (1996); B. J. Danzo, "Environ-

mental Xenobiotics May Disrupt Normal Endocrine Function by Interfering with the Binding of Physiological Ligands of Steroid Receptors
and Binding Proteins," *Environmental Health Perspectives* 105:294–301
(1997); P. V. M. Shakhar, J. Werdell, and V. S. Basrur, "Environmental
Estrogen Stimulation of Growth and Estrogen Receptor Function in
Preneoplastic and Cancerous Human Breast Cell Lines," *Journal of the
National Cancer Institute* 89:1774–782 (1997); M. A. Kettles et al., "Triazine Herbicide Exposure and Breast Cancer Incidence: An Ecologic
Study of Kentucky Counties," *Environmental Health Perspectives*
105:1222–27 (1997). Article gives 23 citations that support this link.

"minor genetic abnormalities . . ." B. S. Hulka, E. T. Liu, and R. A.
Lininger, "Steroid Hormones and Risk of Breast Cancer," *Cancer*
74(3):1111–24 (1994).

"more amenable to prevention . . ." D. L. Davis, H. L. Bradlow, M. Wolff
et al., "Medical Hypothesis: Xenoestrogens as Preventable Causes of
Breast Cancer," *Environmental Health Perspectives* 101:372–77 (1993).

"estrogen can make cancer cells grow . . ." J. Dorgan et al., "Serum Sex
Hormone Levels Are Related to Breast Cancer Risk in Postmenopausal
Women, *Environmental Health Perspectives* 105(3):583–85 (1997).

"More estrogen means the cells . . ." H. Adlercreutz, S. L. Gorbach, B. R.
Goldin, M. N. Woods, J. T. Dwyer, and E. Hamalainen, "Estrogen
Metabolism and Excretion in Oriental and Caucasian Women," *Journal
of the National Cancer Institute* 86:1076–82 (1994).

"increases the risk of breast cancer . . ." S. Preston-Martin et al., "Increased
Cell Division as a Cause of Human Cancer," *Cancer Research* 50:7415–21
(1990); M. C. Pike, D. V. Spicer, L. Dahmoush, and M. F. Press,
"Estrogens, Progestogens, Normal Breast Cell Proliferation, and Breast
Cancer Risk," *Epidemiologic Review* 15:17–35 (1993).

"promoter of breast cancer . . ." G. A. Colditz, "Relationship Between
Estrogen Levels, Use of Hormone Replacement Therapy, and Breast
Cancer," *Journal of the National Cancer Institute* 90:814–23 (1998).

"compared to lean women . . ." S. E. N. Hankinson et al., "Alcohol, Height,
and Adiposity in Relation to Estrogen and Prolactin Levels in Postmenopausal Women," *Journal of the National Cancer Institute*
87:1297–302 (1995); S. Tretli, "Height and Weight in Relation to Breast

Cancer Morbidity and Mortality: A Prospective Study of 570,000 Women in Norway," *International Journal of Cancer* 44:23–30 (1989).

"larger mammary glands . . ." J. Russo et al., "Biology of Disease: Comparative Study of Human and Rat Mammary Tumorigenesis," *Laboratory Investigation* 62:244–78 (1990); L. Hilakivi-Clarke, E. Cho, M. Raygada, and R. Clarke, "How Early Estrogenic Activity Affects Mammary Gland Development to Increase Breast Cancer Risk," from the proceedings of the 86th annual meeting of the American Association for Cancer Research 36:261 (1995).

"DNA to repair any errors . . ." This is why experiments in which cancer-causing substances were given to young virgin rats showed greater breast cancer tumor development than exposing rats who had been pregnant to the same carcinogens. (Dr. Irma Russo Fox, Chase Cancer Center in Philadelphia).

"immature breast cells . . ." D. Trichopoulos, "Hypothesis: Does Breast Cancer Originate in Utero?" *Lancet* 335:939–40 (1990); A. Ekbom and D. Trichopoulos et al., "Evidence of Prenatal Influences on Breast Cancer Risk," *Lancet* 340:1015–18 (1992); K. B. Michels, D. Trichopoulos et al., "Birth Weight as a Risk Factor for Breast Cancer," *Lancet* 348:1542–546 (1996).

"estrogen imprinting . . ." J. A. McLachlan et al., "Environmental Estrogens: Orphan Receptors and Genetic Imprinting," *Advances in Modern Environmental Toxicology* 21:107–13.

"Other research, in 1998 . . ." N. M. Brown et al., "Prenatal TCDD and Predisposition to Mammary Cancer in the Rat," *Carcinogenesis* 19(9):1623–9 (1998).

"exposure to excess estrogen . . ." Devra L. Davis from the World Resources Institute and Susan M. Sieber from the National Cancer Institute, two internationally respected scientists in the field of cancer, say that "for more than 200 years, scientists have appreciated that breast cancer cannot arise without hormonal influences."

"Asian women . . ." A. H. Wu, M. C. Pike, D. O. Stram, "Meta-Analysis: Dietary Fat Intake, Serum Estrogen Levels, and the Risk of Breast Cancer," *Journal of the National Cancer Institute* 91(6):529–34 (1999).

"concentration of estrogen . . ." L. Bernstein and R. K. Ross, "Endogenous Hormones and Breast Cancer Risk, *Epidemiologic Reviews* 15:48–65

(1993); S. E. Hankinson et al., "Plasma Sex Steroid Hormone Levels and Risk of Breast Cancer in Postmenopausal Women," *Journal of the National Cancer Institute* 90:1292–99 (1998); H. V. Thomas, G. K. Reeves, and T. J. Key, "Endogenous Estrogen and Postmenopausal Breast Cancer: A Quantitative Review," *Cancer Causes and Control* 8:922–28 (1997).

"Nurse's Study . . ." S. E. Hankinson et al., "Plasma Sex Steroid Hormone Levels and Risk of Breast Cancer in Postmenopausal Women," *Journal of the National Cancer Institute* 90:1292–99 (1998).

"estradiol levels in postmenopausal women . . ." P. G. Toniolo et al., "A Prospective Study of Endogenous Estrogens and Breast Cancer in Postmenopausal Women," *Journal of the National Cancer Institute* 87:190–97 (1995).

"61 women in Guernsey . . ." J. Cauley et al., "Is Bone Mineral Density a Biological Marker of a Woman's Cumulative Exposure to Estrogen?" Presented at a meeting of the American Epidemiological Society, Rochester, MN (March 13–14, 1997); H. V. Thomas et al., "A Prospective Study of Endogenous Serum Hormone Concentrations and Breast Cancer Risk in Postmenopausal Women on the Island of Guernsey," *British Journal of Cancer* 76:401–05 (1977).

"Research suggests . . ." E. Dewailly et al., "Could the Rising Levels of Estrogen Receptors in Breast Cancer Be Due to Estrogenic Pollutants?" *Journal of the National Cancer Institute* 89(12):888–89 (1997).

"a large-scale human study . . ." P. Pujol, S. G. Hilsenbeck, G. C. Chamness, and R. M. Elledge, "Rising Levels of Oestrogen Receptor in Breast Cancer over Two Decades," *Cancer* 74:1601–06 (1994).

"women with fraternal twins . . ." N. Seppa, "Even Fraternal Twins May Share Cancer Risk," *Science News* 152:389 (1997).

"surgically removing women's ovaries . . ." B. S. Hulka et al., "Steroid Hormones and Risk of Breast Cancer," *Cancer* 74(3):1111–24 (1994).

"Later menopause . . ." B. Rosner and G. A. Colditz, "Nurses' Health Study: Log-Incidence Mathematical Model of Breast Cancer Incidence," *Journal of the National Cancer Institute* 46:796–800 (1990); M. C. Pike et al., "Hormonal Risk Factors, Breast Tissue Age and the Age-Incidence of Breast Cancer," *Nature* 303:767–70 (1983).

"Having one child . . ." B. Rosner, G. A. Colditz, and W. C. Willett, "Reproductive Risk Factors in a Prospective Study of Breast Cancer: The Nurses' Health Study," *American Journal of Epidemiology* 139: 819–35 (1994).

"two to five alcoholic beverages a day . . ." S. A. Smith-Warner et al., "Alcohol and Breast Cancer in Women," *Journal of the American Medical Association* 279(7):535–40 (1998).

"10 years of HRT . . ." I. Persson, E. Thurfjell, L. Holmberg, "Effect of Estrogen and Estrogen-Progestin Replacement Regimens on Mammographic Breast Parenchymal Density," *Journal of Clinical Oncology* 15: 3201–07 (1997); R. C. Marugg et al., "Mammographic Changes in Postmenopausal Women on Hormonal Replacement Therapy," *European Radiology* 7:49–55 (1997).

"Fat consumption . . ." A. H. Wu, M. C. Pike, and D. O. Stram, "Meta-Analysis: Dietary Fat Intake, Serum Estrogen Levels, and the Risk of Breast Cancer," *Journal of the National Cancer Institute* 91:529–34 (1999).

"Framingham Study . . ." Y. Zhang, D. P. Kiel, B. E. Kreger, L. A. Cupples et al., "Bone Mass and the Risk of Breast Cancer Among Postmenopausal Women," *New England Journal of Medicine* 336:611–17 (1997).

"Denser breast on mammograms . . ." N. F. Boyd et al., "Quantitative Classification of Mammographic Densities and Breast Cancer Risk: Results from the Canadian National Breast Screen Trial," *Journal of the National Cancer Institute* 87:670–75 (1995).

"other xenobiotics . . ." S. S. Epstein, "Environmental and Occupational Pollutants Are Avoidable Causes of Breast Cancer," *International Journal of Health Services* 24(1):145–50 (1994).

"genesis of breast cancer . . ." S. Ahamed et al., "Environmental Estrogens Can Activate the Cell Cycle in Breast Cancer Cells," *Poster Session Abstracts* from Estrogens in the Environment IV: Linking Fundamental Knowledge, Risk Assessment, and Public Policy 53 (1997).

"hormone disruptors could increase . . ." D. Christensen, "Breast Cancer and Environmental Estrogens," *New York Times*, July 23, 1997.

"cell and animal studies . . ." J. F. Gierthy et al., "Use of Estrogen-Induced Postconfluent Cell Proliferation and Focus Development in Human MCF-7 Breast Cells as an Assay to Detect and Characterize Xenoestrogens," *Poster Session Abstracts* from Estrogens in the Environment IV: Linking Fundamental Knowledge, Risk Assessment, and Public Policy, 4 (July 21, 1997); W. V. Welshons et al., "Estrogen Receptor Occupancy and Response to Estradiol and Xenoestrogens in MCF-7 Cells," *Poster Session Abstracts* from Estrogens in the Environment IV: Linking Fundamental Knowledge, Risk Assessment, and Public Policy, 12 (July 21, 1997); L. Ren et al., "Effects of Estradiol and Nonylphenol on MUC1 Gene Expression in Normal and Breast Cancer Cells," *Poster Session Abstracts* from Estrogens in the Environment IV: Linking Fundamental Knowledge, Risk Assessment, and Public Policy, 50 (July 21, 1997).

"food packaging materials . . ." S. Jobling, T. Reynolds, R. White, M. G. Parker, and J. P. Sumpter, "A Variety of Environmentally Persistent Chemicals, Including Some Phthalate Plasticizers, Are Weakly Estrogenic," *Environmental Health Perspectives* 103:582–86 (1995).

"bisphenol A is FDA approved . . ." J. Raloff, "Additional Source of Dietary 'Estrogens'," *Science News* 147:341 (1995).

"cause cells to grow . . ." N. Olea et al., "Estrogenicity of Resin-Based Composites and Sealants Used in Dentistry," *Environmental Health Perspectives* 104:298–305 (1996).

"similar to estradiol . . ." C. Dees et al., "Estrogenic and DNA-Damaging Activity of Red No. 3 in Human Breast Cancer Cells," *Environmental Health Perspectives* 105 (3):625–32 (1997); J. S. Foster and J. Wimalasena, "Estrogen and Antiestrogen Regulate Cycling Dependent Kinase 2 (Cdk2) Activity and Retinoblastoma Protein Phosphorylation in MCF-7 Breast Cancer Cells," *Molecular Endocrinology* 10:488–98 (1996).

"one prospective study . . ." J. Greenstein et al., "Risk of Breast Cancer Associated with Intake of Specific Foods and Food Groups," *American Journal of Epidemiology* 141(11) (1996).

"estrogens may program genes . . ." K. Zhu and S. M. Williams, "Methyl-Deficient Diets, Methylated ER Genes and Breast Cancer: An Hypothesized Association," *Cancer Causes and Control* 9:615–20 (1998); S. Li et al., "Developmental Exposure to Diethylstilbestrol Elicits Demethylation of Estrogen-Responsive Lactoferrin Gene in Mouse Uterus," *Cancer Research* 57:4356–59 (1997).

"mammary cancer in adulthood." N. M. Brown, et al, "Prenatal TCDD and Predisposition to Mammary Cancer in the Rat," *Carinogenesis* 19(9):1623–29 (Sept., 1999).

"progesterone resistance . . ." H. W. Simpson, C. S. McArdle, K. Griffiths, A. Turkes, and G. H. Beastall, "Progesterone Resistance in Women Who Have Had Breast Cancer," *British Journal of Obstetrics and Gynaecology* 105:345–51 (1998).

"estrogen metabolites . . ." D. L. David, H. L. Bradlow, M. Wolff et al., "Medical Hypothesis: Xenoestrogens as Preventable Causes of Breast Cancer," *Environmental Health Perspectives* 101:372–77 (1993).

"damage DNA in laboratory tests . . ." With the use of food colorants increasing at a rate of 4 to 5 percent each year since the time of the original survey in 1991, this number is rising rapidly. C. Dees and C. M. Ardies, "Xenoestrogens Significantly Enhance Risk for Breast Cancer During Growth and Adolescence," submitted to *Medical Hypothoses* at time of interview (1999).

"developing breast tissue . . ." C. Dees et al., "Estrogenic and DNA-Damaging Activity of Red No. 3 in Human Breast Cancer Cells," *Environmental Health Perspectives* 105(3):625–32 (1997). The reported intake from young childhood through puberty was actually higher than for the total population.

"scene of the crime . . ." C. Dees, et al. "Are You at Risk?" *The World and I* 156–63 (1996).

"extensive review of women . . ." M. A. Kettles et al., "Triazine Herbicide Exposure and Breast Cancer Incidence: An Ecologic Study of Kentucky Counties," *Environmental Health Perspectives* 105:1222–27 (1997).

"lamppost science . . ." Knight-Ridder Tribune, "Study Finds Breast Cancer Not Linked to DDT," *The New Mexican* A–3 (Oct. 30, 1997).

"Dr. Nancy Krieger . . ." N. Krieger et al., "Breast Cancer and Serum Organochlorines: A Prospective Study Among White, Black and Asian Women," *Journal of the National Cancer Institute* 86(8):589–99 (1994).

"concentrate estrogenic compounds . . ." D. T. Zava and G. Duwe, "Estrogenic and Antiproliferative Properties of Genistein and Other Flavonoids in Human Breast Cancer Cells in Vitro," *Nutrition and Cancer* 27(1):31–40 (1997).

"genetic predisposition . . ." From a personal conversation with Dr. Utian, cochair for the NIH agenda for women's health conferences.

"genetically susceptible . . ." J. Boyd, "Molecular Genetic Analysis of Clear Cell Adenocarcinomas of the Vagina and Cervix Associated and Unassociated with Diethylstilbestrol Exposure in Utero," *Cancer* 77:507–13 (1996).

"metabolized from less to more active . . ." J. A. McLachlan, R. R. Newbold, K. S. Korach, and M. D. Hogan, "Risk Assessment Considerations for the Reproductive and Developmental Toxicity of Oestrogenic Xenobiotics," NIEHS, 187–93.

"fat might be altering . . ." B. E. Walker, "Tumors in Female Offspring of Control and Diethylstilbestrol-Exposed Mice Fed High-Fat Diets," *Journal of the National Cancer Institute* 82(1):50–54 (1990).

"on women in New Zealand . . ." D. C. G. Skegg et al., "Progestogen-Only Oral Contraceptives and Risk of Breast Cancer in New Zealand," *Cancer Causes and Control* 7:512–19 (1996).

"breast (atypias) . . ." F. A. Tavassoli, "The Influence of Endogenous and Exogenous Reproductive Hormones on the Mammary Glands with Emphasis on Experimental Studies in Rhesus Monkeys," *Verhandlungender Deutschen Fur Pathologic* 81:514–20 (1997).

"recent users of birth-control . . ." P. A. Newcomb, "Recent Oral Contraceptive Use and Risk of Breast Cancer (United States)," *Cancer Causes and Control* 7:525–32 (1996).

"breast cancer among birth-control users . . ." C. L. Westhoff, "Oral Contraceptives and Breast Cancer—Resolution Emerges," *Contraception* 54:i–ii (1996).

"Thyroxine . . ." T. Yokoe et al., "Relationship Between Thyroid-Pituitary Function and Response to Therapy in Patients with Recurrent Breast Cancer," *Anticancer Research* 16:2069–72 (1996).

"prevalence of thyroid diseases . . ." P. Fieraci et al., "Breast Cancer and Thyroid Autoimmunity," *Journal of Endocrinological Investigation* 19(6) (1996).

"estrogen and bisphenol A . . ." R. Steinmetz, et al., "The Environmental Estrogen Bisphenol A Stimulates Prolactin Release in Vitro and in Vivo," *Endocrinology* 138:1780–86 (1997).

"insulin-like growth factors . . ." B. A. Stoll, "Western Nutrition and the Insulin Resistance Syndrome: A Link to Breast Cancer," *European Journal of Clinical Nutrition* 53:83–87 (1999)

"amplifying the signal that estrogen . . ." S. Kato et al., "Activation of the Estrogen-Receptor Through Phosphorylation by Mitogen-Activated Protein-Kinase," *Science* 270:1491–94 (1995); G. Bunone, P. A. Briand, R. J. Miksicek, and D. Picard, "Activation of the Unliganded Estrogen Receptor by EGF Involved the MAP Kinase Pathway and Direct Phosphorylation" *EMBO Journal* 15:2174–83 (1996).

"Progesterone: One study showed . . ." L. D. Cowan et al., "Breast Cancer Incidence in Women with a History of Progesterone Deficiency," *American Journal of Epidemiology* 114(2):209–17 (1981).

"protect against DNA damage . . ." D. Christensen, "Breast Cancer and 'Environmental Estrogens'," *New York Times* (July 23, 1997).

"prolactin and melatonin . . ." G. Maestroni and A. Conti, "Melatonin Inhuman Breast Cancer Tissue: Association with Nuclear Grade and Estrogen Receptor Status," *Laboratory Investigation* 75(94):557–61 (1996).

"preventative action . . ." S. Steingraber, "Mechanisms, Proof, and Unmet Needs: The Perspective of a Cancer Activist," *Environmental Health Perspectives* 105(3):685–87 (1997).

CHAPTER 10

"colon cancer, and Alzheimer's disease . . ." A. Paganini-Hill and V. W. Henderson, "Estrogen Replacement Therapy and Risk of Alzheimer's Disease," *Archives of Internal Medicine* 156:2213–17 (1996).

"By the year 2000 . . ." Statistics from program presented by North American Menopause Society (NAMS), (1995). Contact: 216/467-5229.

"estrogen's cancer-causing tendencies . . ." E. R. te Velde, H. van Leusden, "Hormonal Treatment for the Climacteric: Alleviation of Symptoms and Prevention of Postmenopausal Disease," *Lancet* 343(8902):926 (1994).

"Massachusetts Women's Health Study . . . " John McKinlay, Sonja McKinlay, and Donald Brambilla, "Health Status and Utilization Behavior Associated with Menopause," *American Journal of Epidemology*

125(1):110-21 (1987); and John McKinlay et al., "The Relative Contributions of Endocrine Changes and Social Circumstances to Depression in Mid-Aged Women," *Journal of Health and Social Behavior* 28(4):345–63 (1987).

"Premarin . . ." Women, why you should boycott Premarin for estrogen replacement therapy. Physicians Committee for Responsible Medicine, 5100 Wisconsin Ave., NW, Ste. 404, Washington DC 20016.

"horse estrogen is not . . ." I. D. Cox, "Should a Doctor Prescribe Hormone Replacement Therapy Which Has Been Manufactured from Mare's Urine?" *Journal of Medical Ethics* 22:199–204 (1996).

"two thirds of their estrogen production . . ." J. Williams, "Menopause: Planning for 'Second Adulthood'," *Women's Health Concepts* 1(2):3.

"aromatase itself may . . ." H. J. Drenth, C. A. Bouwman, W. Seinen, and M. Vandenberg, *Toxicology and Applied Pharmacology* 148(1):50-55 (1998).

"According to George M. Stancel . . ." G. M. Stancel, "Growth Factor and Steroid Receptor Transcript Expression in Postmenopausal Endometrium." A talk given at IBC's International Symposium on Cutting-Edge Developments in Pharmaceuticals for Women, Scottsdale, AZ (Jan. 25–26, 1999)

"They have children later . . ." P. K. Siiteri and P. C. MacDonald, "Placental Estrogen Biosynthesis During Human Pregnancy," *Journal of Endocriology Metabolism* 26(7):751–61 (1996).

"safest of all the estrogens . . ." F. L. Hisaw, J. T. Velardo, and C. M. Goolsby, "Interactions of Estrogens on Uterine Growth," *Journal of Clinical Endocrinology* 14:1134–43 (1954).

"affecting a variety . . ." P. Hauser et al., "Resistance to Thyroid Hormone: Implications for Neurodevelopmental Research on the Effects of Thyroid Hormone Disruptors," *Toxicology and Industrial Health* 14(1/2):85–105 (1998).

"Lowered levels of vitamin A . . ." D. M. Lithgow and W. M. Politzer, "Vitamin A in the Treatment of Menorrhagia," *South African Medical Journal* 51(7):191–93 (1997). Vitamin A, like vitamin D_3, is considered a hormone and has its own nuclear receptor.

"Thyroid malfunctions . . ." H. Vorherr, "Thyroid Function in Benign and Malignant Breast Disease," *European Journal of Cancer Clinical Oncology* 3:255–57 (1987).

"Dr. Alan Gaby . . ." A. Gaby, "Research Review," *Nutrition and Healing*: 7 (1997).

"Dr. Walter Elger . . ." "Sulfamate Estrogen (ES): A New Principle of Oral Hormone Replacemant Therapy," from IBC's International Symposium on Cutting-Edge Developments in Pharmaceuticals for Women, Scottsdale, AZ (June 25–26, 1999).

"HERS . . ." N. K. Wenger, American College of Cardiology 48th Annual Scientific Session, March 7–10, 1999.

"risk of clots in the vein . . ." D. Grady et al., "Venous Thromboembolic Events Associated with Hormone Replacement Therapy," Letter to the Editor, *Journal of the American Medical Association* 6:477 (1997).

"Studies that have been done . . . selection bias . . ." D. B. Petitti, "Coronary Heart Disease and Estrogen Replacement Therapy: Can Compliance Bias Explain the Results of Observational Studies?" *Annals of Epidemiology* 4:115–18 (1994); K. A. Matthews et al., "Prior to Use of Estrogen Replacement Therapy, Are Users Healthier Than Nonusers?" *American Journal of Epidemiology* 143:971–78 (1996).

"elevated levels of CRP . . ." P. M. Ridker et al., "Hormone Replacement Therapy and Increased Plasma Concentration of C-Reactive Protein," *Circulation* 100:713–16 (1999).

"Oregon Regional Primate Research Center . . ." K. Hermsmeyers et al., "Reactivity-Based Coronary Vasospasm Independent of Atherosclerosis in Rhesus Monkeys," *Journal of the American College of Cardiology* 29:671 (1997).

"The animals on estrogen alone . . ." K. Miyagawa and K. Hermsmeyer, "Medroxyprogesterone Interferes with Ovarian Steroid Protection Against Coronary Vasospasm," *Natural Medicine* 3:324 (1997).

"really dangerous drug . . ." J. Raloff, "Hormone Therapy: Issues of the Heart," *Science News Online* (March 8, 1997).

"investigators from . . ." C. Shairer et al., "Menopausal Estrogen and Estrogen-Progestin Replacement Therapy and Breast Cancer Risk," *Journal of the American Medical Association* 283(4):485–9 (Jan. 2000).

"develop breast cancer . . ." "22 Ns Progestin Adds to Breast Cancer Risk," *Science News* 51:171 (2000).

"A woman who develops cystic breasts . . ." R. Hoover, L. A. Gray, P. Cole, and B. MacMahon, "Amenopausal Estrogens and Breast Cancer," *New England Journal of Medicine* 295:(8):401–05 (1976).

"Nurses' Health Study . . ." F. Gradstein, *New England Journal of Medicine* 336:1769–75 (1997).

"Evidence from mammograms . . ." R. D. et al., "Mammographic Changes in Postmenopausal Women on Hormone Replacement Therapy," *European Radiology* 7:749–55 (1997).

"Studies show . . ." C. Longcope, S. Crawford, and S. McKinlay, "Endogenous Estrogens: Relationship Between Estrone, Estradiol, Nonprotein-Bound Estradiol, and Hot Flashes and Lipids," *Menopause* 3:77–84 (1996); C. B. Johannes, S. L. Crawford, J. G. Posner, and S. M. McKinlay, "Longitudinal Patterns and Correlates of Hormone Replacement Therapy Use in Middle-Aged Women," *American Journal of Epidemiology* 140:439–52 (1994); D. C. Bauer et al., "Factors Associated with Appendicular Bone Mass in Older Women: The Study of Osteoporotic Fractures Research Group," *Annals of Internal Medicine* 118:657–65 (1993).

"better survival rates . . ." L. Bergkvist et al., "Prognosis after Breast Cancer Diagnosis in Women Exposed to Estrogen and Estrogen-Progestogen Replacement Therapy," *American Journal of Epidemiology* 130:221–28 (1989); D. M. Strickland, R. D. Gambrell, C. A. Butzin, and K. Strickland, "The Relationship Between Breast Cancer Survival and Prior Postmenopausal Estrogen Use," *Obstetrics and Gynecology* 80:400–04 (1992); D. B. Willis, E. E. Calle, H. L. Miracle-McMahill, and C. W. Heath, "Estrogen Replacement Therapy and Risk of Fatal Breast Cancer in a Prospective Cohort of Postmenopausal Women in the United States," *Cancer Causes and Control*, 7:449–57 (1996).

"Avrum Bluming . . ." A. Bluming, et al. "Hormone Replacement Therapy (HRT) in Women with Previously Treated Primary Breast Cancer," *Update V Proceedings of the American Society of Clinical Oncology* 18:471 (1999).

"Their rates of recurrence . . ." A. Bluming, personal correspondence with author (2000).

"A seven-year study . . ." A research team headed by Carmen Rodriguez followed 240,073 women for seven years from a study started by the American Cancer Society in 1982.

"Women who had been using estrogen . . ." C. Rodriguez, E. E. Calle, R. J. Coataes, H. L. Miracle-McMahil, M. J. Thun, and C. W. Heath, "Estrogen Replacement Therapy and Fatal Ovarian Cancer," *American Journal of Epidemiology* 141(9):828–35 (1995).

"HRT and Osteoporosis . . ." T. J. Arneson et al., "Epidemiology of Diaphyseal and Distal Femoral Fractures in Rochester, Minnesota 1965–1984," *Clinical Orthopedics* 234:188–194 (1988); R. Lindsay, "The Menopause: Sex Steroids and Osteoporosis," *Clinical Obstetrics and Gynecology* 30:847–59 (1987); R. Lindsay, "Prevention and Treatment of Osteoporosis with Ovarian Hormones," *Annals Chirugerie et Gynaeclogiae* 77:219–22 (1988).

"actually works to restore bone tissue . . ." Osteoporosis actually begins as much as 5 to 20 years before menopause, when ovaries are still functioning and estrogen levels are still high.

"Harvard Medical School . . ." L. Seachrist, "Estrogen Linked to Adult Asthma Risk," *Science News* 148:279 (1995).

"dietary and herbal alternatives . . ." C. Lauritzen, "Results of a 5-Year Prospective Study of Estriol Succinate Treatment in Patients with Climacteric Complaints," *Hormone and Metabolic Research* 19:579–84 (1987).

"reduce the risk of breast cancer . . ." R. R. Recker, K. M. Davies, R. M. Dowd, and R. P. Heaney, "The Effect of Low-Dose Continuous Estrogen and Progesterone Therapy with Calcium and Vitamin D on Bone in Elderly Women," *Annals of Internal Medicine* 130:897–904 (1999).

"Heart disease has declined . . ." P. G. McGovern et al., "Recent Trends in Acute Coronary Heart Disease—Mortality, Morbidity, Medical Care, and Risk Factors: The Minnesota Heart Survey Investigators," *New England Journal of Medicine* 33:884–90 (1996).

"daily multiple vitamin . . ." E. B. Rimm et al., "Folate and Vitamin B_6 from Diet and Supplements in Relation to Risk of Coronary Heart Disease

Among Women," *Journal of the American Medical Association* 279:359–64 (1998).

CHAPTER 11

"1.2 million new cases . . ." D. L. Jacobson et al., "Epidemiology and Estimated Population Burden of Selected Autoimmune Diseases in the United States," *Clinical Immunology and Immunopathology* 84(3):223–43 (1997).

"environmental agents and autoimmune disease . . ." G. G. Cooper et al., "Linking environmental agents and autoimmune diseases," *Environmental Health Perspectives* 107 (Suppl. 5):659–60 (Oct. 1999).

"pesticides do impair immune system . . ." R. Repetto and S. Balina, "Pesticides and the Immune System: The Public Health Risks," World Resources Institute (1996).

"One hypothesis is that NHL. . ." J. Raloff, "PCBs Linked to Rise in Lymph Cancers," *Science News* 152:85 (1997).

"One single dose of dioxin . . ." R. V. House et al., "Examination of Immune Parameters and Host Resistance Mechanisms in B6C3F1 Mice Following Adult Exposure to 2,3,7,8-Tetrachlorodibenzo-p-Dioxin," *Journal of Toxicology and Environmental Health* 31(3):203–15 (1990).

"dolphins along the Eastern U.S. seaboard. . ." http://www.wwfcanada.org/hormone-disruptors

"lifelong immune supression . . ." S. D. Holladay, "Prenatal Immunotoxicant Exposure and Postnatal Autoimmune Disease," *Environmental Health Perspectives* 107 (suppl. 5):687–91 (1999).

"Nurses' Health Study . . ." J. Sanchez-Guerro, "Past Use of Oral Contraceptives and the Risk of Developing Systemic Lupus Erythematosus," *Arthritis & Rheumatism* 40:804–08 (1997).

"The authors of this study . . ." G. S. Cooper et al., "Hormonal, Environmental, and Infectious Risk Factors for Developing Systemic Lupus Erythematosus," *Arthritis & Rheumatism* 41(10):1714-24 (1998).

"Problems with thyroid functioning . . ." M. A. Schmidt and J. S. Bland, "Thyroid Gland as Sentinel: Interface Between Internal and External Environment," *Alternative Therapies* 3(1):78–81 (1997).

"a research team . . ." Z. Limanova et al., "Frequent Incidence of Thy-ropathies in Women with Breast Carcinoma," *Vnitrni Lekarstvi Czech* 44(2):76–82 (1998).

"In a study of twenty-nine women . . ." M. Datta et al., "Thyroid Hormone Stimulates Progesterone Release from Human Luteal Cells by Generat-ing a Proteinaceous Factor," *Journal of Endocrinology* 158(3):319–25 (1998).

"immune function and thyroid . . ." P. Langer, J. Kausitz, M. Tajtakova, J. Kocan, P. Bohov, and E. Hanzen, "Decreased Blood Level of Beta2-Microglobulin in the Employees of a Factory which Produced Polychlo-rinated Biphenyls," *Chemosphere* 34:2595–600 (1997); P. Langer et al., "Increased Thyroid Volume and Prevalence of Thyroid Disorders in an Area Heavily Polluted by Polychlorinated Biphenyls," *European Journal of Endocrinology* 139:402–09 (1998).

"various xenobiotics . . ." S. Lair et al., "Adrenal Lesions in St. Lawrence Estuary Beluga Whale," Poster Session Abstract, Estrogens in the Envi-ronment IV (1997).

"DDT itself was given to some human patients . . ." D. Kupfer, "Effects of Pesticides and Related Compounds on Steroid Metabolism and Func-tion," *Critical Reviews in Toxicology* 4:83–124 (1975).

"abnormal glucose and insulin levels . . ." L. Needham, "Human Health Outcomes Related to Dioxin Exposure," lecture from Environmental Hormones: Past, Present, and Future conference in New Orleans, LA (Oct. 18–20, 1999).

"dioxin accident in Seveso, Italy . . ." P. A. Bertazzi, "Long-Term Health Effects of Dioxin Exposure in a Residential Population," Talk at Key-stone Symposium on Endocrine Disruptors (B5) in Tahoe City, CA (Jan. 31–Feb. 5, 1999).

"International Business Communications . . ." J. E. Cobb, "Novel Potent PPAR Gamma Agonists Derived from L-Tryrosine," Insulin Resistance Symposium, Washington, DC (Mar. 24–25, 1999).

"prenatal exposure to environmental contaminants . . ." E. Reichrtova, et al., "Cord Serum Immunoglobulin E Related to the Environmental Contamination of Human Placentas with Organochlorine Compounds," *Environmental Health Perspectives* 107(11):895–99 (Nov. 1999).

"children are exposed prenatally to methyl mercury . . ." "More evidence of Mercury Effects in Children," *Environmental Health Perspectives* 107(11): A554–A555 (Nov. 1999).

"Changes in liver function . . ." K. Kreiss et al., "Association of Blood Pressure and Polychlorinated Biphenyl Levels," *Journal of the American Medical Association* 245(24):2505–09 (1981).

"history of high blood pressure . . ." J. L. Radomski et al., "Pesticide Concentrations in the Liver, Brain, and Adipose Tissue of Terminal Hospital Patients," *Food and Cosmetics Toxicology* 6:209–20 (1968).

"A preliminary report . . ." S. L. Schantz et al., "Neuropsychological Assessment of an Aging Population of Great Lakes Fish Eaters," *Toxicology and Industrial Health* 12(3–4):403–17 (1996).

"calcium balance in brain nerves . . ." W. Shain, B. Bush, and R. Seegal, "Neurotoxicology of Polychlorinated Biphenyls: Structure-Activity Relationship of Individual Congeners," *Toxicology and Applied Pharmacology* 111:33–42 (1991).

PART III
INTRODUCTION

"and meat products . . ." S. Patandin et al., "Dietary Exposure to Polychlorinated Biphenyls and Dioxins from Infancy until Adulthood: A Comparison Between Breast-Feeding, Toddler, and Long-Term Exposure," *Environmental Health Perspectives* 107(1):45–51 (1999).

"effects on the male offspring of rats . . ." R. M. Sharpe, J. S. Fisher, M. M. Millar, S. Jobling, and J. P. Sumpter, "Gestational Exposure of Rats to Xenoestrogens Results in Reduced Testicular Size and Sperm Production," *Environmental Health Perspectives* 103:2–9 (1995).

"the third generation . . ." R. N. Wine et al., "Reproductive Toxicity of Di-n-butylphthalate in a Continuous Breeding Protocol in Sprague-Dawley Rats," *Environmental Health Perspectives* 105:102–107 (1997).

"Take the case of chlorine . . ." C. Dees and B. Ladd, "It's Time to Get Real About Zero Risk and the Delaney Clause," publication reprint supplied by Dr. Dees, vice president of research and development for GENASE, Inc.

CHAPTER 12

"pus and bacteria . . ." J. Rifken, consumer warning flyer from Rifkin's Foundation on Economic Trends, 1995.

"cows on BGH are given more antibiotics . . ." "Brave New World of Milk," *Time* (Feb. 14, 1994).

"*never* put food covered with cling wrap . . ." M. Burros, "Eating Well," *New York Times* (Jan. 13, 1999).

"Canadian scientists have discovered . . ." J. Raloff, "Pollutant Waits to Smite Salmon at Sea," *Science News* 155:293 (1999).

"You eat small amounts of numerous pesticides . . ." Environmental Working Group report, *Pesticides in Children's Food* (1993).

"with almost one-quarter of this amount . . ." J. Wargo, *Our Children's Toxic Legacy: How Science and Law Fail to Protect Us from Pesticides*, 2d ed.: Yale University Press (1998).

"1,500 ginseng growers . . ." "Wisconsin Growers Nabbed for Pesticide Use," *The New Mexican* (1997).

"In the EWG report . . ." S. Elderkin, R. Wiles, and C. Campbell, "Forbidden Fruit: Illegal Pesticides in the U.S. Food Supply" (1995).

"*Worst First*, published by . . ." "Worst First: High Risk Insecticide Uses, Children's Foods and Safer Alternatives," Consumers Union of U.S., Inc., Washington, DC, 1998. The full analysis is available at http://www.ecologic-ipm.com.

"Another source of pesticides . . ." D. Imhoff, "King Cotton," *Sierra* 84(3):34–36 (May–June 1999).

"Isoflavones . . ." H. Adlercreutz and W. Mazur, "Phyto-oestrogens and Western Disease," Finnish Medical Society DUODECIM *Annals of Medicine* 29:95–120 (1997).

"Asian-Hawaiian men . . ." G. W. Ross et al., "Characterization of Risk Factors for Vascular Dementia: The Honolulu-Asia Aging Study." *Neurology* 53(2):337–43 (1999).

"ductile tissue in the breast . . ." D. T. Zava and G. Duwe, "Estrogenic and Antiproliferative Properties of Genistein and Other Flavonoids in Human Breast Cancer Cells in Vitro," *Nutrition and Cancer* 27(1):31–40 (1997).

"estrogen receptor . . ." B. Blumberg, "Sxr, a Nuclear Receptor Activated by Steroids and Xenophobic Toxicants," a talk at Environmental Hormones: Past, Present, and Future conference in New Orleans, LA (Oct. 18–20, 1999).

"Sales of organic products . . ." S. C. Gwynne, "Thriving on Health Food," *Time* 53 (Feb. 23, 1998).

"royal seal of approval . . ." J. Micklethwait, " 'Genetically Modified' Food Vilified in Britain," *The New Mexican* F-7 (June 13, 1999).

"Danish organic farmers . . ." T. K. Jensen et al., "Semen Quality Among Members of Organic Food Associations in Zealand, Denmark," *Lancet* 347(9018):1844 (1996).

"A review of the literature . . ." V. Worthington, "Effect of Agricultural Methods on Nutritional Quality: A Comparison of Organic with Conventional Crops," *Alternative Therapies* 4(1):58–69 (1998).

"The Associated Press . . ." Associated Press, "Toxic Chemicals Recycled into Fertilizers," reprinted in *The New Mexican* (July 6,1997).

"come from the steel industry . . ." Seattle Times, "270 Million Pounds of Toxic Waste Spread on Fields," reprinted in *The New Mexican* A-3 (March 27, 1998).

"Food Additives." From a Primer on Food Additives posted online by Hopkins Technology, www.hoptechno.com/books27.htm.

"Additives are tested by . . ." Usually, the additive may be used in food at a level that is no more than 1/100th of the highest level at which it did not produce any harmful effects on the test animals.

"because of their known toxicity . . ." from *Nutrition Action Healthletter* 26(2) (March 1999).

"Butylated hydroxyanisole . . ." S. Jobling, T. Reynolds, R. White, M. G. Parker, and J. P. Sumpter, "A Variety of Environmentally Persistent Chemicals, Including Some Phthalate Plasticizers, Are Weakly Estrogenic," *Environmental Health Perspectives* 103:852–86 (1995).

"the food cans in the United States . . ." J. Raloff, "Additional Source of Dietary 'Estrogens'," *Science News* 147:341 (1995).

"Bpa can leach from plastic . . ." J. Raloff, "Lacing Food with an Estrogen Mimic," *Science News* 152:255 (1997).

"growth of human breast cancer cells . . ." J. A. Brotons, M. F. Olea-Serrano, M. Villalobos, V. Pedraza, and N. Olea, "Xenoestrogens Released from Lacquer Coatings in Food Cans," *Environmental Health Perspectives* 103:608–12 (1995).

"cans tested in one study . . ." D. Cadbury, *The Feminization of Nature*, Hamish-Hamilton-London, 1997, p. 156.

"700 chemicals found in . . ." M. Ben, "Is Detoxification a Solution to Occupational Health Hazards?" *National Safety News* (May 1984).

"Environmental Working Group . . ." B. A. Cohen and R. Wiles, "Tough to Swallow: How Pesticide Companies Profit from Poisoning America's Tap Water," Environmental Working Group (1997).

"An earlier EWG study . . ." B. A. Cohen, R. Wiles, and E. Bondoc, "Weed Killers by the Glass: A Citizens' Tap Water Monitoring Project in 29 Cities" (1995).

"Even rainwater contained atrazine. . . ." D. A. Goolsby, "Occurrence of Herbicides and Metabolites in Surface Water, Ground Water, and Rainwater in the Midwestern United States," Proceedings, 1995 Annual Conference: Water Research, American Water Works Association: 588 (1995).

"body metabolizes estrogen . . ." H. L. Bradlow et al., "Effects of Pesticides on the Ratio of 16 Alpha/2-Hydroxyestrone: A Biologic Marker of Breast Cancer Risk," *Environmental Health Perspectives* 103(7):147–50 (1995).

"Ciba-Geigy . . ." D. Fagin, M. Lavelle, and the Center for Public Integrity, *Toxic Deception*, Birch Lane Press, 1996, p. 22.

"chlorinated drinking water . . ." A 1994 report, "Hormone Copycats," from the Great Lakes Natural Resource Center. Reprint by the National Wildlife Federation. Chlorine has been blamed for increases in a variety of cancers such as bladder, breast, and prostate, as well as being incriminated in diseases like endometriosis.

"disinfection by-products . . ." S. Steingraber, *Living Downstream*, Addison-Wesley, 1997, pp. 202–06.

"Dr. Shanna Swan . . ." S. H. Swan and K. Waller, "Drinking Water and Reproductive Outcomes," *Epidemiology* 9(3):358 (May 1998).

"It found that chemicals can survive . . ." M. L. Johnson et al., "Environmental Estrogens in Agricultural Drain Water from the Central Valley of California," *Bulletin of Environmental Contamination and Toxicology* 60:609–14 (1998).

" 'distilled' or 'purified' water . . ." L. Gross, "The Hidden Life of Bottled Water." *Sierra* (May/June 1999) pp. 66–67.

"resveratrol, which protects grapes . . ." B. D. Gehm, J. M. McAndrews, Pei-Yu Chien, and J. L. Jameson, "Resveratrol, a Polyphenolic Compound Found in Grapes and Wine, Is an Agonist for the Estrogen Receptor," Proceedings of the National Academy of Science 94: 14138–43 (1997).

"twelve coffee trees . . ." J. Raloff, "The Environment Upstream of Our Supermarket," *Science News Online* (March 29, 1997).

CHAPTER 13

"One study did try to reduce levels . . ." H. J. Pluim et al., "Influence of Short-Term Dietary Measurements on Dioxin Concentrations in Human Milk," *Environmental Health Perspectives* 102:968–71 (1994).

"process of biotransformation . . ." D. C. Liebler and I. G. Sipes, "Bioactivation: The Role of Metabolism in Chemical Toxicity," Chapter 4 of *Hazardous Materials Toxicology: Clinical Principles of Environmental Health* (eds. J. B. Sullivan and G. R. Krieger), Williams & Wilkins, 1992.

"a process called bioactivation . . ." Ibid.

"a diet too low in protein . . ." A. Melander, D. Lalka, and A. McLean, "Influence of Food on the Presystemic Metabolism of Drugs," *Pharmacology and Therapeutics* 38:253–67 (1988).

"predominately stored in fat . . ." Y. Oschry and B. Shapiro, *Biochimica et Biophysica Acta* 664:210 (1981); a discussion of mobilization and excretion of xenobiotics stored in human fat is available, along with the data produced in this study, in *Reduction of Human Organohalide Body Burdens— Final Research Report* (Foundation for Advancements in Science and Education, Los Angeles, 1983).

"supports liver functions . . ." L. Y. Sheen, C. K. Li et al., "Effect of the Active Principle of Garlic—Diallyl Sulfide—on Cell Viability, Detoxifi-

cation Capability, and the Antioxidation System of Primary Rat Hepato-
cytes," *Food and Chemical Toxicology* 34:971–78 (1996).

"biotransformational enzymes . . ." K. E. Anderson, "Influences of Diet and
Nutrition on Clinical Pharmacokinetics," *Clinical Pharmacokinetics*
14:325–46 (1988).

"Avoid eating too many . . ." J. W. T. Dickerson et al., "Activity of Drug-
Metabolizing Enzymes in the Liver of Growing Rats Fed on Diets High
in Sucrose, Glucose, Fructose or an Equimolar Mixture of Glucose and
Fructose," *Proceedings of the Nutrition Society* 30:27A–28A (1971).

"superfamily of enzymes . . ." D. W. Nebert et al., "The P-450 Superfamily:
Update on Listing of All Genes and Recommended Nomenclature of
the Chromosomal Loci," *DNA* 8:1–14 (1989).

"and even in testicles . . ." J. Rydstrom, J. Montelius, M. Bengtsson (eds.),
Extrahepatic Drug Metabolism and Chemical Carcinogenesis, Elsevier,
1983.

"kinds of fats we eat may also play a role . . ." K. E. Anderson and A. Kap-
pas, "Dietary Regulation of Cytochrome P450," *Annual Review of
Nutrition* 11:141–67 (1991).

"It has known antioxidant effects . . ." L. Galland, *The Four Pillars of Health*,
Random House, 1997, p. 207.

"sulforaphane precursor . . ." J. Raloff, "Anticancer Agent Sprouts Up
Unexpectedly," *Science News* 152:183 (1997).

"The reason adequate protein . . ." E. M. Boyd and E. Carsky, "Kwash-
iorkorigenic Diet and Diazinon Toxicity," *Acta Pharmacologica et Toxico-
logica (Copesh)* 27:284–94 (1969); E. M. Boyd and C. P. Chem, "Lindane
Toxicity and Protein-Deficient Diet," *Archives of Environmental Health*
17:156–63 (1968); E. M. Boyd and C. J. Drignet, "Toxicity of Captan
and Protein-Deficient Diet," *Journal of Clinical Pharmacology* 8:225–34
(1968).

"Vitamin C helps this process, . . ." D. Chakraborty, A. Bhattacharyya, and
J. Chatterjee, *International Journal of Vitamin and Nutrition Research*
48:22 (1978).

"increases the levels of glutathione . . ." C. J. Johnston et al., "Vitamin C
Elevates Red Blood Cell Glutathinone in Healthy Adults," *American
Journal of Clinical Nutrition* 58:103–05 (1993).

"destroy glutathione . . ." D. P. Jones et al., "Glutathione in Foods Listed in the National Cancer Institute's Health Habits and History Food Frequency Questionnaire," *Nutrition and Cancer* 17:57–75 (1992).

"many drugs that rinse out the . . ." Dr. Leo Galland, a leader in the field of parasitology and detoxification. Talk presented at Ark book store in Santa Fe, NM, 1997.

"mix a teaspoonful with honey . . ." S. P. Verma, B. R. Goldin, and P. S. Lin, "The Inhibition of the Estrogenic Effects of Pesticides and Environmental Chemicals by Curcumin and Isoflavonoids," *Environmental Health Perspectives* 106(12):807–12 (1998).

"Do a safe and sensible program . . ." T. G. Randolph and R. M. Wisner, "Detoxification: Personal Survival in a Chemical World," in T. G. Randolph, *An Alternative Approach to Allergies—The New Field of Clinical Ecology Unravels the Environmental Causes of Mental and Physical Ills* Harper & Row, 1988; D. W. Schnare, G. Denk, M. Shields, and S. Brunton, "Evaluation of a Detoxification Regimen for Fat Stored Xenobiotics," *Medical Hypotheses* 9:265–82 (1982).

"optimal activation of the body's detoxification system . . ." T. C. Fagan et al., "Increased Clearance of Propranolol and Theophylline by High-Protein Compared with High-Carbohydrate Diet," *Clinical Pharmacology and Therapeutics* 41(4):402–06 (1987).

"shown in numerous studies . . ." H. A. Salmi, S. Sarna, "Effect of Silymarin on Chemical, Functional, and Morphological Alteration of the Liver: A Double-Blind Controlled Study," *Scandinavian Journal of Gastroenterology*, 17:417–21 (1982).

"Northwest Healing Arts Center . . ." W. J. Crinnion, "Environmental Toxicity and Naturopathic Tissue Cleansing," Northwest Healing Arts Center Information Series 1(1) (1989).

"body's natural excretion of chemicals . . ." D. W. Schnare, M. Ben, M. G. Shields, "Body Burden Reductions of PCBs, PBBs, and Chlorinated Pesticides in Human Subjects," *Ambio* 13(5–6):378–80 (1984).

"The Michigan Seven . . ." M. Wolff et al, "Human Tissue Burdens of Halogenated Aromatic Chemicals in Michigan," *Journal of the American Medical Association* 247:2112 (1982).

"This treatment is currently used in Sweden . . ." D. Schnare, G. Denk, M. Shields, and S. Brunton, "Evaluation of Detoxification Regimen for Fat Stored Xenobiotics," *Medical Hypotheses* 9(3):265–82 (1982).

"United States for a variety . . ." D. Bauer, R. Behrens, and R. C. Warner, "Effective Programs Don't Have to Cost a Bundle," *Employee Health Fitness Newletter* 5(3): 32–4 (1983).

"Electrical Workers . . ." D. W. Schnare and P. C. Robinson, "Reduction of the Human Body Burdens of Hexachlorobenzene and Polychlorinated Biphenyls," *Hexachlorobenzene: Proceedings of an International Symposium* (C. R. Morris and J. R. P. Cabral, eds.), Iarc Scientific Publications 77:597–603 (1986).

"Yugoslavian Capacitor Workers," Z. Tretjak et al., "Xenobiotic Reduction and Clinical Improvements in Capacitor Workers: A Feasible Method," *Journal of Environmental Science and Health* A25(7):731–51 (1990).

"Hubbard detoxification program . . ." L. R. Hubbard, *The Technical Bulletins* 12:3–181 (1980); Other publications reporting reduction in body burden of liophilic chemicals using this technique: D. C. Roehm, "Effects of a Program of Sauna Baths and Megavitamins on Adipose DDE and PCBs and on Clearing of Symptoms of Agent Orange (Dioxin) Toxicity," *Clinical Research* 31:243 (abstr.) (1983). D. W. Schnare, B. Ben, and M. G. Shields, "Body Burden Reductions of PCBs, PBBs, and Chlorinated Pesticides in Human Subjects," *Ambio* 13:378–80 (1984).

"PCBS did *not* elevate . . ." D. W. Schnare and P. C. Robinson, "Reduction of the Human Body Burdens of Hexachlorobenzene and Polychlorinated biphenyls," Iarc Service Publication (77):597–603 (1986).

"higher blood levels of PCBS . . ." M. Imamura, T. C. Tung, "A Trial of Fasting Cure for PCB Poisoned Patients in Taiwan," *Progress in Clinical and Biological Research* 137:147–53 (1984).

"Their fat stores released the drug . . ." R. Warner, "Treatment of PCB Exposure in Narcotics Officers," *Journal of the Fraternal Order of Police* (Winter):18 (1983).

"subtle behavioral changes . . ." K. H. Kilburn et al., "Neurobehavioral Dysfunction in Firemen Exposed to Polychlorinated Biphenyls (PCBS): Possible Improvement after Detoxification," *Archives of Environmental Health* 44:345–50 (1989).

CHAPTER 14

"the typical American home contains 63 . . ." W. Kingsley, "Getting the Chemical Kicks Out of the Kitchen," Proceedings of the Sixth National U.S. EOA Conference on Household Hazardous Waste Management, Seattle, 1991.

"'-cide' in pesticide means 'to kill.' . . ." U.S. EPA website: www.epa/gov/iaq/pesticid.html (June 1998).

"human exposure assessment . . ." W. R. Ott, "Human Exposure Assessment: The Birth of a New Science," *Journal of Exposure Analysis and Environmental Epidemiology* 5(4):449–72 (1995).

"the most important sources of pollution are close . . ." L. Wallace, "Human Exposure to Environmental Pollutants: A Decade of Experience," *Clinical and Experimental Allergy* 25(1):4–9 (1995).

"homes built before April 1988 . . ." For more information, contact W. Sinclair and R. W. Pressinger at the Allergy, Asthma, Immunology, and Airtech Clinic in Vero Beach and Tampa, FL (813/978-1081).

"attention deficit disorder . . ." K. H. Kilburn and J. C. Thornton, "Chlordane Causes Neurological Disorders and ADD Symptoms," *Environmental Health Perspectives* 103:690–94, 1995.

"childhood blood and brain cancers . . ." "Neuroblastoma and Leukemia After Chlordane Exposure," *Teratogenesis, Carcinogenesis, and Mutagenesis* 7:527–40 (1987).

"infertility in mice . . ." K. J. Balash, "Male Infertility after Pesticide Chlordane Exposure," *Bulletin of Environmental Contamination Toxicology* 39:434–42 (1987).

"even obesity . . ." R. A. Cassidy et al, "Overweight—a Symptom of Chlordane Exposure," *Toxicology and Applied Pharmacology* 126:326–37 (1994).

"If you live in an area with construction . . ." H. W. Meilke, "Leaded Dust in Urban Soil Shown to Be Greater Source of Childhood Lead Poisoning Than Leaded Paint," *Lead Perspectives* 28–31 (1997).

"indoor sources of pollution . . ." W. R. Ott and J. W. Roberts, "Everyday Exposures to Toxic Pollutants," *Scientific American* 278(2):86–91 (Feb 1998).

"efficient vacuum cleaners . . ." R. W. Roberts, "Reducing Health Risks from Dust in the Home," in *Training Manual for the Master Home Envi-*

ronmentalist Program (ed. Philip Dickey), American Lung Association of Washington, 1997.

"400 times as much house dust . . ." Ibid.

"Homes treated for termites . . ." Ibid.

"PAHs (polycyclic aromatic hydrocarbons) . . ." Ibid.

"If you're thinking of buying new carpeting . . ." "All about Carpet Fiber": http://www.teleport.com/~jag/fiber.html

"A 1996 study . . ." S. Steingraber, *Living Downstream*, Addison-Wesley, 1997, p. 197.

"Inhaling the steam in an enclosed shower . . ." C. P. Weisel, Wan-Kuen Jo, "Ingestion, Inhalation, and Dermal Exposures to Chloroform and Trichloroethene from Tap Water," *Environmental Health Perspectives* 104:48–51 (1996).

"Infertility in both men and women . . ." B. Rice, "Toxic Dry Cleaning in Your Backyard," *Chlorine-Free* 3(1) (1994).

"According to the EPA . . ." Environmental Protection Agency, "Multi-process Wet Cleaning: Cost and Performance Comparison of Conventional Dry Cleaning and Alternative Process," 1–1 (Sept. 1993).

"An analysis in 1996 . . ." Consumers Union of the United States, the not-for-profit organization that publishes *Consumer Reports* (1996).

"breathing fumes from the perc left in the fabric . . ." D. Fagin, M. Lavelle, and the Center for Public Integrity, *Toxic Deception: How the Chemical Industry Manipulates Science, Bends the Law, and Endangers Your Health*, Birch Lane Press, 1996.

"The EPA has been working with the dry-cleaning industry . . ." C. Wu, "A Green Clean," *Science News* 152:108–09 (1997).

"perc in the water supply . . ." IEPA pilot groundwater protection program needs assessment for Pekin Public Water Supply Facility #1795040 (Springfield, IL: IEPA, Division of Public Water Supplies, 1992), Appendix C, and lengthy 1993 report on Pekin's groundwater: IEPA Pilot Groundwater Protection, 1993.

"Mindy Pennybacker, in . . ." M. Pennybacker, "The Hidden Life of T-shirts," *Sierra* 44–45 (Jan./Feb. 1999).

"The latest Rubbermaid and Tupperware . . ." A. Weil, "Hormone Mimics: An Emerging Threat," *Dr. Andrew Weil's Self Healing Newsletter* (Feb. 1999).

"Secondhand smoke . . ." L. A. Wallace, "Human Exposure to Environmental Pollutants: A Decade of Experience," *Clinical and Experimental Allergy* 25:4–9 (1995).

"Office furniture can emit formaldehyde . . ." K. Erickson, "The Happy Home Office," *Sierra* 18–20 (Jan./Feb. 1998).

"Don't idle the car in the garage. . . ." A. M. Standeven, D. C. Wolf, and T. L. Goldsworthy, "Interactive Effects of Unleaded Gasoline and Estrogen on Liver Tumor Promotion in Female B6C3F1 Mice," *Cancer Research* 54(5):1198–204 (March 1, 1994).

"The EPA pegged U.S. pesticide sales at . . ." *Pesticide and Toxic Chemical News* 25(46):8 (1997).

"homes and lawns and gardens . . ." M. Moses, "Designer Poisons," Pesticide Education Center, San Francisco, CA (1995).

"yet crop losses from pests . . ." D. Pimentel et al., "Insect Loss in Corn: Environmental and Economic Effects of Reducing Pesticide Use," *BioScience* 41:402–9 (1992).

"Integrated Pest Management . . ." Associated Press, "American Scientists Win World Food Prize," reprinted in *The New Mexican* (Oct. 15, 1997).

"The plastic from recycled pesticide . . ." J. Raloff, "Recycling Pesticide Bottles: A Risk?" *Science News* 148:365 (Nov. 25, 1995).

"Even homes in which the herbicide wasn't applied . . ." M. Nishioka et al., "Measuring Transport of Lawn-Applied Herbicide Acids from Turf to Home: Correlation of Dislodgeable 2,4-D Turf Residues with Carpet Dust and Carpet Surface Residues," *Environmental Science and Technology* 30(11) (1996).

"natural wood preservatives . . ." "Wood Preservatives: A Health and Environmental Hazard," EOHSI INFOletter 5(1):1–2 (Jan./Feb. 1991), Environmental and Occupational Health Sciences Institute.

"If you do treat your rugs . . ." R. A. Fenske et al., "Flea Home Treatments Cause High Air Pesticide Levels," *American Journal of Public Health* 80(6):689–93 (1990).

CHAPTER 15

"non-Hodgkin's lymphoma . . ." From "Endocrine Disruptors News" on the Tulane/Xavier website: www.tmc.tulane.edu/ecme/EEHome/newsviews/whatsnew/junnews.html.

"2 million gallons of drinking water . . ." R. Goo, "Do's and Don'ts Around the House," taken from an *EPA Journal* article, EPA-22K-1005 (Nov.-Dec. 1991); http://www.envirosearch.com/housechem.html.

"As a result of its mandate from Congress . . ." 1997 draft of the initial report prepared by EDSTAC. The full report is available at www.epa.gov/opptintr/opptendo/whatsnew.html.

"long-term or delayed effects. . . ." Ibid., Chapter 3, p. 7.

"The World Health Organization . . ." World Health Organization Press Release WHO/31 (20 March 1998). All WHO press releases, fact sheets and features are available on the Internet on the WHO Home Page http://www.who.ch.

"National Religious Partnership for the Environment . . ." *Models of Engagement*, National Religious Partnership for the Environment, 1047 Amsterdam Ave, New York, NY 10025 (Spring 1996).

"the joy of environmental work. . . ." *"The Contemplative Mind in Society: Meeting of the Working Group"* (April 1996) p. 19.

APPENDIX A

"Most abundant man-made environmental pollutants . . ." S. Jobling, T. Reynolds, R. White, M. G. Parker, and J. P. Sumpter, "A Variety of Environmentally Persistent Chemicals, Including Some Phthalate Plasticizers, Are Weakly Estrogenic," *Environmental Health Perspectives* 103(7):582–87 (1995).

"leach or volatilize out as time passes . . ." P. Montague, "Warning on Male Reproductive Health," *Rachel's Environment and Health Weekly* #438. Electronic edition (April 20, 1995).

"sausages have been found to contain phthalates . . ." Ministry of Agriculture, Fisheries, and Food, "Food Surveillance Information Sheet Number 60: Phthalates in Paper and Board Packaging," U.K. Ministry of Agriculture, Fisheries, and Food (1995).

"tested by the ministry in Britain . . ." Ministry of Agriculture, Fisheries, and Food, Food Surveillance Information Sheet number 83, "Phthalates in Infant Formulae," U.K. Ministry of Agriculture, Fisheries, and Food (1996b).

"follow-up study in 1998 . . ." Ministry of Agriculture, Fisheries, and Food, "Phthalates in Infant Formulae—Follow up Survey," Ministry of Agriculture, Fisheries, and Food #168 (Dec. 1998).

"1.6 billion pounds of this bisphenol . . ." J. A. Brotons et al., "Xenoestrogens Released from Lacquer Coatings in Food Cans," *Environmental Health Perspectives* 103:608–12 (1995).

"Six different laboratories . . ." Feldman's lab at Stanford, Mira Ben-Jonathan at the University of Cincinnati Medical School, Ana Soto and her collaborator Nikolea, Kevin Guido at the CIIT lab, vom Saal's lab, and Earl Gray's lab.

"in vivo studies showing . . ." S. C. Nagel, J. A. Taylor, F. S. vom Saal, and W. V. Welshons, "Relative Binding Affinity-Serum Enhanced Access Assay to Predict the Estrogenic Bioactivity of Phytoestrogens and Alkylphenols," In: 77th Annual Meeting of the Endocrine Society (14–17 June 1995) Washington, DC: Endocrine Society: 227. Now published in *Environmental Health Perspectives*; A. V. Krishnan et al., "Bisphenol-A: An Estrogenic Substance Is Released from Polycarbonate Flasks During Autoclaving," *Endocrinology* 132:2279–86 (1993); S. C. Nagel and F. S. vom Saal et al., "Relative Binding Affinity-Serum Modified Access (RBA-SMA) Assay Predicts the Relative *in Vivo* Bioactivity of the Xenoestrogens Bisphenol A and Octylphenol," *Environmental Health Perspectives* 105(1):70–76 (1997).

"Dr. David Feldman from Stanford University . . ." A. V. Krishnan, P. Stathis, S. F. Permth, L. Tokes, and D. Feldman, "Bisphenol A: An Estrogenic Substance Is Released from Polycarbonate Flasks During Autoclaving," *Endocrinology* 132:2279–86 (1993).

"baby formula may contain BPA . . ." D. Cadbury, *The Feminization of Nature*, Hamish Hamilton, London, 1997, p. 158.

"Some 660 million pounds . . ." G. C. Meuller and U. H. Kim, "Displacement of Estradiol from Estrogen Receptors by Simple Aklylphenols," *Endocrinology* 102:1429–35 (1978).

"causing human breast cancer cells to grow . . ." A. M. Soto, H. Justicia, J. W. Wray, and C. Sonnenschein, "P-Nonylphenol, an Estrogenic Xenobiotic Released from Œ Modified 1 Polystyrene," *Environmental Health Perspectives* 92:167–73 (1991).

"spermicides used with contraceptive diaphragms . . ." J. A. Raloff, "The Role of Chlorine—and Its Future," *Science News* 154:59 (1994).

"breakdown compounds persist in rivers . . ." M. Ahel, C. Schaffner, and W. Giger, "Behavior of Alkylphenol Polyethoxylate Surfactants in the Aquatic Environment: Occurrence and Elimination of Their Persistent Metabolites During Infiltration of River Water to Groundwater," *Water Resources* 30:37–46. (1996).

"in vitro and in vivo studies . . ." F. S. vom Saal et al., "A Physiologically Based Approach to the Study of Bisphenol A and Other Estrogenic Chemicals on the Size of Reproductive Organs, Daily Sperm Production, and Behavior," *Toxicology and Industrial Health* 14(1/2):239–60 (1998).

"breakdown products rather than the surfactants . . ." P. Dickey, "Hormones in Your Hair Color?" *Alternatives: Series of Fact Sheets.*, Washington Toxics Coalition Fact Sheet, pdickey@watoxics.org (July 19, 1997).

"drinking water has shown concentrations . . ." L. B. Clark et al., "Determination of Alkylphenol Ethoxylates and Their Acetic Acid Derivatives in Drinking Water by Particle Beam Liquid Chromatography/Mass Spectrometry," *International Journal of Environmental Analytical Chemistry* 147:167–80 (1992).

"Almost 85 percent of the pharmaceuticals . . ." B. Hileman, "Concerns Broaden over Chlorine and Chlorinated Hydrocarbons," *Chemical and Engineering News* 11–20 (April 1993).

"very few naturally occurring organochlorines . . ." G. W. Gribble, "The Diversity of Natural Organochlorines in Living Organisms," *Pure and Applied Chemistry* 68(9):1699–712 (1996).

"A series of PCBs have been shown to . . ." K. S. Korach, P. Sarver, K. Chae, J. A. McLachlan, and J. D. McKinney, "Estrogen Receptor-Binding Activity of Polychlorinated Hydroxybiphenyls: Conformationally Restricted Structural Probes," *Molecular Pharmacology* 33:120–26 (1987).

"and to mimic thyroid, estrogen, and . . ." J. D. McKinney and C. L. Waller, "Polychlorinated Biphenyls as Hormonally Active Structural Analogues," *Environmental Health Perspectives* 102(3):290–97 (1994).

"a thousand-fold higher affinity . . ." "Fitting a PCB into the Lung Millieu," *Science News* 148:312 (Nov. 11, 1995).

"They were, however, produced in Russia . . ." background information on pollutants considered to be hormone disruptors is available at: http://www.wwfcanada.org/hormone-disruptors/

"every area of the global ecosystem . . ." D. G. Patterson et al, "Levels of Non-*Ortho*-Substituted (Coplanar), Mono- and Di-Ortho-Substituted Polychlorinated Biphenyls, Dibenzo-p-Dioxins, and dDibenzofurans in Human Serum and Adipose Tissue," *Environmental Health Perspectives* 102(1):195–204 (1994).

"snow and seawater in the Antarctic . . ." Public Health Statement by the Agency for Toxic Substances and Disease Registry (1989). For more information on PCBS, contact Agency for Toxic Substances and Disease Registry, Division of Toxicology, 1600 Clifton Road, E-29, Atlanta, GA 30333, 1-800-447-1544 or www.atsdr.cdc.gov.

"dioxin in the air in urban regions . . ." "The Problem with Tallying 'Dioxin'," *Science News* 146:206 (Sept. 1994).

"Ninety-five percent of our personal exposure . . ." "Dioxin Health Hazards," *Rachel's Environment and Health Weekly* (Feb. 1995).

"we are exposed to through everyday living . . ." "Putting the Lid on Dioxins," joint report by Physicians for Social Responsibility and the Environmental Defense Fund (1994); J. Raloff, "Those Old Dioxin Blues," *Science News* 151:306–7 (May 17, 1997).

"thyroid hormone regulatory system in infants . . ." S. P. Porterfield, "Vulnerability of the Developing Brain to Thyroid Abnormalities: Environmental Insults to the Thyroid System," *Environmental Health Perspectives* 102(2):125–30 (1994).

"may also disrupt liver enzyme activity . . ." J. D. McKinney, "Multifunctional Receptor Model for Dioxin and Related Compound Toxic Action: Possible Thyroid Hormone-Responsive Effector-Linked Site," *Environmental Health Perspectives* 82:323–36 (1989).

"dioxin was upgraded to a known human carcinogen . . ." "The Report on Carcinogens Subcommittee of the National Toxicology Program's Board of Scientific Counselors," in "NTP's Report on Carcinogens in 1999," *Pesticide and Toxic Chemical News* 4 (Nov. 5, 1997).

"dioxin is one of the most potent carcinogens ever tested . . ." J. Emsley, *The Consumer's Good Chemical Guide*, Chapter 7, Corgi Books, 1994.

"inferred too much from animal studies . . ." "EPA Affirms Health Dangers from Dioxin," *New York Times* A-6 (Sept. 13, 1994); R. Stone, "Dioxin Report Faces Scientific Gauntlet," *Science* 265:1650 (Sept. 16, 1994).

"it binds to the Ah receptor . . ." "The Problem with Tallying 'Dioxin'," *Science News* 146:206 (Sept. 1994).

"Dioxin has a high affinity for this receptor . . ." J. Weinberg and J. Thornton, "Dioxin Paternity Suit: In Search of the Chlorine Donor," *Rachel's Children* 4–5 (Feb. 1995).

"dioxin affects the way the liver . . ." K. Schmidt, "Dioxin's Cellular Siege," *Science News* 141:26–27 (1992).

"International dioxin experts unanimously conclude. . ." M. J. DeVito et al., "Comparisons of Estimated Human Body Burdens of Dioxin-like Chemicals and TCDD Body Burdens in Experimentally Exposed Animals," *Environmental Health Perspectives* 103(9):820–31 (1995).

"The levels of DDT . . ." *Los Angeles Times*, "EPA Pesticide Cleanup to set a Precedent," *The New Mexican* (Mar. 26, 2000).

"properties comparable to those of DDT and chlodecone . . ." A. M. Soto, K. L. Chung, and C. Sonnenschein, "The Pesticides Endosulfan, Toxaphene, and Dieldrin Have Estrogenic Effects on Human Estrogen-Sensitive Cells," *Environmental Health Perspectives* 102(4):380–82 (1994).

"Fatty food is the main route of human exposure . . ." R. Kashyap, L. R. Iyer, and M. M. Singh, "Evaluation of Daily Dietary Intake of Dichloro-Diphenyl-Trichloroethane (DDT) and Benzene Hexachloride (BHC) in India," *Archives of Environmental Health* 49(1):63–66 (1994).

"300 to 500 times greater than in the blood . . ." Accu-Chem Laboratories fact sheet for chlorinated pesticide screening test.

"endocrine disruptive effects include . . ." http://www.wwfcanada.org /hormone-disruptors/list.htm.

"exception of usage for termite control . . ." Molecualr Expressions website: micro.magnet.fsu.edu/pesticides/pages/dieldrin.html.

"promotes endometriosis in rats . . ." A. M. Cummings and J. L. Metcalf, "Effects of Estrogen, Progesterone, and Methoxychlor on Surgically Induced Endometriosis in Rats," *Fundamentals of Applied Toxicology* 27:287–90 (1995).

"Burnt toast, charred steak . . ." J. W. Roberts, "Reducing Health Risks from Dust in the Home," Chapter 6 from the *Training Manual for the Master Home Environmentalist Program*, American Lung Association of Washington, 1997.

"Persistent PAHS can profoundly affect normal brain . . ." A. Brouwer et al., "Interactions of Persistent Environmental Organohalogens with the Thyroid Hormone System: Mechanisms and Possible Consequences for Animal and Human Health, *Toxicology and Industrial Health* 14(1/2) (1998).

"Heavy Metals . . ." M. Warhurst, *Introduction to Hormone Disruption:* http://www.ed.ac.uk/~amw/oestrogenic.html

"Cadmium . . . hormone receptors and receptor activity . . ." P. Garcia-Morales, P. Kenney, and D. S. Salomon et al., "Effect of Cadmium on Estrogenic Activity in Human MCF-7 Breast Cancer Cells," *Proceedings of the Annual Meeting of the American Association of Cancer Research* 34:a1503 (1993).

"medical waste incinerators . . ." "Mercury in Medical Waste," Health Care Without Harm, c/o CCHW, P.O. Box 6806, Falls Church, VA 22040. Also see website: www.noharm.org.

"dental amalgam fillings . . ." P. Herrstrom, A. Holmen, and A. Karlsson, "Immune Factors, Dental Amalgam, and Low-Dose Exposure to Mercury in Swedish Adolescents," *Archives of Environmental Health* 49(3):160–64 (1994).

"Aluminum accumulates and persists . . ." E. Alleva, J. Rankin, and D. Santucci, "Neurobehavioral Alteration in Rodents Following Developmental Exposure to Aluminum," *Toxicology and Industrial Health* 14(1/2):209–21 (1998).

Appendix B

"FDA stamp of approval . . ." J. Needham, *Science and Civilization in China* Vol. 5, Part 5, Cambridge University Press (1983).

"Not all estrogens are created equal . . ." H. M. Lemon et al., "Reduced Estriol Excretion in Patients with Breast Cancer Prior to Endocrine Therapy," *Journal of the American Medical Association* 196:1128–36 (1966); H. M. Lemon, "Pathophysiologic Considerations in the Treatment of Menopausal Patients with Oestrogens: The Role of Oestriol in the Prevention of Mammary Carcinoma," *Acta Endocrinologica* 233:17–27 (1980).

"Testosterone is the major . . ." J. V. Wright and J. Morgenthaler, *Natural Hormone Replacement: For Women over 45*, Smart Publications, 1997, pp. 27–28.

"natural testosterone can reduce the risk . . ." J. Møller, a Danish researcher and leading advocate of testosterone replacement for protecting the heart, wrote, "It is only natural to ask why testosterone is not tried before submitting the patient to the risks of angiography and operation."

"and improve osteoporosis . . ." Anonymous, "Hormone Therapy: Try Estrogen/Androgen in Selected Women," *Modern Medicine* 60:21 (Aug. 1992).

"Studies done during the past decade . . ." Until a few years ago, DHEA was considered a "junk" hormone with no particular significance. Today DHEA has become, according to Dr. William Regelson in *The Superhormone Promise*, Pocket Books (1997), "the superstar of superhormones."

"DHEA does not cause cancer . . ." D. L. McCormick et al., "Exceptional Chemopreventive Activity of Low-Dose Dehydroepiandrosterone in the Rat Mammary Gland," *Cancer Research* 56:1724–26 (1996).

"Para-aminobenzoic acid . . ." W. Ansbacher, W. A. Wisansky, and G. J. Martin, "Para-aminobenzoic Acid and Hormones," *Federal Proceedings* 1:98 (1942); A. R. Gaby, "The Story of PABA: A Little Known but Powerful Vitamin," *Nutrition and Healing* (March 1997), 3–4; B. F. Sieve, "Para-Aminobenzoic Acid and Hormones," *Medical World* (June 1943), 251–53); L. L. Wiesel, A. S. Barritt, and W. M. Stumpe, "The Synergistic Action of Para-aminobenzoic Acid and Cortisone in the Treatment of Rheumatoid Arthritis," *American Journal of the Medical Sciences* (Sept. 1951), 243–48; L. L. Wiesel, "Effect of Para-aminobenzoic Acid on the

Metabolism of Cortisone in Liver Tissue," *American Journal of the Medical Sciences* 227:80 (1954).

"Hrt does not get these results . . ." W. Utian, "Vaginal Function in Post-menopausal Women," Letter to the Editor, *Journal of the American Medical Association* 249(2):194–95 (1983).

"A number of studies . . ." B. B. Rubenstein, "Vitamin E Diminishes the Vasomotor Symptoms of Menopause," *Federal Proceedings* 7:106 (1948). Seventeen women with severe hot flashes following surgical or irradiation menopause who had failed to respond to barbiturates or placebo received 75 mg/day of vitamin E. Fourteen of the 17 women had a marked reduction in hot flashes and six obtained complete relief. H. C. McLaren, "Vitamin E in the Menopause," *British Medical Journal* 2:1378–82 (1949). Dr. Gaby has found that the brand of vitamin E made by the A. C. Grace Company is more effective for some women than are other forms.

"no more effective than a placebo . . ." M. H. G. Blatt, H. Wiesebader, and H. S. Kupperman, "Vitamin E and Climacteric Syndrome: Failure of Effective Control as Measured by Menopausal Index," *Archives of Internal Medicine* 91:792–99 (1953).

"highest dose of flavonoids with Hrt . . ." R. Safati and J. Brux, "Vascular Fragility of the Endometrium Under Estrogen-Progestin Treatment. Treatment by Disodium Flavodate." *Journal de Gynecologie. Obstetrique et Biologie de la Reproduction* (Paris) 2(1):87–94 (Jan.–Feb. 1973).

"double-blind study . . ." E. David, "Purpura hemorrhagica Treated with Vitamin P," *Lancet*, (June 8, 1940), 1063; C. J. Smith, "Non-hormonal Control of Vaso-motor Flushing in Menopausal Patients," *Chicago Medicine* (March 7, 1964).

"pantothenic Acid (pa) . . ." D. Gorrie, M. B. Robertson, and M. B. Glass, "Purpura Hemorrhagica after Arsenic Therapy Treated with Vitamin P," *Lancet*, 1005 (June 1, 1940); P. Matis, "Rutin in Prevention of Vascular Injury Caused by Dicumarol," *Current Medical Literature* 143(14): 1291 (1950); R. Sarfati and J. de Brux, "Administering Vitamin P Can Stop Spotting," *Medical World News* (Oct. 12, 1973); G. Selsman and Steven Horoschak, "The Treatment of Capillary Fragility with a Combination of Hesperidin and Vitamin C," *American Journal of Digestive Diseases* 17:92 (1950).

"Ginseng . . ." M. P. Hopkins, L. Androff, A. S. Benninghoff, "Ginseng Face Cream and Unexplained Vaginal Bleeding," *American Journal of Obstetrics and Gynecology* 159:1121–22 (1988); R. Punnonen and A. Lukola, "Oestrogen-like Effect of Ginseng," *British Medical Journal* 281:1110 (Oct. 25, 1980).

"Soy products . . ." H. Adlercreutz, E. Hamalainen, and S. Gorbach et al., "Dietary Phyto-oestrogens and the Menopause in Japan," *Lancet* 339:1233 (1992). A. Cassidy, S. Bingham, and K. D. R. Setchell, "Biological Effects of a Diet of Soy Protein Rich in Isoflavones on the Menstrual Cycle of Premenopausal Women," *American Journal of Clinical Nutrition* 60:333–40 (1994). Anonymous, "Soy May Cool Down a Hot Flash," *Hippocrates* 15–16 (March 1997).

Appendix C

"Aronson (2000) . . ." K. J. Aronson et al., "Breast Adipose Tissue Concentrations Polychlorinated Biphenyls and Other Organochlorines and Breast Cancer Risk," *Cancer Epidemiology, Biomarkers, and Prevention* 9:55–63 (2000).

"Mendonca (1999) . . ." G.A.S. Mendonca et al., "Organochlorines and Breast Cancer: A Case-Control Study in Brazil," *International Journal of Cancer* 83:596–600 (1999).

"Hoyer (1998) . . ." A. P. Hoyer et al., "Organochlorine Exposure and Risk of Breast Cancer," *Lancet* 352:1816–20 (1998).

"Zheng (1999) . . ." L. T. Zheng et al., "DDE and DDT in Breast Adipose Tissue and Risk of Female Breast Cancer," *American Journal of Epidemiology* 150(5):453–8 (1999); T. Zheng et al., "Environmental Exposure to Hexachlorobenzene (HCB) and Risk of Female Breast Cancer in Connecticut," *Cancer Epidemiology, Biomarkers, and Prevention* 8:407–11 (May 1999).

"Kettles (1997) . . ." M. A. Kettles et al., "Triazine Herbicide Exposure and Breast Cancer Incidence: An Ecologic Study of Kentucky Counties," *Environmental Health Perspectives* 105:1222–27 (1997).

"Helzlsouer (1999) . . ." K. J. Helzlsouer et al., "Serum Concentrations of Organochlorine Compounds and the Subsequent Development of Breast

Cancer," *Cancer Epidemiology, Biomarkers, and Prevention* 8:525–32 (June 1999).

"Dewailly (1994) . . ." E. Dewailly et al., "High Organochlorine Body Burden in Women with Estrogen Receptor-Positive Breast Cancer," *Journal of the National Cancer Institute* 86(3):232–34 (1994).

"Moysich (1998) . . ." K. B. Moysich et al., "Environmental Organochlorine Exposure and Postmenopausal Breast Cancer Risk," *Cancer Epidemiology Biomarkers Preview* 7:181–88 (1998).

"Melius (1994) . . ." J. Melius et al., "Residence Near Industries and High Traffic Areas and the Risk of Breast Cancer on Long Island," New York State Dept. of Health, 1994.

"Hunter (1997) . . ." D. J. Hunter et al., "Plasma Organochlorine Levels and the Risk of Breast Cancer," *New England Journal of Medicine* 337:1253–58 (1997).

"Wolff (1993) . . ." M. S. Wolff et al., "Blood Levels of Organochlorine Residues and Risk of Breast Cancer," *Journal of the National Cancer Institute* 85(8):648–52 (1993).

"Lopez-Carrillo (1997) . . ." L. Lopez-Carrillo et al., "Dichlorodiphenyl-trichloroethane Serum Levels and Breast Cancer Risk: A Case-Control Study from Mexico," *Cancer Research* 57:3728–32 (1997).

"Falck pilot study (1992) . . ." F. Falck et al., "Pesticides and Polychlorinated Biphenyl Residues in Human Breast Lipids and Their Relation to Breast Cancer," *Archives of Environmental Health* 47(2):143–46 (March/April 1992).

"Van't Veer (1997) . . ." P. van't Veer et al., "DDT (Dicophane) and Postmenopausal Breast Cancer in Europe: Case-Control Study," *British Medical Journal* 315:81–84 (July 1997).

"Weston (1990) . . ." J. B. Westin and E. Richter, "The Israeli Breast-Cancer Anomaly," *Annuals of New York Academy of Science* 609:269–79 (1990).

"Adami (1995) . . ." H. O. Adami et al., "Organochlorine Compounds and Estrogen-Related Cancers in Women," *Cancer Causes and Control* 6:551–66 (1995).

"H. Mussalo-Rauhamaa (1990) . . ." H. Mussalo-Rauhamaa et al., "Occurrence of Beta-hexachlorocyclohemane in Breast Cancer Patients," *Cancer* 66:2124–28 (1990).

"Cantor (1995) . . ." K. P. Cantor, P. A. Stewart, L. A. Brinton, and M. Dosemeci, "Occupational Exposures and Female Breast Cancer Mortality in the U.S.," *Journal of Occupational and Emergency Medicine* 37 (3):336-48 (1995).

"Najem (1985) . . ." G. R. Najem et al., "Female Reproductive Organs and Breast Cancer Mortality in New Jersey Counties and the Relationship with Certain Environmental Variables," *Preventive Medicine* (14):620–35 (1985). G. R. Najem et al., "Clusters of Cancer Mortality in New Jersey Municipalities, with Special Reference to Chemical Toxic Waste Disposal Sites and per Capita Income," *International Journal of Epidemiology* 14:528–37 (1985).

"Ahlborg (1995) . . ." U. G. Ahlborg et al., "Organochlorine Compounds in Relation to Breast Cancer, Endometrial Cancer, and Endometriosis: An Assessment of the Biological and Epidemiological Evidence," *Critical Reviews in Toxicology* 25:463–531 (1995).

"Chiazze (1977) . . ." L. Chiazze et al., "Mortality Among Employees of Pvc Fabricators," *Journal of Occupational Medicine* 19:623–28 (1977).

"Krieger (1994) . . ." Krieger et al., "Breast Cancer and Serum Organochlorines: A Prospective Study Among White, Black, and Asian Women," *Journal of the National Cancer Institute* 86(8):589–99 (1994).

"Wasserman (1976) . . ." M. Wasserman et al., "Organochlorine Compounds in Neoplastic and Adjacent Apparently Normal Breast Tissue," *Bulletin of Environmental Contamination and Toxicology* 15(4):478–84 (1976).

"Key (1994) . . ." T. Key and G. Reeves, "Organochlorines in the Environment and Breast Cancer," *British Medical Journal* 308:1520–21 (1994).

Index